Scott Ranson et al
The Quality Book
(Hardcover - Masters
level)

Health Care Quality:
The Clinician's Primer

Edited by
David B. Nash, MD, MBA
Janice L. Clarke, RN
Alexandria Skoufalos, EdD
Melissa Horowitz

D1413414

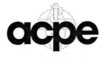

American College of Physician Executives
400 North Ashley Drive
Tampa, Florida 33602

ISBN: 978-0-9787306-7-3

Library of Congress Card Number: 2012935147

Printed in the United States of America by Lightning Source.

Contents

Section I.   Introduction to Quality in Health Care

Section II.   Measuring Quality: Application of Quality Measures

Section III. Evaluating Quality: Diverse Dimensions of the Health Care System

Section IV. Balancing Competing Perspectives: Purchasers, Physicians, Patients

"To clinicians everywhere who ask themselves each day how they might improve."

Foreword

Voltaire—the brilliantly acerbic 18th century writer, philosopher, and satirist—once summarized a wordy missive by England's John Locke in the form of a timeless caution: *"If you desire to speak with me,"* he said, *"... first define your terms."* In health care, the lack of a universally understood definition of "quality" has materially retarded our ability to respond to what is, in reality, a national emergency: The desperate need to drastically improve the performance and cost-effectiveness of medical care.

Although safety and quality are indispensable components of one another, confusion has reigned about them throughout history. A fair question, for instance, is whether "Quality Committees" within hospital boards have actually addressed anything but cost containment versus patient satisfaction. Worse, the recognition that "medical quality" encompasses every aspect of health care delivery (as well as the effectiveness of providers in improving public health) has been obscured by the failure to heed Voltaire's implied warning.

Herculean efforts have been expended over the past decade to heed the alarms, cautions, and warnings inherent in the Institute of Medicine's two pivotal reports (*To Err Is Human* and *Crossing the Quality Chasm*). Indeed, the recent efforts of CMS to force systemic change clearly echo the best thinking on how to rapidly alter what is, in fact, a hidebound culture inherently resistant to change and wedded to the concept that "the way we've always done it" in a cottage industry is as good as it's going to get.

In America alone, up to 30 Americans die each hour on average from a combination of medical mistakes and nosocomial infections. In addition, 17.5 percent of our gross national product (over $2.5 trillion annually) goes to a health care non-system producing less than 50 percent of the quality and effectiveness of other industrialized nations.

We do not have the luxury of relying on casual or apocryphal definitions. The need for immediate, clear, detailed, and authoritative *operational* understanding of precisely what medical quality is, and must be, is too important to be left to esoteric or casual interpretation.

This is the primary reason why *Health Care Quality: The Clinician's Primer*, is such an important and universally needed work. Within the following pages are the very definitions we've long needed, stated in direct and clear essays by top authorities, and assembled to provide (as the title promises) a handbook for understanding each and every major facet of medical quality.

After all, to provide it, you have to have an unequivocal understanding of it. Jan Clarke, David Nash, Melissa Horowitz, and Alexis Skoufalos have done a world-class job of bringing clarity out of chaos in what should be required reading by every clinician.

I urge you to dive into this work with the intent of reading it at least twice, ear-marking appropriate sections, and testing yourself on your depth of ability to understand both the macro and the micro of medical quality. Indeed, getting it right—this emergency drive to creating a true health system—is far too important not to have a harmonized and universal understanding.

John J. Nance, JD
American College of Health Care Executives' 2009 Book of the Year Award Winner for *Why Hospitals Should Fly.*

Preface

In the second decade of the 21st Century, our nation is engaged in a transformation of one of the largest industries in our country; namely the health care system. Indeed, this transformation has been under way, in earnest, for several years. It has highlighted some uncomfortable realities, some truths that we find unsettling. Among these truths is the fact that our nation spends the most for health care, and the value we obtain from the dollars spent is low. We find ourselves at a crossroads—a crossroads that makes clear we could do better, we could improve quality and safety of the care we deliver and we could deliver this care at a more competitive price. In a word, we could do more to achieve higher *value* for the health care system. This, then, is our call to arms and the reason we have edited this new book. *Health Care Quality: The Clinician's Primer* is designed for clinicians of all types and for others who yearn for a single-volume overview of the quality and safety challenges facing the nation.

Why another text on quality, especially one coming from a school of population health? Although the Jefferson School of Population Health remains the only such school in the nation, it is an idea whose time has come. Population health sends an undeniably strong signal that we must take a broader perspective if we are truly to improve the health of the public. We must explicitly recognize the nature of care within our system. We must strive for better understanding of the evidentiary basis of what we do every day at the bedside and across every setting where care is provided. We must be take responsibility as stewards of the vast public resources for which we are accountable to our citizens. A school of population health, then, is perfectly situated to produce a new volume, organized in such a way as to give clinicians a deeper understanding of the challenges we face in creating a health care system that will be patient-centered—and one that will achieve value for the services delivered. By improving the quality and safety of the care delivered, we will most certainly improve the health of the population.

How is this book organized?

The book is organized into six sections. In Section I, the contributors provide a comprehensive background of the scholarly nature of the field of quality and safety, including useful definitions, key terms, and concepts. Following a deep dive into the legal and regulatory aspects of the field, the section concludes with an overview of the current policy environment as it relates to the quality and safety agenda.

Section II focuses on how the measures that were reviewed earlier are applied. It is highlighted by contributions devoted to data collection and process improvement at the national level.

Section III presents diverse dimensions of the quality and safety agenda—including where care might be delivered, such as the inpatient, ambulatory, and long-term care settings. It delves into quality at the health plan level and, importantly, quality and safety with regard to the delivery of pharmaceutical services.

Section IV, "Balancing Competing Perspectives," ties together the previous three sections as it elucidates the notion of value-based purchasing. We are fortunate to have chapters contributed by several public policy leaders on topics such as the public reporting of quality measures and the design and organization of a statewide patient safety authority. The section concludes with the introduction of emerging organizational issues that might impact quality and safety moving forward.

Section V centers on the national agenda, with chapters highlighting such concepts as Six Sigma, the role of information technology, and, importantly, the ongoing challenges in changing clinician education to focus more clearly on the quality and safety agenda. Finally, Section VI forecasts future directions for this vitally important field.

Who should read this book?

Clinicians recognize that their central responsibility is to deliver care that is safe, effective, timely, efficient, and patient-centered. As citizens we recognize that we must find solutions to help the nation deliver care of greater value. As persons, we recognize that each of us will one day be a patient. Because of the foregoing, the editors believe all clinicians should have a core understanding of the issues around the quality and safety of health care services. The conversation is not limited exclusively to physicians—it must encompass all persons who touch patients. For clinicians seeking a single, multi-authored authoritative compendium that summarizes the field of quality and safety, this primer is the ideal resource.

In addition to the core clinician audience, the editors also believe that this book is appropriate and useful for graduate work in health care quality and safety in various settings, including schools of public health, health administration, medicine, nursing, and pharmaceutical sciences. Each chapter contains learning objectives and key review questions. In addition, each chapter is thoroughly referenced and has numerous suggested websites and other sources of additional information to enrich understanding of these complex issues.

Many persons played keys role in the genesis of this book. As the Senior Editor, I would particularly like to thank our university leadership, including Michael Vergare, MD, Senior Vice-President for Academic Affairs at Thomas Jefferson University, and Thomas J. Lewis, Chief Executive Officer of our university hospital. This duo has been extremely supportive of our work as a school and of me personally during my more than two-decade tenure at Thomas Jefferson University. We also say goodbye to the out-going university President, Robert L. Barchi, MD, PhD, and recognize his early support for the creation of our school.

I want to especially thank my co-editors, Janice Clarke, Melissa Horowitz , and Alexis Skoufalos, for their dedication to keeping this complex undertaking on track. I would be remiss if I did not also recognize our colleagues Bill Steiger, Susan Quinn and Debi Marsh at the American College of Physician Executives. This was truly a team effort, and I am very proud of our collective efforts.

All multi-authored, edited texts share certain limitations. It is the responsibility of the editors to weave together disparate chapters into a coherent tapestry. I want to especially thank all of our contributors from across the nation. They were drawn from a leadership cohort and represent the best thinking in our field. We are grateful for their contributions and recognize their collective central role in creating a new health care system for the future. We are responsible, in turn, for any errors of omission or co-mission. As editors, we greatly value feedback from readers and would appreciate hearing from you as fellow travelers on the still bumpy road toward a high-quality and safe health care system.

As Senior Editor, I want to thank the leadership of the American College of Physician Executives. For more than 20 years I have had the distinct privilege of leading the College's educational efforts in the quality and safety arena. For example, our course, The Three Faces of Quality, during its initial 20-year run, was presented to more than 5,000 ACPE members, both in-person and online. This makes The Three Faces of Quality the most highly subscribed course on Quality and Safety for physicians in the world. I am very appreciative of the feedback I received over many years from these attendees who helped form the basis of this primer. It was a privilege to work with so many colleagues from across the country over so long a period of time, and their collective wisdom contributed greatly to the design and execution of this book. I can never really repay that debt.

One of the hallmarks of good leadership is to help prepare the next generation of leaders. I am confident that—*"Health Care Quality: The Clinician's Primer"*—will help you to become a more effective, compassionate, and capable clinician, ready to contribute to a system that puts quality and safety at the core of everything we do. I am also confident that this book will help us to deliver care of higher value, care that the nation can be proud of, and care that we will want as patients one day in the future. When you are done reading this book, pass it along to a colleague so that he or she can participate in this journey with us together.

David B. Nash, MD, MBA
Dean
Jefferson School of Population Health

Contributors

Jaya Agrawal, MA, MHSA
Director Transfer Center and Clinical Research Office
Mercy Health

Evan M. Benjamin, MD, FACP
Senior Vice President
Chief Quality Officer
Baystate Health, Inc.
Associate Professor of Medicine
Tufts University School of Medicine

Bettina Berman, RN, CPHQ, CNOR
Project Director for Quality Improvement
Jefferson School of Population Health
Thomas Jefferson University

Eric J. Berman, DO, MS
Regional Chief Medical Officer
Northern Division Managed Care
AmeriHealth Mercy Family of Companies

John Caruso, MD, FACP
Associate Dean, Graduate Medical Education
Jefferson Medical College

Donald E. Casey Jr., MD, MPH, MBA, FACP, FAHA
Chief Medical Officer and Vice President of Quality
Chief Research Officer and Chief Academic Officer
Atlantic Health

Amanda Cornett, MPH
Associate Director
NC Center for Public Health Quality

Laura Cranston, RPh
Executive Director
Pharmacy Quality Alliance

Dave Davis, MD, CCFP, FCFP
Senior Director, Continuing Education and
Performance Improvement,
Association of American Medical Colleges

Susan DesHarnais, PhD, MPH
Former Professor
Jefferson School of Population Health
Thomas Jefferson University

Yosef D. Dlugacz, PhD
Senior Vice President and Chief of Clinical Quality,
Education and Research
Krasnoff Quality Management Institute a division of
North Shore-LIJ Health System

Michael C. Doering, MBA
Executive Director
Pennsylvania Patient Safety Authority

David Domann, MS, RPh
Director Health Care Quality
Strategic Customer Group
Johnson & Johnson Health Care Systems Inc.

Michael J. Dowling
President and Chief Executive Officer
North Shore-LIJ Health System

Karen Drenkard, PhD, RN, NEA-BC, FAAN
Executive Director
American Nurses Credentialing Center

Neil I. Goldfarb
Executive Director
Greater Philadelphia Business Coalition on Health

Stephen R. Grossbart, PhD
Senior Vice President and Chief Quality Officer
Center for Patient Safety and Clinical Transformation
Catholic Health Partners

Judith Hibbard, DrPH
Professor Emerita and Senior Researcher, Institute for
Policy Research and Innovation, University of Oregon

Peter J. Katsufrakis, MD, MBA
Vice-President, Assessment Programs
National Board of Medical Examiners

David E. Longnecker, MD, FRCA
Director, Health Care Affairs
Association of American Medical Colleges

Mary Lou Manning, PhD, CRNP
Associate Professor
Director, Doctor of Nursing Practice Program
Thomas Jefferson University Jefferson School of
Nursing

Rick May, MD
CEO
Ascent Clinical Quality Improvement

Karen E. Michael, RN, MSN, MBA
Vice President, Corporate Medical Management
AmeriHealth Mercy Family of Companies

Mary Minniti, CPHQ
Program and Resource Specialist
Institute for Patient- and Family-Centered Care

Tina Morton RN, BSN, CCM, CPHQ, CHCQM
Sr. Director Quality Management
Keystone Mercy Health Plan

David B. Nash, MD, MBA
Dean
Jefferson School of Population Health
Thomas Jefferson University

David Nau, RPh, PhD, CPHQ
Senior Director of Quality Strategies
Pharmacy Quality Alliance

Alon Peltz, MD, MBA
Vanderbilt University School of Medicine
Owen Graduate School of Management

Valerie Pracilio, MPH, CPPS
Project Director for Quality Improvement
Jefferson School of Population Health
Thomas Jefferson University

Rangaraj Ramanujam, PhD
Associate Professor of Management
Owen Graduate School of Management
Vanderbilt University

Greg D. Randolph MD, MPH
Director, NC Center for Public Health Quality
Associate Professor, Department of Pediatrics
Adjunct Associate Professor, Gillings School of
Global Public Health
University of North Carolina at Chapel Hill

Martha C. Romney, RN, JD, MPH
Assistant Professor
Jefferson School of Population Health
Thomas Jefferson University

Harm J. Scherpbier, MD
Vice President and Chief Medical Information Officer
Main Line Health

Adrianne Seiler, MD
Associate Medical Director
Division of Health Care quality
Baystate Medical Center
Assistant Professor of Medicine
Tufts University School of Medicine

Richard G. Stefanacci, DO, MGH, MBA, AGSF, CMD
Chief Medical Officer
The Access Group

Carolyn Sweetapple, RN, CPA, MBA
Vice President, Finance and Business Operations
Krasnoff Quality Management Institute a division of
North Shore-LIJ Health System

Edward A. Walker, MD, MHA
Professor, Psychiatry & Health Services
Schools of Medicine and Public Health, University of
Washington

Flossie Wolf
Director, Health Policy Research
Pennsylvania Health Care Cost Containment Council

Bonnie L. Zell, MD, MPH
Principal
Zell Community Health Strategies, LLC
Strategic Advisor, Community Health
Contra Costa Health Services

Section I.

Introduction to Quality in Health Care

Chapter 1

Background

By Neil I. Goldfarb

Executive Summary

This book is intended to provide clinicians with an understanding of how quality can be measured and improved in clinical settings. The topic is important because many studies have identified ongoing problems with care quality. In its 2001 seminal report, *Crossing the Quality Chasm*, the Institute of Medicine delineated the quality challenge facing the United States health care system, and called for a system that is safe, timely, effective, equitable, patient-centered, and efficient. Although efforts continue to be made to advance the science of quality measurement and improvement, much work remains to be done, as evidenced by national and international quality-tracking systems.

Learning Objectives

1. Become familiar with major milestones in the U.S. quality movement.

2. Understand the components of an ideal health system as articulated by the Institute of Medicine (IOM).

3. Recognize that, in most measures of performance, there remains much room for improvement.

Key Words: Quality, Institute of Medicine, World Health Organization, Commonwealth Fund

Introduction

This book is all about quality measurement and improvement, with an emphasis on the critical role clinicians can and should play in the quality movement. Before going about fixing a problem, one has to recognize that the problem exists. This chapter reviews the evidence that there is significant room for improvement in health care quality and safety in the U.S. health care system.

What is Quality?

The Institute of Medicine (IOM) defines quality as "the degree to which health services for individuals and populations increase the likelihood of desired health outcomes and are consistent with current professional knowledge."[1] This definition emphasizes the importance of population health—not only individual patient health—in delivering quality care, and the ever-changing evidence base regarding what constitutes quality. Because much of the care commonly delivered today is not evidence-based (i.e., confirmed as effective based on published research), clinicians often rely on what they were taught, what has worked in the past, or what their colleagues advise them to do. As knowledge and guidelines change, what we view as high-quality care, and how we measure it, may change as well.

The Quality Measurement Movement

Quality measurement in health care is not a new concept. The modern era of performance measurement can be traced back to Ernest Codman, MD, a Massachusetts surgeon who became interested in measuring surgical outcomes for his patients.[2] Codman kept a log of how his patients fared in the post-operative period and sought to identify factors associated with patient mortality. Dr. Codman was not popular with his peers when he first suggested that they should be tracking their outcomes as well. Yet today, Dr. Codman is revered as one of the founders of the quality measurement movement.

Moving forward nearly 100 years, the IOM issued a clarion call for improvement in health care quality and safety. *To Err Is Human,* issued in 1999 by the IOM, reported that as many as 98,000 deaths occur in hospitals each year due to medical error.[3] Whether the actual number is 98,000 or 36,000, the number is alarming, especially since that is just the number of errors resulting in death, and not the total number of errors. Since that report, much effort has gone into identifying ways to improve patient safety and implement evidence-based safe practices; however, most quality experts believe that medical errors continue to be both common and deadly.

As a follow-up to *To Err Is Human,* the IOM issued *Crossing the Quality Chasm,* a call for radical change in delivery of care in the United States.[4] The report identified six key elements that are essential to a strong health system:

- Safe: As noted above, the IOM had already called attention to medical error as a major issue.

- Timely: Numerous studies document delays in diagnosis and treatment and the impact on patient outcomes and costs of care.

- Effective: Numerous studies demonstrate that many services that are commonly delivered are not effective, i.e., do not significantly impact outcomes in a positive way and may even produce harm.

- Equitable: Numerous studies show that access to care, quality of care, and treatment patterns are influenced by patient age, geographic location, gender, socioeconomic status, insurance status, and other factors.

- Patient-centered: National surveys of consumers show growing dissatisfaction with access to care and with navigating an increasingly complex, provider-centric system.

- Efficient: Data available through international comparative studies, as well as local resources such as the Dartmouth Atlas (which analyzes geographic differences in use of Medicare services), suggest that much of our utilization is wasteful.

Where Do We Stand Today?

We have many examples from the research literature and policy-monitoring organizations to support the need for improvement in our health system's performance. The Commonwealth Fund's *National Scorecard on U.S. Health System Performance,* most recently updated in the fall of 2011, shows significant opportunity for improvement (www.commonwealthfund.org). Across 42 performance indicators, largely mirroring the system elements identified by the IOM, the U.S. scored 64 out of a possible 100 when actual performance was compared with national and international benchmarks.

While key quality of care indicators have shown modest improvement since the first report in 2006, access to care actually showed worsening, due to economic factors and erosion of health insurance and health care affordability. Data available through both the Commonwealth Fund and the World Health Organization[5] demonstrate that while the United States spends more (both per capita and as a percentage of gross domestic product) than any other western nation (and, in comparison to most nations, spends twice as much) on measures of quality, including life expectancy at birth and healthy life expectancy, the U.S. ranks beneath most of those nations.

In a seminal study on health care quality in the U.S., Elizabeth McGlynn and colleagues at the RAND Corporation conducted a national chart review (2003), examining preventive, acute care, and chronic care delivery against established care guidelines.[6] The overall finding was that patients received care that was delivered in accordance with the guidelines just 54% of the time. The results were remarkably similar for both adult and pediatric populations, although findings varied depending on the condition being examined (e.g., for hypertension, the guidelines adherence rate was 65 percent whereas it was 45 percent for diabetes). Even acknowledging that patient behavior plays a role in performance on process and outcomes measures of care for these conditions, it's clear that there is much room for improvement in performance.

While the RAND study largely documented underuse of preventive services, the system also faces problems with overuse. Examples of services that have been found to be commonly overutilized are Cesarean-section deliveries and diagnostic CT scans. Overutilization may result from defensive medicine (i.e., practicing so as to reduce the risk of malpractice), higher reimbursement under fee-for-service medicine for these procedures, lack of clinical knowledge about appropriateness, patient demand, or all of the above. Overutilization is not only a cost issue, but also a quality issue. In the C-section example, the patient may be exposed to higher risk of infection and other complications, and several recent studies show that repeat CT scans expose patients to unacceptably high levels of radiation.

Where Are We Going?

The U.S. Department of Health and Human Services released the "National Quality Strategy" in early 2011.[7] The strategy emphasizes the "Triple Aim" of better care, healthy people and communities, and affordable care. In brief, the strategy calls for: improving the health of the U.S. population through both health care and the surrounding behavioral, social, and environmental systems; making sure that, when people do need health care, it is accessible, high-quality, safe, and patient-centered; and lowering the costs of care for purchasers (i.e., employers and government) and consumers.

The six priorities outlined in the plan include: 1) making care safer and reducing harm; 2) engaging consumers as partners in their care; 3) promoting effective care coordination and communication between patients and providers and between providers on behalf of their patients; 4) promoting effective care, with an emphasis on leading causes of morbidity and mortality; 5) partnering with communities to support healthier lifestyles; and 6) improving the affordability of care. Admittedly, these are very broad goals, but they represent a broad consensus among stakeholder groups. The challenge now will be translating these broad goals and priorities into specific programs that advance health care quality and safety and the population's health.

Conclusion

Despite the IOM's call for radical change in the U.S. health care system 10 years ago, little has changed, and we continue to be faced with the challenge of how best to improve performance. Few, if any, clinicians want to deliver poor quality of care, so the questions to be asked are, why are we not doing better as a health care system, and what can we do moving forward? Clearly, any effort to transform the system will rely on clinicians—nurses, physicians, pharmacists, and the many other professionals who deliver care. As you read this book, we hope to give you more insight into the tools for practicing care that meets the IOM challenge.

Study and Discussion Questions

1. When people say "The U.S. has the best health care in the world," what does this mean?

2. If you were the U.S. policy czar, what would you do to start to address the quality issues identified in this chapter?

3. Almost all clinicians want to deliver good care and believe that they do so; can this belief be reconciled with the data provided in this chapter?

References

1. *Medicare: A Strategy for Quality Assurance.* Kathleen N. Lohr (ed); Committee to Design a Strategy for Quality Review and Assurance in Medicare. Institute of Medicine, Washington, DC: National Academies Press,1990.

2. "Ernest Amory Codman, 1869-1940," *N Engl J Med,* 224(7):296-299, Feb. 13, 1941.

3. *To Err Is Human: Building a Safer Health System.* Kohn L, Corrigan J, Donaldson M (eds.) Committee on Quality of Health Care in America, Institute of Medicine. Washington, DC: National Academies Press, 1999.

4. *Crossing the Quality Chasm: Shaping the Future for Health.* Institute of Medicine, Washington, DC: National Academies Press, 2001.

5. World Health Statistics 2011. World Health Organization. http://www.who.int/gho/publications/world_health_statistics/EN_WHS2011_Full.pdf

6. McGlynn EA, and others. The quality of health care delivered to adults in the United States. *N Engl J Med,* 348(26):2635-45, Jun 26, 2003..

7. *Report to Congress: National Strategy for Quality Improvement in Healthcare.* U.S. Department of Health and Human Services. March 2011. http://www.healthcare.gov/law/resources/reports/quality03212011a.html#es

Chapter 2

Conceptualization and Definitions of Quality

By Stephen R. Grossbart, PhD and Jaya Agrawal, MA, MHSA

Executive Summary

For far too long, the health care industry approached quality with an inconsistent definition and was hampered by a lack of consensus around assessment methodologies. In two path breaking reports issued between 1999 and 2001, the Institute of Medicine (IOM) presented a new conceptualization that began to reframe the industry's understanding of both quality and safety in health care.

The science of health care improvement had advanced dramatically through the work of pioneers such as Avedis Donabedian and health care providers who championed systematic use of evidence-based medicine. This work helped lay the groundwork for an emerging body of consensus measures based on evidence that provided important tools for assessing the care delivered by health care providers. However, it was not until after the publication of the IOM reports that a paradigm shift began to emerge, one that provided new frameworks for assessing quality and safety and for initiating the overdue transformation of a care delivery system that still fails to provide safe and effective care.

Learning Objectives

1. Understand quality as defined in *Crossing the Quality Chasm.*

2. Understand the interrelationship between quality and patient safety and how this relationship has evolved since the publication of *To Err Is Human*.

3. Describe the Donabedian Quality Triad and its relationship to the practice of evidence-based medicine, quality improvement, and cultural transformation in health care settings.

Key Words: Donadbedian Quality Triad, National Quality Forum, Institute for Medicine Reports, Institute for Health Care Improvement, Affordable Care Act, Value-Based Purchasing, Evidence-Based Medicine

Introduction

In September 1999, the Institute of Medicine (IOM) released *To Err Is Human: Building a Safer Health System*.[1] Attributing 44,000-98,000 needless deaths in U.S. hospitals to medical errors, this groundbreaking report challenged health care providers by calling for a 50 percent reduction in errors by 2004. Although the report was preceded by a series of studies that raised concerns about the safety of patients in our health care system, it alone captured the broad attention of the American people and the health care industry.[2,3] Within two weeks of publication, congressional hearings were initiated and the President called for studies to determine how the report's recommendations could be implemented.

The report was not greeted warmly by the health care provider community; one editorial response described the work as "...hot and shrill. It shouts about death and disability in U.S. hospitals."[4,5] Less emotionally, in the pages of the *New England Journal of Medicine*, Troyen A. Brennan disputed the meaning of the word "error," arguing that the actual number of patients needlessly harmed or maimed by health care providers was much lower.[6] In a study of physician attitudes, Robert J. Blendon *et al.* reported survey results indicating that, although 35 percent of physicians had personally experienced a medical error during their own care or care of a family member, "only 5 percent of physicians...identified medical errors as one of the most serious problems" in our hospitals. The majority of physicians believed that the IOM report grossly overestimated deaths due to errors and thought 5,000 per year to be a more reasonable estimate. The physicians perceived that other entities should be held accountable for the few errors that occurred and that more effective error reduction solutions should be aimed at "requiring hospitals to develop systems for preventing medical errors, e.g., information technology (55 percent) and increasing the number of nurses in hospitals (51 percent)."[7]

The IOM publication led to an intense period of national performance measurement development (e.g., The Joint Commission, the Center for Medicare & Medicaid Services) and their subsequent endorsement as national consensus measures by the National Quality Forum (NQF). Patient safety training programs were developed by the American Hospital Association (AHA), the National Patient Safety Foundation (NPSF), and the Institute for Healthcare Improvement (IHI). As early adopter hospitals worked to understand and address the problems outlined in *To Err Is Human,* a second IOM report, *Crossing the Quality Chasm*, laid out a blueprint for action.[8]

Although the IOM reports led to profound policy recommendations during the late 20th and early 21st centuries, the health care provider community demonstrated only limited interest in tackling the transformation needed to provide safe and affordable care.[9] Five years after the publication of *To Err Is Human,* Drew Altman *et al.* surveyed a sample of Americans and found that, "Unfortunately, despite 5 years of focused attention, people do not seem to feel safer. More than half (55 percent) of the respondents in our survey said that they are currently dissatisfied with the quality of health care in this country"[10] Two of the most visible champions of the patient safety movement, Lucien L. Leape, MD and Donald M. Berwick, MD, were prompted by such reports to reflect on the positive but largely unfulfilled goals of *To Err Is Human*.[11]

With over a decade behind us since *To Err Is Human*, and with the Department of Health and Human Services steadily implementing the Patient Protection and Affordable Care Act (ACA), the inability of the health care industry to transform itself has become even more evident. Although our awareness of error is far greater—today, no well-read health care provider challenges the IOM's findings—errors have not declined significantly.

Christopher P. Landrigan *et al.* systematically analyzed records from a sample of hospitals to see whether the frequency and severity of medical errors had decreased in the post *To Err Is Human* decade. They found a nonsignificant one percent reduction, with "no significant change over time in the rate of harms identified by internal reviewers." The authors theorized that this failure to improve was due to "the penetration of evidence-based safety practices being quite modest... only 1.5 percent of hospitals in the United States have implemented a comprehensive system of electronic medical records, and only 9.1 percent have even basic electronic record-keeping in place; only 17 percent have computerized provider order entry."[12]

In November 2010, the Office of the Inspector General (OIG) issued *Adverse Events in Hospitals: National Incidence among Medicare Beneficiaries*, a scathing indictment of the industry that reported 13.5 percent of "hospitalized Medicare beneficiaries experienced adverse events during their hospital stays." An astounding 15,000 deaths a month were attributed to these events. At least 44 percent of the reviewed events were preventable and such failures are estimated to result in $4.4 billion in waste annually.[13]

Despite good intentions, there is overwhelming evidence that U.S. health care quality is substandard, patient safety is lacking, the definition of quality remains ambiguous, and the cultural barriers to developing high-reliability systems often seem insurmountable. Even at the most elementary level, health care providers appear to be unwilling to reduce health care-associated infections by simply washing their hands, removing their ties, dressing naked below the elbow, and getting rid of their lab coats.[14] Most surgical teams refuse to use simple yet effective checklists or to adhere to evidence-based standards for eliminating preventable perioperative complications[15,16]

A clear indication that the industry has not consistently embraced the need for cultural change is evident in recently released data on preventable harm in our hospitals. CMS reported that, among Medicare fee-for-service patients, nearly 1 in every 10,000 who underwent surgery in the United States had an object accidentally left in his or her body after surgery (foreign object retained after surgery).[17] Yet, high-reliability hospitals that use checklists and have a standardized process to account for sponges and other objects can prevent virtually 100 percent of these events. Apparently, such cultural resistance in the face of common sense and a significant body of evidence keeps health care providers from achieving breakthrough performance levels.

As we reflect upon the "patient safety movement" and the substantial quality improvement work that has occurred, one thing is striking. Hospitals and providers have not culturally accepted the existence of a "quality chasm," and thus we routinely fail to provide safe evidence-based care that is centered on healing the patient.

One important concept for quality and safety leaders can be found in Thomas S. Kuhn's *The Structure of Scientific Revolutions*.[18] Though not a common reference in the bibliographies of most health services research, Kuhn's concept of a "paradigm shift" has seeped into the popular culture since it was first published in 1962. Kuhn emphasizes that, rather than being incorporated in a continuous and linear process, scientific knowledge is marked by episodic scientific revolutions that disrupt the understanding of the scientific community. Typically met by resistance and skepticism, such revolutions ultimately have the capacity to shift the scientific community's paradigm of understanding.

To Err Is Human may be to health care delivery what Nicolaus Copernicus's *Commentariolus* was to astronomy. Copernicus's work—questioned, challenged, and dismissed when it appeared—ultimately led to Galileo Galilei's work and the collapse of the existing Ptolemaic system. The lukewarm reception of the health care industry to quality and patient safety improvement is strikingly similar. Through our inaction, the health care industry demonstrates a lack of understanding and acceptance of the findings contained in *To Err Is Human*. Yet its influence is episodic, and we appear to be witnessing a paradigm shift despite a majority of "Ptolemaics" in our industry who are unwilling to acknowledge that anything is wrong with the existing health care delivery system.

The culture of patient safety first articulated in *To Err Is Human* is beginning to emerge, and, within this new paradigm, we are better able to conceptualize and define quality.

Definitions of Quality Improvement

Donabedian Triad: The old paradigm

Writing in the 1960s, Avedis Donabedian pioneered a framework for understanding and evaluating quality improvement work in heath care[19,20] that continues to resonate with many clinicians today. His body of work helped lay the foundation for recognizing that health care quality is measurable and that quality assessment depends on looking at three key components known as the Donabedian Quality Triad.

The Triad rests on the assumption that health care quality is the product of two factors, science and technology, and the practical application of these in the health care industry. The Triad explores quality as a balance of the three dimensions: 1) structure (the tools and resources available to providers and their physical and organizational settings), 2) process (the normative behaviors of providers and the interactions between them and their patients), and 3) outcome ("changes in a patient's current and future health status"). As originally presented by Donabedian, the Triad appeared in a linear relationship as follows: *Structure → Process → Outcome.*

Because Donabedian theorized that all the elements are linked, a more appropriate schematic follows:

Figure 1. Donabedian Triad

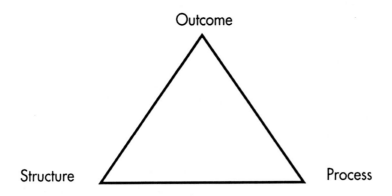

Insight into just one component of the Triad is insufficient to measure and evaluate quality. As summary views of quality, outcome measures were the most prevalent indicators of success. However, recent research has shown that process metrics provide increased detail and are more sensitive to incremental changes in performance.[21] Beginning in the late 1980s, an emphasis on assessing all elements in the Triad has helped create the conditions for a focus on process redesign. Outcomes alone are recognized as lying "too far down the stream of production of care to be efficient detectors of quality problems." In the 1980s and 1990s, the industry attempted to move toward measuring structure and processes in addition to outcomes, thus avoiding what Berwick described as the "tyranny of outcomes."[22, 23]

Donabedian emphasizes the critical role of health care *structure*, a prerequisite for process and outcome.[24] Structure includes physical infrastructure (e.g., facilities, equipment, supplies) and the structure of organizational capability (e.g., provider qualifications). Increasingly, it is believed that structure should include organizational operational capability since "leadership, human capital, information management systems and group dynamics...are essential structural elements of quality improvement in a health care organization and serve as primary catalysts for process change."[25]

Process includes all activities that take place between direct and indirect organizational health care providers and patients. These are categorized into technical and interpersonal processes. Technical processes deal with clinical activities focused primarily on individual health and reduction of associated clinical risk. In contrast, interpersonal processes focus on the social and psychological interactions between individual health providers and the patient. Donabedian emphasized the technical skill of providers, and, therefore, process is the primary focus of quality improvement initiatives addressing intra- and inter-profession activities and closely examining the culture of collaboration and cooperation between them.[26]

Describing the *outcome* leg of the Triad, Donabedian wrote that, "Outcome means a change in a client's current and future health status that can be attributed to antecedent health care."[24] The Triad elements lead to the identification of four broad clusters of outcomes that can be identified, measured, and categorized as: 1) behavioral 2) experiential 3) clinical, and 4) financial. This area contains the effect (outcomes) of processes and available structure elements—for example, the impact of the change initiative on mortality, hospital readmissions, or patient experience.[27]

While the Triad provided a basic framework for understanding quality improvement, it overlooks certain areas, such as cost and efficiency.[28] In addition, Donabedian's work fails to incorporate culture—particularly the culture of patient safety called for by the IOM—and places undue emphasis on technical skill without considering systems of care and the culture of high-reliability teams.

Evidence-Based Care and the Role of Guidelines

When Donabedian described *process* in the 1960s, his focus was on the "appropriateness, completeness, and redundancy of information obtained through clinical history, physical examination and diagnostic tests; justification of diagnosis and therapy; technical competence in the performance of diagnostic and therapeutic procedures, including surgery; evidence of preventive management in health and illness; coordination and continuity of care; [and] the acceptability of care to the recipient."[23] Since that time, the terminology has shifted to "adherence to evidence-based care and clinical practice guidelines."[29]

The number of clinical guidelines grew rapidly in the 1990s. Research dating back to the early 1970s, much of it led by John E. Wennberg, MD at Dartmouth University, demonstrated unexplained variation in health care.[30] The industry's failure to standardize its processes was seen as resulting in both under- and overutilization. Although guidelines, in theory, should have helped clinicians to standardize care and reduce such variation, it became increasingly clear that "the accelerated pace of development…led to an abundance of guidelines created by different organizations with different methods and different objectives."[31] Moreover, guidelines did not consistently adhere to the evidence, or they became outdated long before they were widely adopted.[3, 32, 33]

In the 1990s, the Veterans Administration (VA) defined clinical practice guidelines as "recommendations for the performance or exclusion of specific procedures or services derived through a rigorous methodological approach that includes the following:

- Determination of appropriate criteria, such as effectiveness, efficacy, population benefit, or patient satisfaction; and

- Literature review to determine the strength of evidence (based in part on study design) in relation to these criteria."[34]

Although the VA's *Clinical Practice Guideline Primer* stressed that guidelines must be evidence-based, providers in the 1990s were slow to adopt the evidence. One of the most striking examples of this was prescribing aspirin for heart attack patients. In 1988, clear evidence emerged from clinical trials that heart attack victims without contraindications benefited from timely administration of aspirin. Three years following the release of this evidence, researchers reported that aspirin use following acute myocardial infarction (AMI) had increased from 39 to 72 percent for patients in 106 North American hospitals.[3, 35]

In 2002, The Joint Commission began collecting data on aspirin use upon arrival at the hospital for AMI patients. CMS began reporting this information publicly in 2004, ultimately linking the data to payment. With CMS's first release of data, the national average rate of administering aspirin within 24 hours of admission for AMI patients was a respectable 94 percent; however, variation remained high. Nearly 5 percent of the 2,817 hospitals treating more than ten AMI patients in the first two quarters of 2004 administered aspirin to less than 80 percent of eligible patients. Fewer that 90 percent of eligible AMI patients received aspirin within 24 hours at over 20 percent of the nation's hospitals, while nearly half of these hospitals administered aspirin within 24 hours to less than 95 percent of their eligible AMI patients.[36]

After years of public reporting, these numbers have improved. In the 12-month period ending September 2010, all but 11 percent of the 2,665 hospitals treating more than ten patients administered aspirin to over 95 percent of their AMI patients, while only 4 percent of the nation's hospitals administered aspirin to less than 90 percent of their eligible patients; less than 1 percent of hospitals administered aspirin to less than 80 percent of their patients.[37]

Historically, providers have been slow to accept evidence, providing face validity to the research of Everett M. Rodgers, who argued that the adoption of innovation follows a normal distribution. In his work, *Diffusion of Innovation*, Rodgers demonstrated that it took 15 years for Iowa farmers to adopt the use of superior hybrid seed corn in the 1920s and 1930s.[38] The timeline for a nearly full implementation of the use aspirin upon arrival for AMI patients (1988 to 2010) is only slightly behind the pace of the Iowa farmers.

The industry's slow rate of adopting evidence-based guidelines and the growing demand for valid process measures to identify compliance with the evidence has significantly transformed health care. The IOM's *Crossing the Quality Chasm Report* specifically pointed out that "…in the current health care system, scientific knowledge about best care is not applied systematically or expeditiously to clinical practice. An average of about 17 years is required for new knowledge generated by randomized control trials to be incorporated into practice."[12]

The *Chasm Report's* findings dovetailed well with work under way elsewhere. In 1999, the NQF was created as a not-for-profit membership organization. This public-private partnership includes national, state, regional, and local groups representing consumers, public and private purchasers, employers, health care professionals, provider organizations, health plans, accrediting bodies, labor unions, supporting industries, and organizations involved in health care research or quality improvement. Through its efforts to build consensus across various stakeholder groups, the NQF created a common and relatively non-controversial approach to measuring health care quality. Increasingly, the NQF is recognized as a critical force for reviewing and endorsing performance measures for public accountability. Several major organizations, including The Joint Commission, CMS, and the National Committee for Quality Assurance (NCQA), have aligned with NQF standards. Thus, the NQF has brought a level of stability to performance measurement.

Another force driving the industry toward adoption of evidence-based guidelines is the Institute for Healthcare Improvement (IHI). Founded in 1991, the IHI focused attention on improving the safety of hospital care with the launch of its *100,000 Lives Campaign* on December 14, 2004. With over 3,000 hospitals participating, this voluntary campaign became a *de facto* national standard. Regardless of their participation in the campaign, hospitals faced significant legal incentives to adopt the 6 recommended evidence-based interventions proposed by the IHI to reduce avoidable inpatient deaths.[39] The *100,000 Lives Campaign* was followed by the IHI's *5 Million Lives Campaign*, with a focus on additional interventions aimed at reducing patient harm.

While the NQF developed consensus measures to help assess quality, the IHI supplied tools and methods to help providers implement evidence-based practices to improve care. At the same time, both organizations helped to accelerate the regulatory changes first proposed in the IOM's *Chasm Report* and recently embedded in the Affordable Care Act. The approval of consensus measures by the NQF ensured that CMS could implement regulatory changes that would enable it to increase transparency with respect to quality performance and to transition its remuneration structure to pay for quality rather than procedures. We now know that all health care providers will be included in CMS's "pay for reporting" requirements and, with the launch of value-based purchasing initiatives, NQF-endorsed measures will be used by CMS as well as other regulatory agencies and many commercial payers to enforce accountability.[40]

The IHI provides a learning laboratory for a small but energetic cohort of providers who have demonstrated that care can be dramatically improved through systematic interventions. In part because of the IHI's focus, early adopters in the provider community were able to reduce harm near to zero for patients receiving central lines or being placed on ventilators.[41] Thus, the IHI helped eliminate the industry's ability to challenge the direction of CMS by making the pursuit of perfection a realistic and attainable goal.

In turn, CMS rapidly incorporated IHI's recent work into its reform and payment strategies. Critics are increasingly on the defensive in challenging the findings of the IOM reports and policies built upon the reports' foundations.

The industry's unwillingness to adhere to evidence-based practice has further opened the door for a regulatory environment that intends to enforce adherence, whether or not providers agree. Once The Joint Commission began to collect process measures in 2002, CMS followed (in 2004) and quickly linked payment to reporting. The ACA adds significant regulatory oversight with respect to guideline adherence. The value-based purchasing rule issued by CMS on May 6, 2011, includes 12 process measures consistent with evidence-based guidelines.[42] Hospitals that fail to perform at acceptable levels will experience a loss of Medicare reimbursement.

The list of process measures is likely to grow. The proposed CMS Inpatient Prospective Payment System rule (2012) includes a total of 35 evidence-based clinical process measures, while another 20 process measures are included in the current Outpatient Prospective Payment System rule. These measures will likely be added in the future to value-based purchasing rules.[43, 44] Use of evidence-based guidelines are now, and will increasingly become, a requirement for payment by both public and private payers.

Crossing the Quality Chasm Report

Moving beyond simple outcome measurement, Donabedian provided a framework for assessing quality by focusing on process measures and, to a lesser extent, structural measures, thus helping to create a common understanding that quality is measurable. Evidence-based medicine and its incorporation into clinical practice guidelines laid the groundwork for developing clearly defined performance measures and a more meaningful standard for identifying high-quality providers.

Ultimately, it was the IOM's *Chasm Report* that provided a new framework for assessing and improving quality. With its publication, the health care industry finally had a sufficiently broad and comprehensive definition of quality that moved us beyond the Triad. Appearing in March 2001, the report was a strategy for reinventing the entire health care delivery system. After boldly stating that, as currently organized, the United States health care delivery system could not provide high-quality care, the report created a blueprint for its restructuring. The report was embraced rapidly by health policy leaders—many aspects have been incorporated into public policy—and it is slowly being adopted by health care providers as they develop their quality improvement strategies.

Immediately, the *Chasm Report* began to change the conversation among health policy makers—CMS, employers, business coalitions, and increasingly commercial payers. Publication of the report was truly a transformative event; nine years later, much of the report was embedded in the PPACA signed into law by President Barack Obama on March 23, 2010. In contrast, hospital staff and health care providers were often the last to read and comprehend the *Chasm Report* and have been slow to adopt its recommendations for developing quality improvement strategies.

One cannot begin to conceptualize and define health care quality without understanding the *Chasm Report*. The report laid out 6 aims for improvement of health care that we quote at length:

- *Safe*—avoiding injuries to patients from the care that is intended to help them.
- *Effective*—providing services based on scientific knowledge to all who could benefit and refraining from providing services to those not likely to benefit (avoiding underuse and overuse).
- *Patient-centered*—providing care that is respectful of and responsive to individual patient preferences, needs, and values and ensuring that patient values guide all clinical decisions.
- *Timely*—reducing waits and sometimes harmful delays for both those who receive and those who give care.
- *Efficient*—avoiding waste, including waste of equipment, supplies, ideas, and energy.
- *Equitable*—providing care that does not vary in quality because of personal characteristics such as gender, ethnicity, geographic location, and socioeconomic status.[12]

In effect, quality is determined by the ability to accomplish the six aims of the *Chasm Report*. The report also provided a framework for achieving the report's aims by focusing on four specific levels of improvement in the following areas:

A) The experience of patients and communities.

B) Improving and redesigning microsystems of care—the small units where value for a patient or consumer is actually created. This calls for a fundamental shift from old models of care with the articulation of 10 simple rules:

    1. Care based on continuous healing relationships

    2. Customization based on patient needs and values

    3. The patient as the source of control

    4. Shared knowledge and free flow of information

5. Evidence-based decision making

6. Safety as a system property

7. The need for transparency

8. Anticipation of needs

9. Continuous decrease in waste

10. Cooperation among clinicians

C) Redesign of health organizations, with a focus on: (1) "robust and persistent systems for finding best practices and assuring that the best-known clinical models...become organizational standards"; (2) information technology; (3) investment in and development of the health care workforce; (4) team-based care; (5) improved care coordination; and (6) measurement systems that accurately capture performance around all six IOM aims.

D) Changes to the external health care environment, including but not limited to regulatory, accreditation, litigation, and policy changes.[12, 45]

The IOM aims contained in the *Chasm Report* do not neatly fit into Donabedian's structure-process-outcome framewoık. Certainly, effective and timely care is aligned with process, while safe and patient-centered care can be considered outcomes. Efficiency was not tightly tied to the Donabedian Quality Triad and equity did not play a prominent role. The major divergence, explicit in *Chasm Report,* is a recognition that a "higher level of quality cannot be achieved by further stressing current system of care. The current care system cannot do the job. Trying harder will not work. Changing systems of care will."[12] Moreover, changing systems of care requires new methods and approaches. The *Chasm Report* did not call for tweaking structure; rather, it called for a reinvention of the way care is delivered, thus providing a new paradigm for understanding quality and safety.

The *Chasm Report* and *To Err Is Human* were direct assaults on the health care delivery system that fundamentally changed the way innovative health providers approached quality improvement. In the aftermath of these publications, quality improvement followed two complementary but different paths. As already noted, process measurement and adoption of evidence-based practices matured rapidly due, in part, to regulatory pressure. Yet simple measurement was not sufficient to achieve the IOM aims. Improvement in process measures *did not* transform health care providers into high-reliability organizations.

The most significant change in health care in recent years is only partly due to more aggressive adoption of evidence-based medicine and the transparency associated with public reporting of provider performance. High-reliability health care providers are differentiating themselves by recognizing that cultural transformation is required to change our "current care system [that] cannot do the job."[12]

The need for profound cultural transformation was implicit in both IOM reports. In his keynote address at the 12th Annual IHI National Forum on Quality Improvement in Healthcare, Berwick captured this challenge by calling for "deep change—change in what we do and change in what we think."[46] Since Berwick spoke in 2000, a significant driver of this change has been story telling. Story telling gained popularity through the IHI's *5 Million Lives Campaign*, which included a plank for "Getting the Board on Board." The campaign called for hospital boards of trustees to get data and hear stories. Boards, the IHI argued, should "select and review progress toward safer care as the first agenda item at every board meeting, grounded in transparency, and putting a 'human face' on harm data."[47,48] Telling stories is important because stories help hospitals and providers to construct a safety knowledge. Through the social interaction of story telling, caregivers can make sense of safety events. When appropriately used, stories become a form of organizational learning that can move the culture of an institution to a level of higher reliability.[49]

While Donabedian moved the industry away from measuring rare outcomes (e.g., mortality) and emphasized process, the changes emerging in the post-*Chasm Report* decade are harking back to "outcomes." Rather than as a systematic way to measure quality, the focus is increasingly on how organizations culturally respond to harm events. In this new model, harm rates per 1,000 patients are a less important measure than how an organization responds to failures and redesigns care, one patient at a time.

Conclusion

The conceptualization and definition of quality is undergoing a dramatic change. Since Donabedian first provided a framework for assessing quality, our conceptualization and definition of quality has matured. The *Chasm Report*, coming on the heels of *To Err Is Human*, provides a conceptualization that has already been embraced by many within the industry, in particular policy makers. In order for health care providers to influence the direction of health care quality, they too must comprehend and embrace the *Chasm Report's* conceptualization of quality and continue to adopt tools and approaches to implement change as outlined in the report and as embodied in the implementation of health care reform.

Study and Discussion Questions

1. What are the key components of the definition of quality contained in *Crossing the Quality Chasm*?

2. How did the publication of *To Err Is Human* change the industry's understanding of patient safety and harm?

3. Describe Donabedian Triad and its relationship to the practice of evidence-based medicine, quality improvement, and cultural transformation in health care settings.

Suggested Reading and Web Sites

Berwick DM. *Escape Fire: Designs for the Future of Health Care.* San Francisco: Jossey-Bass, 2004.

Donabedian A. *The Definition of Quality and Approaches of its Assessment.* Volume 1: Explorations in Quality Assessment and Monitoring. Ann Arbor, MI. Health Administration Press, 1981.

Gwande A. *The Checklist Manifesto: How to Get Things Right.* New York: Metropolitan Books, 2010.

Institute of Medicine. *Crossing the Quality Chasm: A New Health System for the 21st Century.* Washington, DC: National Academy Press, 2001.

Kohn LT, Corrigan JM, and Donaldson MS, eds. *To Err Is Human: Building a Safer Health System.* Washington, DC: National Academy Press, 2000.

Millenson ML. *Demanding Medical Excellence: Doctors and Accountability in the Information Age.* Chicago: University of Chicago Press, 1997, 1999.

Institute for Healthcare Improvement. (http://www.ihi.org)

Agency for Healthcare Research and Quality (http://www.ahrq.gov)

The Joint Commission (http://www.jointcommission.org)

The National Quality Forum (http://www.qualityforum.org/Home.aspx)

References

1. Kohn LT, Corrigan JM, and Donaldson MS, eds. To Err Is Human: Building a Safer Health System. Washington, DC: National Academies Press, 2000.

2. Bates DW et al. Incidence of adverse drug events and potential adverse drug events: Implications for prevention. *JAMA*, 274(1):29-34, July 5, 1995.

3. Advisory Commission on Consumer Protection and Quality in the Health Care Industry. Quality First: Better Health Care for All Americans: Final Report to the President of the United States. Washington, DC: U.S. Government Printing Office, 1998.

4. McDonald CJ, et al. Deaths due to medical errors are exaggerated in Institute of Medicine report. *JAMA*, 284(1):93-5, July 5, 2000.

5. Hayward RA, Hofer TP. Estimating hospital deaths due to medical errors: preventability is in the eye of the reviewer. *JAMA,* 286(4):415-20, July 5, 2001.

6. Brennan TA. The Institute of Medicine report on medical errors—Could it do harm? *N Engl J Med,* 343(9):663-5, April 13, 2000.

7. Blendon RJ, DesRoches CM, Brodie M, et al. Views of practicing physicians and the public on medical errors. *N Engl J Med*, (24):1933-40, Dec. 12, 2002.

8. Institute of Medicine. Crossing the Quality Chasm: A New Health System for the 21st Century. Washington, DC: National Academies Press, 2001.

9. Brennan TA, Gawande A, Thomas E, Studdert D. Accidental deaths, saved lives, and improved quality. *N Engl J Med*, 353(13):1405-9, Sept. 29, 2005.

10. Altman DE, Clancy C, and Blendon RJ. Improving patient safety--Five years after the IOM Report. *N Engl J Med*, 351(20):2041-3, Nov. 11, 2004.

11. Leape LL, Berwick DM. Five years after To Err Is Human: What have we learned? *JAMA*, 293(19):2384-90, May 18, 2005.

12. Landrigan CP, Parry GJ, Bones CB, *et al*. Temporal trends in rates of patient harm resulting from medical care. *N Engl J Med*, 363(22):2124-34, Nov. 25, 2010.

13. Levinson DR. *Adverse Events in Hospitals: National Incidence Among Medicare Beneficiaries.* Washington, DC: Office of Inspector General, 2010.

14. For the reaction of the American Medical Association to suggestions that dirty lab coats not be worn in the hospital see Yao, L. AMA: White coats need more study. *Wall Street Journal*, June 16, 2009 http://blogs.wsj.com/health/2009/06/16/ama-the-white-coats-are-going-the-white-coats-are-going. Accessed March 20, 2011.

15. Gwande A. *The Checklist Manifesto: How to Get Things Right*. New York: Metropolitan Books, 2010, pp.136-157.

16. Haynes AB, Weiser TG, Berry WR, et al. A surgical safety checklist to reduce morbidity and mortality in a global population. *N Engl J Med*, 360(5):491-9, Jan. 29, 2009.

17. HANYS DataGen. Medicare Hospital-Acquired Condition (HAC) Rate Analysis (April 2011). https://www.datagen.info/ (subscription required). Accessed April 19, 2011.

18. Kuhn TS. *The Structure of Scientific Revolutions*. 2nd ed. Chicago: University of Chicago Press, 1962, 1970.

19. Donabedian A. Evaluating the quality of medical care. *Milbank Memorial Fund Quarterly*, 44(3):166-206, July 1966; rpt. *Milbank Quarterly*, 83(4):691–729, 2005.

20. Donabedian A. *The Definition of Quality and Approaches of its Assessment*. Volume 1: Explorations in Quality Assessment and Monitoring. Ann Arbor, MI: Health Administration Press, 1981.

21. Hammermeister KE, Shroyer LA, Sethi GK, Grover FL. Why it is important to demonstrate linkages between outcomes of care and processes and structures of care. *Medical Care*, 33(10):OS5-OS16, Oct. 1995.

22. Berwick DM. Toward an applied technology for quality measurement in health care. *Med Decis Making*, 8(4):253-8, Oct-Dec 1988.

23. Berwick DM. Continuous improvement as an ideal in health care. *N Engl J Med*, 320(1):53-6. Jan 5, 1989.

24. Kunkel S, Rosenqvist U, Westerling R. The structure of quality systems is important to the process and outcome, an empirical study of 386 hospital departments in Sweden. *BMC Health Serv Res*, 7(104):1-8, July 8, 2007.

25. Glickman SW, Baggett KA, Krubert CG, Iet al. Promoting quality: The health-care organization from a management perspective. *Int J Qual Health Care*, 19(6):341-348, Dec. 2007.

26. Postema T. Quality assessment: Process or outcome? The use of performance indicators for quality assessment in Dutch health care. *Quality Digest*, 2005. http://timpostema.nl/Quality%20Digest%20Magazine.htm. Accessed June 22, 2011.

27. Runciman WB, Baker GB, Michel P et al. Tracing the foundations of a conceptual framework for a patient safety ontology. *Qual Saf Health Care*, 19(6):1-5, .Dec. 2010. http://qualitysafety.bmj.com/content/early/2010/08/10/qshc.2009.035147.abstract. Accessed on June 22, 2011.

28. Ransom SB, Griffith JR, Campbell DA, Ransom ER. Conceptualizing and improving quality: An overview. In Nash DB, Goldfarb NI, eds. *The Quality Solution: The Stakeholder Guide to Improving Health Care.* Sudbury, MA: Jones and Bartlett, 2006:49-72.

29. Weingarten S. Assessing and improving quality of care. In Williams, SJ, Torrens, PR. *Introduction to Health Services*, 6th ed. Albany, NY: Delmar Publishers, Inc., 2002, pp.373-391.

30. Wennberg J, Gittelsohn A. Small area variations in health care delivery. *Science,* 182(117):1102-8, Dec. 14, 1973..

31. Weingarten S. Using practice guideline compendiums to provide better preventive care. *Ann Intern Med*, 130(5):454-8, Nov 2, 1999.

32. Weingarten S. Practice guidelines and prediction rules should be subject to careful clinical testing. *JAMA*, 277(24):1977-8, June 25, 1997.

33. Shekelle PG, Ortiz E, Rhodes S, *et al*. Validity of the Agency for Healthcare Research and Quality clinical practice guidelines: how quickly do guidelines become outdated? *JAMA*, 286(12):1461-7, Sept. 16, 2001.

34. *Clinical Practice Guidelines.* Boston, MA: Management Decisions and Research Center; Washington, DC: VA Health Services Research and Development Service in collaboration with Association for Health Services Research, 1998.

35. Lamas GA, Pfeffer MA, Hamm P, *et al*.. Do the results of randomized clinical trials of cardiovascular drugs influence medical practice? *N Engl J Med*, 327(2):241-7, July 23, 1992.

36. Center for Medicare & Medicaid Services. Hospital Compare Database, April 2005 release. http://www.medicare.gov/download/downloaddb.asp. Accessed January 8, 2007.

37. Center for Medicare & Medicaid Services. Hospital Compare Database, June 2011 release. http://www.medicare.gov/download/downloaddb.asp. Accessed July 10, 2011.

38. Rogers EM. *Diffusion of Innovations*. 4th ed. New York: The Free Press, 1995, pp. 252-266.

39. Gosfield AG, Reinertsen JL. The 100,000 lives campaign: crystallizing standards of care for hospitals. *Health Aff*, 24(6):1560-70, Nov.-Dec. 2005.

40. Berwick DM, James B, Coye MJ. Connections between quality measurement and improvement. *Med Care*, 41(Suppl 1): I-30–I-38, Jan. 2003.

41. Pronovost P, Needham D, Berenholtz S. *et al*. An intervention to decrease catheter-related bloodstream infections in the ICU. *N Engl J Med*, 355(26):2725-32, Dec. 28, 2006.

42. Department of Health and Human Services. Centers for Medicare and Medicaid Services. Medicare program; Hospital inpatient value-based purchasing program. *Federal Register*. 76 (88): 26490-547, May 6, 2011. http://www.gpo.gov/fdsys/pkg/FR-2011-05-06/pdf/2011-10568.pdf. Accessed July 10, 2011.

43. Department of Health and Human Services. Centers for Medicare and Medicaid Services. Medicare program; Proposed changes to the hospital inpatient prospective payment systems for acute care hospitals and the long-term care hospital prospective payment system and fiscal year 2012 rates. *Federal Register.* 76 (87): 25788-6084, May 5, 2011. http://www.cms.gov/AcuteInpatientPPS/IPPS2012/itemdetail.asp?filterType=none&filterByDID=-99&sortByDID=1&sortOrder=ascending&itemID=CMS1246629&intNumPerPage=10. Accessed July 10, 2011.

44. Department of Health and Human Services. Centers for Medicare and Medicaid Services. Medicare program; Hospital outpatient prospective payment system and CY 2011 payment rates; Ambulatory surgical center payment systems and CY 2011 payment rates; Payments to hospitals for graduate medical education costs; Physician self-referral rules and related changes to provider agreement regulations; Payment for certified registered nurse anesthetist services furnished in rural hospitals and critical access hospitals; Final. *Federal Register.* 75 (226):71800-2580, Nov. 24, 2010. http://edocket.access.gpo.gov/2010/pdf/2010-27926.pdf. Accessed July 10, 2010.

45. Berwick DM. A user's manual for the IOM's 'Quality Chasm' report. *Health Aff,* 21(3): 80-90, May-June 2002.

46. Berwick DM. "Dirty words and magic spells." in *Escape Fire: Designs for the Future of Health Care.* San Francisco: Jossey-Bass, 2004, pp. 211-238.

47. 5 Million Lives Campaign. Getting Started Kit: *Governance Leadership "Boards on Board" How-to Guide.* Cambridge, MA: Institute for Healthcare Improvement, 2008. http://www.ihi.org/knowledge/Pages/Tools/HowtoGuideGovernanceLeadership.aspx

48. Conway J. Getting boards on board: engaging governing boards in quality and safety. *Jt Comm J Qual Patient Saf,* 34(4):214-20, April 2008.

49. Waring JJ. Constructing and re-constructing narratives of patient safety. *Social Science & Medicine,* 69(12):1722-31, Dec. 2009.

Chapter 3

Legal and Policy Issues in Quality

By Martha C. Romney, RN, JD, MPH

Executive Summary

"Quality" as defined by the Institute of Medicine is "the degree to which health services for individuals and populations increase the likelihood of desired health outcomes and are consistent with current professional knowledge."[1] For more than a decade, federal and state governments, health care systems, and quasi-regulatory and professional organizations have implemented policies and initiatives aimed at improving the quality of the nation's health outcomes and reducing unsustainable costs of health care.[2] Currently, key strategies for improving patient outcomes while reducing costs include: adopting value-based health economic models through implementation of nationwide interoperable electronic technology to support transparent, coordinated, evidenced-based care; enhancing communication with patients by adopting culturally and linguistically appropriate language and health literacy techniques; and disclosing medical errors that are also associated with better outcomes.

The framework for achieving current and future strategies for bending the cost curve is based upon myriad laws and policies. However, the complexity and fluidity of health care governance at federal, state, and local levels, as well as professional and organizational standards and policies, are challenging to interpret and implement. Keeping abreast of and compliant with legal and regulatory requirements is necessary to avoid significant financial and other penalties.

This chapter provides an overview of the laws related to governmental, organizational, and professional initiatives and recommendations on compliance with the mandates. Physicians are encouraged to consult with their legal counsels, insurers, and compliance officers for timely and relevant legal and policy changes impacting their practices and health care delivery organizations.

Learning Objectives

1. Describe the complexities of the U.S. legal foundations of health care quality.

2. Highlight examples of current key quality initiatives associated with legal mandates.

3. Identify opportunities and challenges associated with engaging in quality initiatives.

Key Words: Physician Quality Reporting System, Medical errors, Disclosure statutes, HITECH Act, Apology statutes, Health literacy

Introduction

The spectrum of health care quality is expansive, encompassing patient-centered coordinated care; application of evidence-based guidelines to drive clinical decisions; implementation of standard procedures to reduce, disclose, and remedy medical errors; and protection of the privacy and security of patient data supported through interoperable electronic health records. Linguistic and culturally appropriate communications that follow health literacy principles to improve patient engagement in their care are another component of quality of care.

While the focus of this chapter is primarily on federal programs implemented by the U.S. Department of Health and Human Services (DHHS), the issues are relevant to all health care providers. Efforts to control costs through implementing quality measures, reducing medical errors, and improving communication with patients are also in place at the state level and through non-governmental organization (NGO) accreditation and professional and insurance organizations.

The complexity of the U.S. legal environment is due, in part, to the structure and organization of our constitutional government that distributes powers across three branches—legislative, executive and judicial—to create an intricate system of checks and balances. Adding to the complexity, the 10th Amendment to the U.S. Constitution grants states authority to exercise powers not directly delegated to Congress, provided they do not conflict with federal law.

Our health care delivery system operates through a multitude of legislative, administrative, and judicial mandates from federal, state, and local authorities; quasi-regulatory accreditation and licensing standards and; organizational policies. Laws may be complex, difficult to interpret and implement, and inconsistent with other laws. Regulations developed by administrative agencies establish the rules for implementing statutes, including professional licensure, certification and practice standards, conduct of research, and reporting requirements. In addition, NGOs develop, endorse, and/or monitor quality and safety standards—for example, the Joint Commission's accreditation and patient safety standards; the National Quality Forum's (NQF's) endorsed quality measures, which have been adopted by the Centers for

Medicare and Medicaid Services (CMS); and other federal and state entities as legal standards, as well as the initiatives of the Leapfrog Group and other organizations.[4-7]

The failure of these measures to reduce the prevalence and severity of adverse events associated with mortality and unsustainable costs, particularly with respect to preventable medical errors, has led to more stringent requirements. For the past decade, the government's strategy for improving quality in health care has focused on: reporting and analyses of patient outcomes, institutionalization of evidence-based clinical guidelines, improvement of communication to engage and inform patients, and adoption of interoperable electronic health infrastructure to support coordination of care.

To illustrate the breadth and complexity of laws directed at improving quality of care through changes in the delivery of health services, this chapter highlights four current initiatives:

1. The Physician Quality Reporting System

2. The HITECH Act's 'Meaningful Use' electronic health record initiative, and expanded HIPAA privacy and security protections

3. Medical error reporting, disclosure, and apology statutes

4. Improving patient health literacy

These initiatives reflect evolving strategies pursued by the federal government to bend the cost curve through iterative laws and policies with greater intricacy and penalties for noncompliance.

Physician Quality Reporting Initiatives

There is an urgent need to improve patient quality reporting and to lower preventable medical errors, mortality, and costs through adopting a value-based purchasing model. In the wake of its report *To Err Is Human,*[3] the Institute of Medicine (IOM) recommended demonstration projects with coordinated models of care, electronic repositories for voluntary and mandatory reporting of endorsed quality measures and unanticipated outcomes at the federal and state level, and the establishment of interoperable health information technology (HIT).[3] Unfortunately, mandatory licensure and accreditation standards and medical error and quality reporting statutes have not significantly impacted patient outcomes or costs.[8]

Over the past decade, insurers have been shifting from traditional fee-for-service economic models to value-based pay-for-reporting and pay-for-performance (P4P) programs that reward and motivate high-quality care.[9,10] These initiatives vary in focus, structure (e.g., mandatory, voluntary), sources of reporting (e.g., health care systems, health care professionals, patients), quality measures (e.g., outcomes, satisfaction, costs, process medical errors, readmissions, hospital-acquired infections, efficiency), and financial incentives/disincentives.[10]

Federally sponsored initiatives to engage physicians in the value-based model have included the Physician Voluntary Reporting Program; the Physician Group Practice Demonstrations; the eRX Incentive Program; and, most recently, the Physician Quality Reporting Initiative/System.[11-14] While these programs impact health care delivery to Medicare and Medicaid beneficiaries, private insurers and health care business coalitions have adopted similar quality improvement (QI) and value-based approaches.

The Physician Quality Reporting Initiative (PQRI) was launched in 2007 by CMS as a mandate of the 2006 Tax Relief and Health Care Act.[14] PQRI is a voluntary, Medicare pay-for- reporting demonstration program for improving care by means of clinical evidence-based guidelines.[15] Incentives are paid to "eligible physicians for reporting endorsed quality measures codes for services covered under the Medicare B Physician Fee Schedule either individually or through a group."[14]

The quality indicators are developed through an iterative, consensus-based process involving specialty medical groups and the American Medical Association Physician Consortium for Performance Improvement, subsequently endorsed by the NQF and ultimately approved by CMS.[15] Each program year, CMS publishes the proposed measures in the *Federal Register* and the finalized indicators in the annual Physician Fee Schedule Final Rule.[15]

To enroll in PQRI, eligible physicians report the Current Procedural Terminology Category 2 (CPTII) codes on three listed quality measures for eligible patients.[9] Currently, physicians reporting specific claims measures must submit codes for 50 percent of eligible patients, whereas codes for 80 percent of eligible patients are required for submission to registries.[14] CMS analyzes the data and provides individual quality reports to participating physicians.[14] Eligible physicians who meet the specified reporting period criteria receive bonus payments.[9]

Congress re-authorized the PQRI program and expanded the criteria for reporting eligibility (individual, group), quality measures, and financial incentives through the Medicare, Medicaid, and SCHIP Extension Act of 2007; the Medicare Improvements for Patients and Providers Act of 2008; and the Patient Protection and Affordable Care Act (ACA).[16-18]

Under the Patient Protection and Affordable Care Act of 2010 (ACA), the program was made permanent and renamed the Physician Quality Reporting System (PQRS).[18] Significant changes included an increase in the number and stringency of individual quality measures and the creation of an informal appeals process.[18] The percentages associated with incentive payments were reduced to one percent in 2011 and will be further reduced to 0.5 percent in 2012-2014.[18] Physicians also may receive an enhanced incentive through 2013 for participating in a Maintenance of Certification (MoC) Program, completing a MoC practice assessment, and reporting quality measures for a 12-month period.[18] Beginning in 2015, participation will be mandatory and penalties of 1.5 percent will be imposed on eligible providers who do not satisfactorily report quality data measures.[18] The penalty will increase to two percent in 2016.[18]

Studies show that the impact of physician quality reporting on patient outcomes is inconsistent.[10,15, 19] Proponents of PQRS argue that preliminary data reflect quality improvement that will become more apparent when outcome data are submitted and the system evolves to a P4P model.[8] In studies showing either limited or no improvement in quality,[15,19,21] researchers have attributed the results to practice burdens, inadequate computer training and support, and confusion with program requirements.[15,19,21] Still other critiques speak to the size of the financial incentive relative to the effort required and whether the paradigm contributes to improving quality of care.[15,19]

In addition to federal initiatives, at least 25 states, NGOs, and professional specialty organizations have instituted quality reporting programs.[21] For example, the Joint Commission, the Leapfrog Group, and the NQF have incorporated hospital-based quality and patient safety reporting programs into accreditation standards, computer physician-ordered standards, and endorsed quality measures respectively. These, in turn, have been adapted by federal and state governments, health plans, hospitals, and private organizations.[4,7,5,20,22] Other states have contracted with organizations to administer data collection and reporting procedures.[20,21]

Despite the reported challenges, financial and pragmatic considerations support physician involvement in the programs prior to mandatory participation beginning in 2015. Providers should consider adopting electronic technology and becoming familiar with the program requirements and procedures while it is possible to receive feedback and bonuses from CMS.[18] Reporting requirements will become more stringent and clinicians need to be prepared to participate and to avoid penalties in 2015.[19]

Health Information Technology for Economic and Clinical Health (HITECH) Act

The era of paper patient records maintained by individual providers and health care systems is drawing to a close. The use of electronic health records (EHR) facilitates efficient transmission of patient care information to support timely and accurate diagnoses and treatments. In turn, it enables evaluation of patient outcomes to inform the development of evidence-based practice guidelines for delivering better care and lowering costs. Since 1991, proponents of information technology (including the IOM) have advocated an electronic health infrastructure to support medical records, physician and medication orders, transmission of diagnostic results, and communication among providers, and to serve as a vehicle for disseminating patient information.[21] Adoption of information systems has been slow and uneven, particularly for smaller health organizations and practices.[8] To further the federal government's strategy for a nationwide interoperable health information infrastructure, Congress passed the HITECH Act, as part of the American Recovery and Reinvestment Act of 2009.[22]

The next iteration of the federal government's voluntary pay-for-reporting program, HITECH authorizes "incentive payments to participating Medicare and

Medicaid eligible providers (EP), eligible hospitals (EH), and critical access hospitals (CAH) that report and subsequently demonstrate "meaningful use of certified EHR technology."[22] The meaningful use criteria were developed to advance the following objectives: "improving the quality, safety, and efficiency of care while reducing disparities; engaging patients and their families in their care; promoting public and population health; improving care coordination; and promoting the privacy and security of EHRs."[22]

To date, $27 billion has been authorized for initiatives to support the adoption of electronic infrastructures by providers, entitlement programs, hospitals, and state governments through 2016.[23] Eligible providers must select whether to receive incentive payments from Medicare or Medicaid, and may earn up to $44,000 between 2011 and 2015 (Medicare) or up to $63,750 between 2011 and 2021 (Medicaid).[23,24] HITECH provides $650 million for the creation of 70 regional technology support centers to assist providers in setting up EHR systems and $560 million for state governments to develop inter-and intra-state information exchange capabilities.[23]

The program is being implemented in three stages. In December 2010, DHHS published the proposed regulations for Stage 1, which defined "eligible" participants, provided the initial criteria for meaningful use and quality measures, and defined the reporting timelines for 2011 and 2012.[23] In addition, interim final regulations were issued with the standards for "certifying" EHR technology and formulas for calculating the annual incentives.[23] To meet the 2011 meaningful use criteria, providers must report on meeting 15 core objectives and 5 non-core criteria, including one 'clinical decision support' rule.[24,25]

Over the next 5 years, providers will be required to submit data to meet the clinical quality measures meaningful use criteria for Stages 2 and 3 published in the *Federal Register* with the reporting requirements.[23, 24] Congress has mandated that the meaningful use criteria become increasingly more stringent and the monetary incentives will decrease with each stage.[23] Beginning in 2017, penalties will be imposed on participating providers who do not become "meaningful users."[23,24]

HITECH presents opportunities and challenges for health care providers who must understand the current and future EHR program requirements, including the meaningful use and reporting criteria. Physician participants in the meaningful use program have experienced difficulties implementing EHR systems and collecting, calculating, and reporting Stage 1 quality measures. Some have questioned the adequacy of the certification requirements identified through serious medication errors identified in CPOE system simulation.[10]

Improvements in care have been reported by large health care organizations that use individually designed EHR systems to support coordinated care and provide aligned incentives.[10] In smaller organizations and practices, meaningful use outcomes have varied, with some reporting benefits and others reporting minimal impact.[21,25] Providers are encouraged to develop HIT strategic plans that include pre-implementation, pilot, and annual EHR system evaluations; self-assessments of the technology by the users; and crisis management plans for system emergencies.[10,26,27]

To protect against increased risks to unprotected patient health information (PHI) resulting from the broader use of electronic technology, HITECH expanded privacy and security provisions and added breach notifications to the Health Insurance Portability and Accountability Act of 1996 (HIPAA).[22] Privacy and security compliance with HIPAA provisions are key components of meaningful use certification. The most significant changes to HIPAA include:

- Expansion of the scope and applicability of the Privacy and Security Rules;[27]

- Expansion of the HIPAA regulations to include "business associates;"[28]

- New and increased penalties and enforcement provisions;[29]

- Addition of a federal breach notification law.[30]

HITECH imposed stricter rules for documentation of disclosures, marketing restrictions, and "minimum necessary" disclosure standards.[31] Also, it entitles consumers to an electronic copy of their medical records when a covered entity uses or maintains electronic health records.[32] HIPAA privacy and security provisions, previously applicable only to covered entities, have been expanded to cover their business associates.[33] Business agreements between covered entities, business associates, and their subcontractors must document compliance with the privacy and security provisions, including notification of breaches of unsecured PHI.[33]

HITECH requires notification of breaches by covered entities and business associates.[34] A "breach" is "the unauthorized acquisition, access, use, or disclosure of PHI that compromises the security or privacy of such information.[35]There are three exceptions to the definition of "breach":

1. "Unintentional acquisition, access, or use of PHI by an employee or individual authorized by a covered entity or business associate, if the activity use was made in good faith and within the course and scope of employment or other professional relationship and there is not further activity with the PHI;

2. Inadvertent disclosure from an individual authorized to access PHI at a facility operated by a covered entity or business associate to another similarly situated individual at same facility;

3. PHI received as a result of a disclosure that is not further acquired, accessed, used, or disclosed without authorization by any person."[36]

The law specifies the content and timelines of notifications to individuals, the media, and the DHHS Secretary as well as posting on the DHHS website.[37] Notifications of breaches must be provided "to each individual whose unsecured PHI has been, or is reasonably believed to have been accessed, acquired, or disclosed during such breach" within 60 days and annually to DHHS.[38] The law excludes notification where an "unauthorized person to whom such information is disclosed would not reasonably have been able to retain such information."[38] Notifications of breaches involving 500 or more individuals also must be made to DHHS and through a media outlet.[39]

To increase enforcement of HIPPA, HITECH expanded the Office of Civil Rights' (OCR's) enforcement authority. Effective February 9, 2012, OCR will conduct mandatory periodic audits and investigations and impose increased penalties for violations.[40] Civil monetary penalties are tiered on the basis of the nature of the violations, level of defined culpability, and other factors including history of violations and responses to the breach.[41] The range of penalties is from $100 to $50,000 per violation with annual aggregated fines of $1.5 million.[41] HIPAA also authorizes criminal penalties for "knowingly obtaining and disclosing PHI" ranging from $50,000 and/or one-year imprisonment to $250,000 and/or 10-year imprisonment.[42] Although individuals cannot bring legal action against health care providers, HITECH extended authority to state attorney generals who may initiate civil suits on behalf of their residents.[43]

Regulations issued periodically by DHHS and the Federal Trade Commission define and refine the implementation of the HITECH provisions. At this writing, the Final Breach Notification Rule is on hold and the Interim Breach Notification Rule of October 2009 is in effect.[44] In addition to the federal statute, 46 states have enacted different data protection laws.

The significant expansion of HIPAA scope and enforcement requires that health care providers take steps to understand and stay informed regarding new laws and regulations in order to avoid risks and penalties associated with noncompliance. Health care providers should consult with clinical practice and health system attorneys and health system compliance/privacy officers to receive timely notices about changes to the HITECH Privacy, Security, Enforcement and Breach Notification Rules. Collaborative reviews and updates of policies, procedures, systems, and risk management strategies for staff and business associates include ongoing training to ensure compliance, preparedness, and timely response if necessary.

Medical error reporting, disclosure, and apologies

Physician and hospital failure to disclose medical errors adds to the exorbitant costs of health care delivery, fosters patient distrust of and anger with the health system, and contributes to endemic litigation. In 1991, the IOM estimated that 98,000 annual deaths—in addition to hundreds of thousands of preventable nonfatal injuries[45]—were due to medical errors.[3] Estimates of the associated costs are $37.6 billion, with $17 billion attributable to preventable medical errors.[46] Preventable medication errors alone account for $21 billion.[47]

Factors contributing to medical errors include incomplete patient information, miscommunication of and misunderstanding of medication orders, and systems-related issues.[46] Despite myriad public and private initiatives to understand and mitigate the underlying factors, patient and economic outcomes have not improved.[46] Initiatives include mandatory and voluntary reporting with financial incentives and disincentives, confidentiality protections, root cause analyses, new accreditation and endorsed quality standards, and litigation.

With the exception of the Department of Defense and the Veterans Health Administration, there is no national mandatory medical error reporting system to date.[48] In 2005, Congress passed the Patient Safety and Quality Improvement Act (PSQIA) to address the issue of under-reporting and to encourage voluntary physician reporting of patient safety information.[49] Under PSQIA, information about patient safety events communicated to a certified Patient Safety Organization is considered confidential and privileged, hence protected from discovery in litigation.[49] However, "patient safety work product" is narrowly defined and does not entirely eliminate legal reporting or other obligations under federal, state, or local laws and accrediting and licensing requirements.[49]

The Joint Commission has included review of organizational responses to sentinel events as part of the accreditation process since 1998.[50] The National Committee on Quality Assurance (NCQA), the American Hospital Association (AHA), the American College of Physician (ACP), and many other organizations have developed programs for reporting errors.[48] The NQF's list of 27 serious reportable "never events"(2002) was expanded to 29 in June 2011 and adopted by a majority of states.[51] As of 2009, 27 states have mandatory reporting systems, which vary extensively by reportable incidents, procedures and timing, levels of legal protections, enforcement authority, and penalties for noncompliance.[52] Other states contract with NGOs to analyze their medical error data.[52]

Another approach to reducing medical errors is termination of insurance payments for treatment of preventable conditions. The Deficit Reduction Act of 2005 mandated the Secretary of DHHS to identify preventable high-volume and/or high-cost conditions resulting in higher payment DRGs.[53] In October 2008, CMS terminated Medicare and Medicaid payments for care linked with 10 identified preventable conditions.[54] Private insurers in at least 7 states no longer cover certain corrective procedures.[52]

Despite these efforts, the rate of physician error reporting is estimated to be only 1 in 4. Studies have shown there is no accepted definition of error nor any consensus around the necessity to disclose error without injury to patients.[55,56,57] Some of the known barriers to provider reporting include embarrassment and shame; concern about professional discipline, loss of clinical privileges, licensure, and reputation; lack of training about disclosure, anonymity, and immunity; and fear of litigation.[55,56,57] To increase reporting rates, many states mandate physician disclosures and/or apologies for medical errors to patients through statutes, accreditation standards, and other administrative procedures.[52,55,56] Legal protections for physicians vary from state to state and across federal, professional, and organizational standards.[52] Providers who lack understanding and informed guidance from appropriate legal counsel may fail to comply with and/or create exposure for themselves through their communications.[52]

Patients expect their physicians to inform them about medical errors with explanations of the underlying causes and events.[57] Patients also expect physicians to convey their apologies, accountability, and plans for remediation.[57] The percentage of actual disclosures is low despite ethical, professional, and legal principles supporting disclosures of error.[53,55] In addition to professional obligations for honest communication with patients, disclosure of errors provides opportunities to improve care, enhance clinical practice standards, and either reduce legal claims or contribute to lower and faster settlements.[56]

There are distinctions between the medical and legal concepts and statutory provisions for statements of disclosure and apology.[55 56] To increase reporting of physician disclosures and/or apologies for medical errors to patients, statutes, accreditation standards, and other administrative procedures have been developed.[58] The Joint Commission's disclosure standard and the NQF's endorsed but voluntary safe-practice guidelines require that patients be informed of all outcomes of care, including unanticipated outcomes.[58] Nine states have enacted disclosure laws and 34 states and the District of Columbia have apology laws.[56] Six states have both types and 13 states do not have disclosure or apology laws.[52] Disclosure statutes generally require physicians to provide explanatory information to patients about the unanticipated outcomes.[55] Provisions governing the disclosure of the triggering event—the required content to be communicated; the covered providers; their voluntariness, form, and timing of the communication; and the protected content—varies from state to state.[55] Apology statutes also differ with respect to required and protected expressions of sympathy.[55] In states with "sympathy-only" laws, any explanation of the unanticipated outcome or accountability for the error will be admissible in court. Other jurisdictions may require explanations, statements of accountability, and steps to "make amends" to the patient.[55]

In the absence of national tort reform, concerns about malpractice litigation remain a deterrent to affirmative disclosures by physicians.[55] Professional standards and ethics promote disclosures of errors to patients, and federal law encourages and protects specific incident-related information. However, it is critical that providers know the current provisions of the PSQIA as well as their respective state disclosure and apology statutes' requirements and limitations to fulfill professional obligations to patients while complying with current legal and policy mandates.

Health Literacy as a Quality Measure

Communication is an essential component of high-quality physical and mental health care. Delivery of care, patient engagement, and compliance depend on effective exchange of information. Individuals with sensory impairments, as well as those who do not speak, understand, or read the language being conveyed orally and/or in writing, experience communication barriers. While services are available to individuals with sensory limitations, unrecognized language barriers are a critical issue as the demographics of the U.S. population undergoes change. An estimated 23 million Americans experience limited English proficiency (LEP), defined as "individuals who do not speak English as their primary language and/or who have a limited ability to read, write, speak, or understand English."[59,60] Research shows that the average reading level for American adults is 8th or 9th grade; however 1 in 5 adults reads at 5th grade level or lower.[61] LEP has been associated with underutilization of preventive services, delays and denials of care, poor self-care, and higher rates of chronic illness and mortality.[62] In addition to LEP, an estimated 90 million adults have difficulty reading and comprehending health information, calculating medication dosages, and following recommendations.[62]

The IOM defined health literacy as "the degree to which individuals have the capacity to obtain, process, and understand basic health information and services needed to make appropriate health decisions."[63] Research reveals that health literacy is a stronger predictor of individual health status than income, education, employment, race, or ethnicity.[64] Low health literacy is associated with higher rates of medication errors resulting in readmissions, the inability to manage chronic illness, and higher rates of mortality.[65] The estimated costs associated with low health literacy are reported to be $106 billion to $238 billion annually.[65]

The legal foundations for reducing communication barriers and providing access to language services are contained in federal and state statutes, regulations, and policy guidance to ensure equal access to language services for consumers whose low English proficiency (LEP), limited literacy, innumeracy, and cultural differences create potential barriers to safe and high-quality care. The Civil Rights Act of 1964 prohibits discrimination, exclusion from participation, or denial of benefits from federally funded programs on the basis of "race, color, or national origin."[66] Language is considered a proxy for national origin.[67] Federal agencies, including the DHHS, have issued policy guidelines requiring recipients of federal funding to take responsible steps to ensure access to language services by LEP persons."[68] DHHS guidelines apply to all providers, including physician offices, hospitals, community clinics, nursing homes, pharmacies, state agencies, and managed care plans involved with federal programs.[69]

Improving health literacy is an objective of the Healthy People 2020 strategies: "to develop appropriate written materials for audiences with limited literacy" and "to improve patients' reading skills."[69] In addition, the Office of Minority Health has proposed enhanced Culturally and Linguistically Appropriate Service (CLAS) standards in health care.[70]

All 50 states require access to language services in health care settings.[71,72] The provisions for accessing services, reimbursement for services from public and private insurers, continuing education for health care providers, certifications of medical interpreters, and mandates for language translations including forms, interpreters, and patient education vary across the states.[71,72] Some states require language services as a condition for facility licensure."[71,72] At least 46 states require special language services addressing mental health services.[71,72] Quality standards for health literacy have been adopted by the majority of health care organizations and professional associations, including the Joint Commission, NQF, the Leapfrog Group, NCQA, and many medical associations, including the AMA and the ACP.[4,5,7,64,74.75]

Health care professionals have a legal and ethical duty to ensure that their patients understand verbal and written communications. With an increasingly diverse population, knowledge of patients' cultural, ethnic, religious, and educational values that influence their lifestyles, health care behaviors, and practices is essential. Lack of provider understanding and respect for language and cultural differences is associated with patient noncompliance, mistrust, shame, and avoidance of health systems.

Effective communication is necessary for clinicians to obtain complete and accurate family and medical histories, discern meaningful differential diagnoses, determine appropriate treatments, and assess patient outcomes. To comply with accreditation and professional standards, health care systems are conducting assessments of: health literacy in facility signage, legal and medical documentation, availability of interpreter services, and mandatory staff orientation and annual trainings.

Studies show that more than half of the medical information patients receive is forgotten immediately, and that retained is incorrect.[75] The incorporation of best practices to support more effective communications between clinicians and patients is critical to improve safe and effective care. While many literacy assessment tools exist, the "universal precautions" approach is recommended to avoid creating patient shame and embarrassment as well as assuming a level of health literacy that does not exist.[76]Using plain language, with minimal medical jargon, accompanied by colorful materials written at a 5th grade reading level with graphics, makes health information more accessible.[76] In addition, communication techniques such as "Ask Me 3" and "Teach Back" encourage patients to ask questions about their health and treatment and enable clinicians to verify each patient's comprehension of important information.[76]

Every provider can bolster patient health literacy, improve outcomes and reduce costs by taking time to communicate with—and ensure comprehension of—his/her patients. Governmental, professional, and private organizations offer free trainings, Webinars, patient education information, and materials. To support communication with individuals with LEP, community services may be available and many health institutions subscribe to telephonic interpreter services. Physicians can significantly improve their quality of care with professional commitment and the investment of time to:

- Understand current laws, guidelines, and professional standards;

- Know their clinical setting's policies, practices, and resources;

- Arrange for access to qualified interpreters/translators relative to the patient population;

- Ensure that patient written and electronic documents meet recognized health literacy standards;

- Adopt a universal precautions approach, including techniques to ensure patient understanding.

Conclusion

A review of past decades' policies and initiatives designed to improve the nation's poor health outcomes and reduce unsustainable costs reflects limited success. Participation in voluntary tracking and reporting programs, institutionalization of nationwide interoperable health information infrastructure systems, provision of safer and more effective health care delivery through adherence to evidence-based clinical guidelines, and improved communication with and engagement of patients has shown disappointing results. Driven by the economic imperative to bend the cost curve, governmental, NGO, and professional policies and initiatives targeting improved quality and lower priced care are being transformed into government mandates with penalties for noncompliance. Reporting requirements across a spectrum of domains will increase in volume, criteria, and stringency. Pay-for-reporting initiatives are in place to encourage provider participation in preparation for value-based purchasing programs. And health care providers will need to carefully navigate the conflicting world of medical error reporting and disclosures/apologies until a more equitable tort reform system is in place.

In the current environment, health care providers face tremendous opportunities and challenges. Providers must keep abreast of health-related laws and policies, particularly those that directly impact their practices. Many resources are available to support health care professionals meet the challenges of the ever-changing health care environment. Among these are attorneys with health law expertise, who can provide timely, accurate, and insightful updates and guidance for complying with the multitude of complex requirements impacting health care. From deciphering statutes to interpreting regulatory requirements for practice, to drafting HIPAA-compliant policies, procedures, and documents, to advocating and negotiating with health care institutions, government officials, other health care professionals, insurers, and business associates, attorneys can help navigate the turbulent waters ahead.

Study Questions

1. Which factors should physicians consider when developing strategies for implementing electronic health records and participating in CMS quality reporting programs?

2. What considerations should clinicians keep in mind when instructing patients about complex medication regimens?

3. As chief medical officer of a health care organization, what recommendations would you make to the Board of Directors about physician disclosure and apology policies?

References

1. Lohr K. Committee to Design a Strategy for Quality Review and Assurance in Medicare (Eds). *Medicare: A Strategy for Quality Assurance,* Vol. 1. Washington, DC: National Academies Press, 1990.

2. Chantrill C. Total Budgeted Government Expenditure. 2011. http://www.usgovernmentspending.com/index.php. Accessed November 5, 2011.

3. Kohn LT, Corrigan JM, Donaldson MS (Eds). *To Err is Human: Building a Safer Healthcare System.* Washington, DC: National Academies Press, 1999

4. The Joint Commission. The Joint Commission History. http://www.jointcommission.org/assets/1/18/Joint_Commission_History_20111.PDF. Accessed November 5, 2011.

5. National Quality Forum. About NQF. http://www.qualityforum.org/About_NQF/About_NQF.aspx. Accessed November 5, 2011.

6. Centers for Medicare and Medicaid Services. Physician Quality Reporting Initiative. http://www.cms.hhs.gov/pqri. Accessed November 5, 2011.

7. The Leapfrog Group. http://www.leapfroggroup.org/ Accessed November 5, 2011.

8. Chaudhry B, Wang, J, Wu, S, *et al.* Systematic review: impact of health information technology on quality, efficiency, and costs of medical care. *Ann of Intern Med,* 2006 May 16;144(10):742-52, May 16, 2006.

9. Stulberg J. The Physician Quality Reporting Initiative – a gateway to pay for performance: what every health care professional should know. *Q Manage Health Care,* 17(1):2-8, Jan-Mar. 2008.

10. Rosenthal MB, Fernandopulle R, Song HR, et al. Paying for quality providers' incentives for quality improvement. *Health Affairs,* 23(2):127-41, Mar.-Apr. 2004

11. CMS. Physician Voluntary Reporting Program. https://www.cms.gov/MLNMattersArticles/downloads/MM4183.pdf. Accessed November 5, 2011.

12. CMS. Physician Group Practice Demonstration Projects. 2011. https://www.cms.gov/DemoProjectsEvalRpts/01_Overview.asp#TopOfPage. Accessed November 5, 2011.

13. CMS. Electronic Prescribing (eRx) Incentive Program. 2011. http://www.cms.gov/ERxIncentive. Accessed November 5, 2011.

14. CMS. Physician Quality Reporting System. 2011. https://www.cms.gov/PQRS/. Accessed November 5, 2011.

15. Harolds JA, Merrill JK. The Physicians Quality Reporting Initiative: What is it, will it increase health care quality, and should wide participation be encouraged? *Clinical Nuclear Medicine,* 36(2):118-20, Feb. 2011.

16. Medicare, Medicaid and SCHIP Extension Act of 2007 (Pub. L. 110-275)

17. Medicare Improvements for Patients and Providers Act of 2008 (Pub. L. 110-275)

18. Patient Protection and Affordable Care Act (ACA) (Pub L. 111-148) http://www.cms.gov/pf/printpage.asp?ref=http://www.cms.gov/PRQI). Accessed November 5, 2011.

19. Gavagan TF, Du H Saver BG, *et al.* Effect of financial incentives on improvement in medical quality indicators for primary care. *JABFM,* 23(5):622-31, 2010 Sep-Oct.

20. Ross JS, Sheth S, Krumholz HM. State-sponsored public reporting of hospital quality: results are hard to find and lack uniformity. *Health Affairs,* 29(12):2317-22, Dec. 2010.

21. Buntin MB, Burke MF, Hoaglin MC, *et al.* The benefits of health information technology: a review of the recent literature shows predominantly positive results. *Health Affairs,* 2011 Mar;30(3):464-71 Mar. 2011.

22. HITECH Act, American Recovery and Reinvestment Act of 2009 (PL 111-5). http://frwebgate.access.gpo.gov/cgi-bin/getdoc.cgi?dbname=111_cong_bills&docid=f:h1enr.pdf. Accessed November 5, 2011.

23. Blumenthal D. Launching HITECH. *N Engl J Med,* 362(5):382-5, Feb. 4, 2010.

24. Blumenthal D, Tavenner M. The "Meaningful Use" Regulation for electronic health records. *N Engl J Med,* 363(6):501-4, Aug. 5, 2010.

25. Clausen DC, Bates DW. Finding the meaning in meaningful use. *N Engl J Med,* 365(9):855-8, Sept. 1, 2011.

26. Robinson JC, Casalino LP, Gillies RR, et al. Financial incentives, quality improvement programs, and the adoption of clinical information technology. *Medical Care,* 47(4):411-7, Apr. 2009.

27. HITECH, Section 13401(a). 2009. http://frwebgate.access.gpo.gov/cgi-bin/getdoc.cgi?dbname=111_cong_bills&docid=f:h1enr.pdf. Accessed November 5, 2011.

28. HITECH, Sections 13401(a), (b), 13402, 13404. http://frwebgate.access.gpo.gov/cgi-bin/getdoc.cgi?dbname=111_cong_bills&docid=f:h1enr.pdf. Accessed November 5, 2011.

29. HITECH, Sections 13410. http://frwebgate.access.gpo.gov/cgi-bin/getdoc.cgi?dbname=111_cong_bills&docid=f:h1enr.pdf. Accessed November 5, 2011.

30. HITECH, Section 13402, 13407. http://frwebgate.access.gpo.gov/cgi-bin/getdoc.cgi?dbname=111_cong_bills&docid=f:h1enr.pdf. Accessed November 5, 2011.

31. HITECH, Section 13405(a), (c), (d), (b). http://frwebgate.access.gpo.gov/cgi-bin/getdoc.cgi?dbname=111_cong_bills&docid=f:h1enr.pdf. Accessed November 5, 2011.

32. HITECH, Section 13405(e). http://frwebgate.access.gpo.gov/cgi-bin/getdoc.cgi?dbname=111_cong_bills&docid=f:h1enr.pdf. Accessed November 5, 2011.

33. HITECH, Section 13401, 13404, 13408. http://frwebgate.access.gpo.gov/cgi-bin/getdoc.cgi?dbname=111_cong_bills&docid=f:h1enr.pdf. Accessed November 5, 2011.

34. HITECH, Section 13402. http://frwebgate.access.gpo.gov/cgi-bin/getdoc.cgi?dbname=111_cong_bills&docid=f:h1enr.pdf. Accessed November 5, 2011.

35. HITECH, Section 13400(1)(A). http://frwebgate.access.gpo.gov/cgi-bin/getdoc.cgi?dbname=111_cong_bills&docid=f:h1enr.pdf. Accessed November 5, 2011.

36. HITECH, Section 13400(1)(B). Accessed November 5, 2011. http://frwebgate.access.gpo.gov/cgi-bin/getdoc.cgi?dbname=111_cong_bills&docid=f:h1enr.pdf.

37. HITECH, Section 13402(d), (e)(1), (e)(2), (e)(3), (e)(4) http://frwebgate.access.gpo.gov/cgi-bin/getdoc.cgi?dbname=111_cong_bills&docid=f:h1enr.pdf. Accessed November 5, 2011.

38. HITECH, Sections 13402(e). http://frwebgate.access.gpo.gov/cgi-bin/getdoc.cgi?dbname=111_cong_bills&docid=f:h1enr.pdf. Accessed November 5, 2011.

39. HITECH, Section 13402(2). http://frwebgate.access.gpo.gov/cgi-bin/getdoc.cgi?dbname=111_cong_bills&docid=f:h1enr.pdf. Accessed November 5, 2011.

40. HITECH, Sections 13411, 13410. http://frwebgate.access.gpo.gov/cgi-bin/getdoc.cgi?dbname=111_cong_bills&docid=f:h1enr.pdf. Accessed November 5, 2011.

41. HITECH, Section 13410(d). http://frwebgate.access.gpo.gov/cgi-bin/getdoc.cgi?dbname =111_cong_bills&docid=f:h1enr.pdf. Accessed November 5, 2011.

42. HIPAA. Pub. L. 104-191. Section 1320D.-6. http://www.law.cornell.edu/uscode/usc_ sec_42_00001320---d006-.html. Accessed November 5, 2011.

43. HITECH, Section 13410(e). http://frwebgate.access.gpo.gov/cgi-bin/getdoc.cgi?dbname =111_cong_bills&docid=f:h1enr.pdf. Accessed November 5, 2011.

44. DHHS. Final breach notification rule on hold. July 30, 2010. http://www.healthcarein-fosecurity/.com/articles.php?art_id=2801. Accessed November 5, 2011.

45. Rowin EJ, Lucier D, Pauker SG. Does error and adverse event reporting by physicians and nurses differ? *Joint Commission Journal on Quality and Patient Safety,* 34(9):537-45, Sept. 2008.

46. Vantage Professional Education. A Guide to Medical Errors Prevention and Reporting. (#093322). 2009. http://www.vantageproed.com/mederrors/mederrorsc.htm. Accessed November 5, 2011.

47. National Priorities Partnership. 2010. Preventing medication errors: A $21 billion op-portunity. http://www.nationalprioritiespartnership.org/. Accessed November 5, 2011.

48. Karlsen KA, Hendrix TJ, O'Malley M. Medical error reporting in America: A chang-ing landscape. *Q Manage Health Care,* 18(1):59-70, Jan.-Mar. 2009.

49. Patient Safety and Quality Improvement Act of 2006 (Pub. L. 109-41). Tax Relief and Health Care Act of 2006 (Pub. L. 109-432).

50. Joint Commission. 2011. Sentinel Events. http://www.jointcommission.org/assets/ 1/6/2011_CAMOBS_SE.pdf. Accessed November 6, 2011.

51. National Quality Forum. Serious Reportable Events. http://www.qualityforum.org/Pu-lications/2008/10/Serious_Reportable_Evnts.aspx. Accessed November 5, 2011.

52. Yale Editorial Staff. A national survey of medical error reporting laws. *Yale Journal of Health Policy, Law and Ethics,* 9(1):201-86, Winter 2009.

53. Deficit Reduction Act of 2005 (Pub. L. 109-171) Section 5001 (c). http://frwebgate. access.gpo.gov/cgi-bin/getdoc.cgi?dbname=109_cong_bills&docid=f:s1932enr.txt. pdf. Accessed November 5, 2011.

54. CMS. Hospital-Acquired Conditions. 2008. https://www.cms.gov/hospitalacqcond/. Accessed November 5, 2011.

55. Kaldjian LC, Jones EW, Wu BJ, *et al.* Reporting medical errors to improve patient safety: A survey of physicians in teaching hospitals. *Arch Intern Med,* 168(1):40-6, Jan. 14, 2008.

56. Saitta NM, Hodge SD. Is it unrealistic to expect a doctor to apologize for an unfore-seen medical complication? A primer on apologies laws. *Philadelphia Bar Association Quarterly,* 93-110, 2011.

57. Mastroianni AC, Mello MM, Sommer S, et al. The flaws in state "apology" and "disclosure" laws dilute their intended impact on malpractice suits. *Health Affairs,* 29(9):1611-9, Sept. 2010.

58. Gallagher TH, Studdert D, Levinson W. Disclosing harmful medical errors to patients. *NEngl J Med,* 356(26):2713-9, June 28, 2007.

59. Youdelman MK. The medical tongue: U.S. laws and policies on language access. *Health Affairs,* 27(2):424-33, Mar.-Apr. 2008.

60. Department of Justice. Limited English Proficiency. A Federal Interagency Website. Accessed November 6, 2011. http://www.justice.gov/crt/lep/faqs/faqs.html#OneQ1.

61. National Patient Safety Foundation. Health literacy: statistics at-a-glance. http://www.npsf.org/askme3/pdfs/STATS_GLANCE_EN.pdf. Accessed November 5, 2011.

62. Powers BJ, Trinh JV, Bosworth HB. Can this patient read and understand written health information? *JAMA,* 304(1):76-84, July 7, 2010.

63. Nielsen-Bohlman, Panzer AM, Kindig DA. (Eds). *Health literacy: A Prescription to End Confusion.* Washington, DC: National Academies Press, 2004.

64. American Medical Association. Health Literacy. 2011. http://www.ama-assn.org/ama/pub/about-ama/ama-foundation/our-programs/public-health/health-literacy-program.page. Accessed November 5, 2011.

65. Vernon JA, Trujillo A, Rosenbaum S, et al. 2007. Low health literacy: implications for national health policy. http://www.npsf.org/askme3/pdfs/Case_Report_10_07.pdf. Accessed November 5, 2011.

66. Civil Rights Act of 1964 (PL 88-352). http://www.eeoc.gov/laws/statutes/titlevii.cfm. Accessed November 5, 2011.

67. "Guidance to Federal Financial Assistance Recipients Regarding Title VI, Prohibition Against National Origin Discrimination Affecting Limited English Proficient Persons: Final Guidance." *Federal Register,* 69(7):1763-8, 2004.

68. Limited English Proficiency. A Federal Interagency Website. Federal Agency LEP Guidance & Language Access Plans. http://www.lep.gov/guidance/guidance_index.html. Accessed November 5, 2011.

69. Department of Justice. Limited English Proficiency. A Federal Interagency Website. http://www.justice.gov/crt/lep/faqs/faqs.html#OneQ1. Accessed November 6, 2011.

70. US DHHS. Healthy People 2020. Health Communication and Health Information Technology. Objectives HC/HIT-1 Improve health literacy of population. http://healthypeople.gov/2020/topicsobjectives2020/objectiveslist.aspx?topicId=1. Accessed November 5, 2011.

71. US DHHS. Office of Minority Health.National Standards on Culturally and Linguistically Appropriate Services. http://minorityhealth.hhs.gov/templates/browse.aspx?lvl=2&lvlID=15. Accessed November 5, 2011.

72. Perkins J, Youdelman M. Summary of State Law Requirements: Addressing Language Needs in Health Care. 2008. National Health Law Program. http://www.healthlaw.org/images/stories/issues/nhelp.lep.state.law.chart.final.0319.pd. Accessed November 5, 2011.

73. Au M, Taylor EF, Gold M. Policy Brief: Improving Access to Language Services in Health Care: A Look at National and State Efforts.Mathematica Policy Research Inc. 2009: 1-10. www.mathematica-mpr.com. http://www.mathematica-mpr.com/publications/PDFs/health/languageservicesbr.pdf. Accessed November 5, 2011.

74. National Committee for Quality Assurance. Multicultural Health Care Distinction. http://www.ncqa.org/tabid/1195/Default.aspx. Accessed November 5, 2011.

75. American College of Physicians.ACP's Focus on Health Literacy. 2011. http://www.acpfoundation.org/health_lit.htm. Accessed November 5, 2011.

76. Weiss BD. *Health literacy: A Manual for Clinicians.* Chicago, IL: American Medical Association/American Medical Association Foundation. 2003.

77. DeWalt DA, Callahan LF, Hawk VH, et al. Health Literacy Universal Precautions Toolkit. (Prepared by North Carolina Network Consortium, The Cecil G. Sheps Center for Health Services Research, The University of North Carolina at Chapel Hill, under Contract No. HHSA290200710014.) AHRQ Publication No. 10-0046-EF) Rockville, MD.Agency for Healthcare Research and Quality. April 2010. http://www.ahrq.gov/qual/literacy/healthliteracytoolkit.pdf. Accessed November 6, 2011.

Chapter 4

Patient Safety and High Reliability Organizations

By Edward A. Walker, MD, MHA

Learning Objectives

1. Articulate the characteristics of a high-reliability organization focused on patient safety.

2. Compare and contrast the cultures of health care and high-reliability industries such as commercial aviation and nuclear power.

3. Define and give examples of Root Cause Analysis and Failure Modes and Effects Analysis.

4. Describe the principal components of the Just Culture Algorithm.

5. List 10 things that you can do tomorrow to make your patient care more safe and reliable.

Key Words: Reliability, patient safety, error, adverse event, error disclosure, root cause analysis, failure modes and effects analysis, Just Culture Algorithm, standardization, *TeamSTEPPS®*

Introduction

Patient safety is our prime directive as physicians. In this chapter, I have chosen to depart from the usual structured textbook format to engage your emotions and seek your commitment to the most important thing we do as physicians. This chapter begins with a fictional letter from a man whose spouse was seriously injured due to a lapse in patient safety. The writer, a Boeing industrial engineer, sits for weeks at the bedside of his injured wife trying to understand what has happened to her by applying his knowledge of industrial engineering to medical care. He gently confronts and educates the doctor who made the error, channeling his loss into a productive effort to help the physician understand how to be a high-reliability practitioner. I can think of no better format than this letter to help communicate what is necessary to be a committed proponent of patient safety—that is, knowledge of the tools of high reliability coupled with a burning desire to eliminate error.

As the writer considers his engineering world and compares it to what he sees in the hospital, he realizes that U.S. medicine has evolved as a cottage industry focused on individual outcomes with little attention to standardization. Observing the hospital at work, he sees one opportunity after another to apply the tools of standard work and high reliability—checklists, root cause analyses, failure mode and effects analyses, simulation, standardized communication strategies, teamwork and crew resource management among others—to achieve superior, error-free outcomes. He advances models from industrial engineering and commercial aviation that have been perfected over decades and invites the physician to a new way of practicing in a blame-free but accountable culture focused on doing things right the first time.

I hope that at the end of this chapter you will be inspired to change your practice and become a patient safety leader. The letter is a work of fiction yet the content is real and uncomfortably familiar. Too many physicians can describe the concepts and tools of patient safety yet lack the burning desire to make the changes necessary for care that is reliable and safe. We know how to do this. We still need the resolve and personal commitment to make it happen. Harry Driscoll will explain it all to you.

Dear Doctor Williams,

I don't know if you remember me, but 6 months ago you were one of the physicians in charge of the care of my wife, Agnes Driscoll, at Baker Memorial. Agnes is a 50-year-old woman who was admitted for unclear abdominal pain and underwent an exploratory laparotomy. We had planned on a short, uncomplicated hospital stay but, due to a medical error during surgery that involved similar drug names, she experienced a stroke that led to her remaining in the hospital for a stressful and difficult six weeks. We were unsure Agnes would pull through. Keeping a lonely, day-and-night vigil by her bedside as she slowly regained consciousness, I had ample time to reflect and think about what had happened and why.

I doubt that you know this, but I am an industrial engineer for Boeing as well as a private pilot. Over time, I became increasingly preoccupied with the remarkable differences between the cultures of medicine and the high-reliability world of aerospace engineering and aviation that is so familiar to me. After considerable thought, I decided to write a letter to you outlining what I see as a serious gap. I have moved past my anger about this and am now focused on making a difference so that it never happens again.

Although I appreciated that you personally disclosed the error, I was surprised at how long it took, how defensive and uncomfortable you appeared, and how unsatisfied I felt. Several nurses on the unit told me that the doctors (and nurses too) frequently do not feel comfortable with this disclosure process. I surmised that doctors who deal with life and death situations may have a need to feel that they are right all the time. Mistakes must be threatening to that self-image. I wondered if the real or perceived arrogance we associate with doctors stems from their keeping feelings at bay to maintain focus in situations that demand heroic efforts.

These traits are very different from those of my engineering colleagues. Nevertheless, I thought you might like an article I read on how doctors should disclose errors in which they are involved.[1] It gives guidelines on how to do a meaningful disclosure, and I would have appreciated your doing it this way for me.

As I briefed myself on the topic, I discovered some amazing facts about medical error. I was astounded to learn that most physicians over the age of 30 had no formal training about patient safety or medical error reduction as part of their medical school or residency! It took a series of very public errors in the mid 1990s to get a national focus on this area. Before then, doctors were so fearful of punishment that they repressed their mistakes or tried to hide them. I know that physicians are not amoral people, but human nature tends to minimize responsibility for bad outcomes, especially when the responsible person is in a high-risk profession with unavoidable complications.

I ended up reading *To Err Is Human,*[2] an impressive book in which the Institute of Medicine summarized a decade of converging evidence that medical error was much more widespread than previously appreciated. Two doctors who looked at a large number of hospital discharge records in the mid 1990s found that somewhere between 44 and 98 *thousand* people die *each year* as the result of medical care. If there are about 6000 hospitals in the U.S., this means that between 7 and 16 people, on average, die in each of our hospitals each year as the result of medical care! And that doesn't even consider people like Agnes who didn't die but were severely harmed by the care. If Boeing or United Airlines had an aircraft or pilot failure rate that high, the public and Congress would be up in arms.

One of the best books I read on this subject was titled *Why Hospitals Should Fly*[3]—I could barely put it down! Written by John Nance, a former airline pilot and attorney who is now a patient safety advocate, the story is a fictional account of a visionary doctor who decides that the error rates at his Denver hospital are too high. He redesigns the entire hospital on the basis of aviation safety practices. Bravo! At least someone else is making the connection I am seeing.

The most memorable passage in the book was the comparison of death rates. From 2002 until 2006, there were *zero* deaths attributable to commercial aviation and between 250 and 600 *thousand* patient deaths attributable to medical care. That's like flying 1400 fully loaded 747s into the ground for no reason. How did this discrepancy get to be so large?

Growing up, I remember the ex-WWII and Korean War fighter pilots who later became airline pilots. They had a swagger akin to what I observe in some doctors today. Nance recounts the wake-up call for the aviation industry when, in 1977, two fully loaded 747s crashed into each other on a foggy Tenerife runway. After 582 people died due to a series of errors, the culture of aviation changed forever. In a way, U.S. health care is right where aviation was before that accident.

The airlines' and the FAA's response is where my specialty comes into play. They began to think of commercial aviation as a *high-reliability* enterprise. Another high-reliability business taking shape at that time was nuclear power. Even though nuclear engineers take reactors and their operations very seriously, there were events like Three Mile Island and Chernobyl—nothing in this work is perfect, and not even the science of high reliability is flawless.

In my work as an industrial engineer, I try to design error and waste out of processes. Waste, the less troubling of the two, is just inefficiency. But in nuclear engineering, commercial aviation, and medicine, error can get people hurt. I wondered why only two of these three industries "got it." Part of the problem comes back to the way doctors think about bad outcomes.

First, let me make some important distinctions between the definitions of errors, adverse outcomes, and complications. A complication is usually an unavoidable outcome that is very difficult to control in a medical procedure. It's the "process variability" we cannot completely control and that is likely to occur in a certain percentage of cases no matter how skilled or careful the doctor. For a doctor, it's "the cost of doing business."

Error and adverse outcomes have an interesting relationship. An error can be either the failure of a plan or the choice of a wrong plan. In contrast, an adverse outcome is an unanticipated result that involves harm. So, some errors result in adverse outcomes; for instance, prescribing too much medicine results in the patient's experiencing an overdose. However, some errors do not result in adverse harm; for instance, a nurse administering a scheduled pain medication an hour late. Technically, this is an error, but it's probably not important. Likewise, adverse events are usually preceded by error but some are not. Think of a patient who was unaware of a drug allergy who was prescribed an antibiotic to which she had an anaphylactic reaction. Clearly this was an adverse event, but not one preceded by physician error since the doctor asked and the patient gave what she thought was a truthful answer.

I got to know some other spouses during Agnes' time in the hospital, and one morning we decided to do a little experiment. We drew up a checklist to keep track of things we understood to be part of routine, safe patient care for our spouses—things like hand sanitization as doctors and nurses entered and left the room, nurses checking for two pieces of identification prior to administering a medication, and making sure the right medication was being given. Sharing our checklists after a week, we were disappointed to see how often lapses occurred. An excellent book on this topic—the *Checklist Manifesto*[4] by Dr. Atul Gawande—makes a convincing case for importing checklists from aviation and other high-reliability industries to effectively reform medical safety.

As a result of our observations, we started to remind the doctors and nurses of what they needed to do. At first they seemed shocked or nonplussed about being questioned, but, once they recognized it was the right thing to do, the lapses decreased dramatically.

How many family members are at the patient's bedside all the time, and how many have the training I have? We cannot have safe patient care by simply relying on the vigilance of family members (although, I'm now convinced we should be partners in this care). We need to have procedures that work even when no one is looking—standard ways of doing things that don't depend on individuals.

For example, remember the day you told me that you needed to put in a "central line" so that Agnes could get some of her medications more easily? I watched what seemed like a pretty complicated procedure that didn't appear to move in a well-sequenced manner. After you told me that the lung puncture was a complication of the procedure, I went on line (Institute for Healthcare Improvement [ihi.org]) and found a central line procedure in which a group of smaller reliable processes are "bundled" into a high-reliability set. A bedside ultrasound device is recommended to correctly find the vein. Please don't think I'm raising another issue with your care. I'm just letting you know that there's an emerging culture about medical error and safety that I wasn't aware of.

As an industrial engineer in training, I read a paper by psychologist James Reason[5] in which he described system failure using the aptly named *"Swiss Cheese"* model. Imagine a laser aimed at a target. If the laser hits the target, bad things happen. To prevent the laser from hitting the mark, we put a barrier between the laser and the target. But we soon learn that this barrier isn't as effective as we first thought. Its imperfections occasionally allow the laser beam through. So we put up more barriers, hoping that their combined effects will stop the laser beam. The more barriers, the better, right?

While duplication and redundancy will get additional reliability, each new barrier has potential weaknesses as well (the holes in the Swiss cheese) that will permit the beam to get through and the error to occur. Redundancy is not as good as we might think. The chances of any one barrier failing is small and doubling your defenses repeatedly makes the chances even smaller—but never zero.

Why is that? Even low probability events can occur when the "N" is high enough and, given how busy hospitals are, it happens sooner than people expect. Furthermore, unlike with Swiss cheese, the holes move and change in size—that is, the weaknesses of systems are dynamic and exhibit a property known as emergence. Sometimes the complex system goes into a state that nobody anticipated and the laser hits the mark. This is because barriers are designed to do a certain thing well (high specificity) but it's hard to get the system to trap every error (simultaneous high sensitivity).

Why are the holes so difficult to pin down? Human factors research has shown that we are imperfect creatures—easily fatigued, easily distracted, "creative," and often surprised by things we don't expect. We're not always the best communicators and are sometimes too autonomous for our own good. We suffer from all sorts of psychological misperception problems; that is, our brains are wired to try making sense out of information, even when the "information" is nonsense. Systems engineers and information scientists worry as much about attributing false meaning to noise as they do about missing true signals.

I made some observations of communication during Agnes' hospitalization. As a pilot, I rely on hearing important information in a standard format and a structured manner. I am required to read the information back to be sure I heard it correctly. I noticed that you and your colleagues spend a lot of time talking with each other, particularly around the frequent handoffs. On at least two occasions, I witnessed doctor-nurse conversations where the message clearly didn't get through because it was neither written nor communicated in a standardized template. Such miscommunication must be particularly prevalent as shifts change and people go from one part of the hospital to the other.

To me, your conversations with colleagues appear to be telegraphic, reactive, and impromptu. This suggests that there's an opportunity to improve the accuracy of what you say. You might take a look at a program called *TeamSTEPPS*[R6] that originated in military hospitals to increase the clarity and openness of communication. They have designed a low-cost and effective "train the trainer" program that focuses on paying attention to important information, communicating it clearly, and standing up to authority when you feel something is wrong.

The other improvement I'd suggest in this area is applying "systems thinking." People who use systems thinking tend to see the integrated whole rather than a bunch of contributory parts. They understand how information flows, how decisions are made, how to maintain mindfulness of what is transpiring, and how to keep an eye on the big picture. Being a physician forces you to focus on a series of relatively small decisions, and it's probably easy to get lost in the detail. Systems thinking is particularly important in error-prone environments. A good systems thinker sees the potential for error and marshals a three-stage process to deal with it.

First, some errors can be prevented by *good engineering design:* for example, it is impossible to plug a 110 volt appliance into a 220 outlet. I read that anesthesiologists have done something similar with their machines so that oxygen and nitrous oxide inputs don't get mixed up. Although this error-proofing is very common in engineering, medicine doesn't seem to have caught on as much as I would have hoped. If a process can't be physically re-engineered to make it impossible to do the wrong thing, at least steps can be taken to make it more difficult to create an error. For instance, you explained to me that Agnes was injured because you picked up a syringe from your anesthesia tray with a drug name similar to what you needed, but which was a very different drug. Didn't anyone ever think about that happening and try to avoid it by discriminating those syringes or setting up the tray so that it is less likely to happen? Isn't there some labeling process that could be regulated by the pharmacy with colors or other visual or tactile clues that signal the right choice? In airplanes, the landing gear handle has a little wheel on the end of it, and the flap indicator looks like a small wing. This makes it just a little more difficult to get it wrong.

The second error reduction strategy is more cultural. In airline cockpits for the past 30 years, there has been a flattening of the hierarchy to create high-performing teams. In the old culture the captain was the boss and multiple airline accidents, including the one that happened in John Nance's book, were attributed to subordinates not speaking up when they knew something important. Today, the captain has become a team leader, first among equals in modern commercial aviation. From my conversations with doctors and nurses, I got the distinct impression that there is still a pecking order in medicine. Authority tends to make people tense, guarded, and self-protective. I saw many examples of this in your doctor and nurse colleagues. *Collegial teams* provide a level of redundant focus where people are watching each others' backs and feel free to detect and report errors as they occur. I would much prefer having a doctor who says, "Thank you for pointing that out" just before an error, than to have a silent set of witnesses to some awful mistake that could have been prevented. The *TeamSTEPPS*® communication training process really helps here, because it encourages this kind of free communication and vigilance.

The third component is the process of *mitigation*—if something goes wrong there is already a backup plan and it is swiftly executed. The prevention either failed or was not possible, the team didn't catch the error despite vigilance, and the error occurred anyway. This is not the time for improvisation. The recovery plan is defined and you just do it. Did you know that the Space Shuttle has *three* completely redundant and independent hydraulic systems to power its control surfaces? Engineers are very serious about safety!

You looked terrible when you came to see me on the day of the medical error. Of course you were embarrassed and upset, but I noticed that you were not looking well in general. You told me that you had come to work with a cold, had been up all day and into the night, and that you were extremely tired. I had wondered how the hospital would function at 3 a.m. when Agnes had her surgery. I expected that there would be work rules and limits to what a physician was allowed to do—the way the FAA limits pilots to duty shifts. I read that the New York State legislature enacted a law that paved the way for national rules that limit the number of hours doctors in training can serve without rest. I can understand that, both as an engineer and a pilot—both Three Mile Island and Chernobyl occurred in the wee hours of the morning when we're not at our best due to sleep cycle issues.

As an industrial engineer, I spend a lot of time thinking about what can go wrong. We have two processes that really help with this. The first is called Failure Modes and Effects Analysis, or FMEA. We consider potential untoward states of the system and figure out how likely it is for those things to occur. For example, we'd like to know about something that is very likely to happen, is very bad, and is nearly undetectable until it happens. So, we give ratings to all three of those characteristics on a scale of 1 to 10. If something is very likely, very bad, and can sneak up on you, we give each a high number and multiply them together, e.g., 10 x 10 x 10 = 1000. Likewise, something that is highly unlikely, isn't very damaging if it occurs, and you can see coming a mile away, gets a much lower score. Once you've ranked all the worrisome outcomes you can think of, the computer spits out a spreadsheet of things you might want to prioritize.

As an engineer, I probably would have visited your workstation and thought all the bad thoughts I could about how things might go awry. I'd also interview you and ask what you worry about most, as well as the worst outcomes you could think of. I'd say chances are good that I would have figured out that the event that harmed Agnes could have happened once I looked at the syringes. The interesting question is why this never occurred to you. If you knew this error was likely, you'd do everything you could to avert it by marking the medications, arranging the tray differently, or some other strategy. But because you work with this tray every day, you developed a kind of blindness to the safety issues. The error never happened before, so it's natural to feel more and more comfortable. It's like what happened with that O-ring on the Challenger space shuttle. They kept launching at lower and lower temperatures and getting closer to the edge of the safety margin while not experiencing a failure (a process called *normalization of deviance*) until finally their luck ran out.

Interestingly, the O-ring failure was not judged to be the ultimate cause of the accident, because NASA did another safety process called a Root Cause Analysis or RCA. The O-ring failure was important, and clearly the *proximal* cause of the explosion, but the investigators found something that was even more worrisome. The RCA process keeps asking *"why?"* until you run out of causes in the event chain and get to the "root" cause. Similarly, the FMEA process has a formal way to do this, but often you can get to the right answer just by asking *"why?"* over and over until you get to the principal cause.

Sometimes two or more causal chains combine into a final common pathway. Interestingly, the NASA investigators finally came up with their ultimate contributory problem—the safety and management cultures of NASA itself! It turns out that the management culture was more hierarchical than anyone realized. Engineers who were worried about the launch and had correctly identified potential problems were not encouraged to speak up. Sound familiar? It's déjà vu with the Nance book I mentioned earlier. Cockpits and NASA management structures had the same oppressive hierarchical gradient and people died because of it.

After you apologized for this error, I wondered what happened next. I knew that this moment of inattention was due to forces not completely under your control. One of the reasons I didn't press the issue with you was that I felt your heart was in the right place. But that's also why I decided to write to you again. Did your system forgive you, counsel you, punish you....what happened?

One of the best things to happen at Boeing was the development of what is known as the *Just Culture Algorithm*.[7] David Marx, another engineer friend of mine, finally figured out that a just culture would think carefully about how errors occurred and adjust the consequences appropriately. You've probably heard the saying that one way to judge a culture is by how it treats its animals. The same can be said about how an organization treats those who make mistakes. After creating the *Just Culture Community*, Marx travels throughout the country preaching an important gospel—not all errors are created equal, and it's time to stop treating them as if they were.

Marx has good instincts when it comes to balancing the need to fix the system versus the need to fix the person. He defines *errors* as the products of poorly engineered systems. If you scold a medical student on rounds and she gets anxious and then she mislabels two blood samples, you have two problems: a blaming culture and the lack of an error-proofing system. Don't blame the med student— you invited the error. Fix the system by making the culture safe and supportive, and then simultaneously insist on standardization. In the Just Culture world, one is encouraged to *console the error, not blame the person who made it*. You know that the student feels bad, so help her see how to fix the system that let her down.

So, you say, is this just a weak, non-accountable culture that condones bad actions? Not at all—remember, not all bad outcomes are equal, and there are other situations requiring higher levels of consequences.

Sometimes people are a bit careless or lazy or give incomplete reports. This is different from error in that the person has some complicity through inattention to detail. This *at-risk behavior* is partially the person's fault, so you *counsel* this behavior. A poor sign out that leaves the covering doctor without the big picture is asking for trouble. It might happen once due to some "Swiss cheese" event, but, if there is a pattern, it's time to counsel the person to shape up and to hold the person to an improvement plan.

Finally, people who are reckless or who deliberately flaunt rules are a hazard to safe care. They need to be punished. Because recklessness and rule-bending imply forethought, it's important to act in accord with the institution's values in making offenders accountable. When you put all this together, you simply *console the error, counsel the at-risk, and punish the reckless*.

As far as I can tell, you were a victim of your institution's failure to build a safe system. You seem to be an honest, forthright man who got caught in bad system design and was never taught how to move the system in the right direction. Safety is a leadership issue. Certainly you need to lead from where you are, but I hope that you will also have a talk with your senior leaders about the culture of this hospital. The hospital has a long way to go, but people like you can make a difference tomorrow if you just decide to do it.

Well, this went on much longer than I had intended. All those days of sitting and pondering what went wrong was, quite literally, an education for me. Agnes is up and about with just a few functional limitations, but she considers herself lucky to be alive and we are enjoying our time together.

I hope this letter ignites a spark in you. You can change how you think about care, and you can influence those around you as well. You asked me once if there was anything you could do to make a difference for us. I believe I have just given you my answer. I hope you can continue to practice your craft as one who heals your profession as well as your patients.

Respectfully,

Harry Driscoll

Although fictional, this letter speaks for itself in describing a fairly typical patient safety scenario that occurs in multiple hospitals every day. After more than a decade of focus on patient safety, events like this are still happening on a regular basis. I do not know of any physician who actively chooses to harm a patient, but we all have to understand that the "business as usual" practice of medical care continues to harm patients in a predictable manner. We have been reading and talking about patient safety for more than 10 years, but things are only marginally better. My challenge to you is to stop and think, and to make an action plan to prevent this from happening in your practice with your patients.

Medical error and harm both result from the very things that make us human. We don't like to face things that are unpleasant, and we don't like to think that all our training focused on excellence and patient advocacy can still result in unintentional harm. The first step in an action plan must be to overcome denial. Medical errors do not occur to poorly trained or careless physicians. Most physicians are well-trained, busy individuals who try to do their best work. The human factor issues outlined by James Reason can eventually catch up with even the best of us.

As medical care becomes more complex, it is easy to become overloaded. A state of constant multitasking inevitably leads to mistakes. In order to avoid these errors the first requirement is that you admit to yourself that, even at your best, you will make mistakes. Fortunately, most of the errors we will make as physicians are small and do not involve harm. Rather than seeing these as "the cost of doing business," we must begin to see them as warning signs of potentially harmful near misses and harm events. So, step number one is to admit, "It can happen to me." Actually, let me rephrase that: "It *will* happen to me."

"Mindfulness"—a state of combined self-awareness and situational awareness—is one of the best ways to inoculate oneself against harm events. I am oriented to how I'm feeling, with whom I am working, what I am required to do, and how much focus I must maintain on what I'm doing. It's a state of minimal distraction and vigilance at critical moments of procedures and patient interactions accompanied by the realization that constant, perfect vigilance is unsustainable. It is also an awareness of what could go wrong at any given time, my own personal biases and emotional distractions, as well as the quality of the doctor-patient relationship. Mindfulness decreases as we become fatigued, irritable, rushed, or preoccupied with life events outside our role as a physician. Fortunately, mindfulness is something that can be learned and practiced, either alone or with a coach or friend, until it becomes second nature. What are you willing to do to increase your mindfulness? Who will help you develop those habits of situational awareness?

The next step is greater reliability. Mindfulness is a state of semi-sustained vigilance. Unfortunately, we are hardwired to detect widespread environmental change, not for sustained attention to one task. One way to mitigate this normal human limitation is to depend on reliable, structured procedures. Recall that reliability is simply doing the same thing the same way over and over to achieve a standardized outcome. Whether this is something complex such as putting in a central line, or relatively simple such as thoroughly sanitizing your hands, a high-reliability process achieves a uniform outcome.

Having said this, we must be realistic about the limits of this concept as it applies to patient care. A Toyota factory can place and correctly torque all the bolts on a vehicle with something close to 100 percent reliability. But we know that medical care does not take place in highly regulated Toyota factories where every operation can be standardized. Corollas do not loosen their own bolts, nor do they refuse to allow the bolts to be inserted in the first place. Patients, on the other hand, choose not to follow or undo the therapeutic advice and treatment we give. Nevertheless, we frequently have more control than we choose to assert. Patient safety requires that we standardize to remove unnecessary variability —the variations in care that are arbitrary, idiosyncratic, and personal. We still need variability in care, but only that which is required to provide good treatment of an individual patient.

The action item here is a call to standardizing what we do. For example, when you prescribe a drug from a class of similar drugs (e.g., antidepressants), is there a protocol that you follow in the sequence of your choices? Are you using the best evidenced-based algorithm that is available to guide your choice and dose, or are you allowing yourself to be influenced by the success or failure of the last patient you treated? Are you systematic in your diagnostic processes using checklists, measurement scales, and quantitative assessments of your patient's symptoms and signs, or are you more likely to go with impressionistic hunches? Reliability does not rule out creativity or intuition. It just allows these non-rational forces to interplay with systematic rational assessments and algorithms. High-reliability systems are safer because they're standardized. Where in your practice are you willing to begin using standardized assessments and treatment algorithms? Where are you doing procedures that need to be turned into standardized protocols? Where is there a role for evidence in driving your practice to achieve more reliable outcomes?

The next step is to admit that you're not the only person taking care of your patient, and that you need to pay close attention to the other clinicians and systems from which your patients receive care. Communication is at the heart of a significant number of quality problems and harm events, and it presents another opportunity for standardization. One of the main hazard areas is at the boundaries of care: admission, discharge, transfer to another part of a hospital, transfer to diagnostic services, and referrals to other specialists in ambulatory care. These are times at which clear and standardized transfer communications are essential. Are you mindful of these transitions? Do you standardize your handoff communications with your colleagues and expect the same from them? Even within the consulting room (where you are handing off care to the patient for self-care), patients don't always clearly understand the education and instructions we give them. Do you take the time to have them repeat what you have told them in their own language (e.g., to check the accuracy of the dosing of a new medication or its potential side effects)?

Another thing that you can do is to become a master at systems thinking. Try to view your whole medical practice from the 30,000 foot level. When you go to work every day, it is very easy to slip into a routine and become so focused on the trees that you rarely appreciate the forest. A useful exercise is to mentally stand outside of your practice and view your actions as a detached observer with respect to the efficiency, mindfulness, standardization, and risk avoidance of your work. One good way to do this is to mentally walk through a typical day and note areas of high harm potential—these might be procedures, handoffs, diagnostic interventions, medication reconciliation moments, or anything where less than full attention might result in direct harm.

It's also important to recognize opportunities for indirect harm where it is not an act, but the *absence* of an act, that is creating the potential for a harm event. This is best done by viewing your work both as an individual and as a contributing member to a team. Sometimes harm events occur because critical information was not documented or communicated, or because a team member was unable or unwilling to speak up. The self-assessment action item here is to think about your practice as a system from a crew resource management perspective. Does everybody have the information they need to provide good care? Is team communication crisp, accurate, and timely? Are there planned huddles to share critical information, particularly in acute care environments like ICUs and emergency departments?

The challenge here is to reengineer your practice the way you might reengineer a physical system to avoid harm. Anesthesiology has come a long way in designing equipment that is nearly impossible to set up in a manner that would harm a patient (e.g., crossed oxygen and nitrous oxide lines), standardizing medication trays, and using lean methodology to prevent harmful events. Nevertheless, even anesthesiologists make errors, and the majority of errors cannot be prevented. Think about how you could change the structure of your practice so that errors would be either prevented or trapped as they occurred. What is the status of the treatment team to which you belong? Are you truly a team? What do you need to get you to the next step? You might want to review the *TeamSTEPPS*® reference at the end of this chapter to learn more about what's possible in your setting.

You also need to worry more. What? That's not something you want to hear given the anxiety you are probably already experiencing your practice. But there are certain things you really should worry about more than you do. The key here is to worry about the *right things*. Imagine sitting down with your team once a week to pick a common practice in your clinic and imagine all the ways in which it could go wrong. As you think through these possibilities, you could use the *Failure Modes and Effects Analysis* tool described above to rank the probabilities of what could go wrong for a patient. Additionally, you could take a recent medical error and do a thorough root cause analysis to see how the process could be improved. Teams that do these exercises change their practices and make their care safer. Are you willing to commit to something like this?

The next step is to think about *Just Culture Algorithm*. Visit the Just Culture web site and reflect on how refreshing it might be to have this broader spectrum of responses to error. Are you too quick to blame the individual, deemphasizing the system components of error? Or are you unlikely to hold a culpable individual responsible, seeing the person as a victim of a poorly designed process? The *Just Culture Algorithm* helps to clarify the appropriate response to any adverse outcome and helps to achieve the right proportions of redesign and accountability. Are you willing to sit with your peers and discuss this? Will this become the driving principle of how you deal with adverse events in a reliable manner?

The purpose of this chapter was to let Harry Driscoll introduce to you patient safety. There are a lot of things he would have liked to explain to you that you can learn in the next few months and years to understand the mechanisms by which unsafe care occurs. Nevertheless, until you make a personal commitment to change your behavior and the behavior of your teammates, the unacceptably high rates of medical error will continue. Even if you commit to doing just one thing in this chapter on a regular basis, you will be taking a positive step to safer patient care. Read everything you can, stay focused and mindful, and give the high-quality care that you expect to receive for you and your loved ones.

So, what will be your commitment to patient safety?

Study and Discussion Questions

1. Many physicians have attended Grand Rounds presentations on patient safety during the past decade, yet in the 10 years since the publication of *To Err Is Human*, there has been only low to moderate progress in reliably attaining patient safety outcomes.[8,9,10] Why do you think that has occurred? What needs to change to make more physicians effective in this area?

2. The disclosure article[1] mentioned in this letter outlines a set of best practices for disclosing an error. Try to list them, and then check out the article to see how many you got.

3. How high do you think high-reliability can get? Is a "zero-defects" culture possible in health care? If so, in what areas? If not, give examples of kinds of errors and adverse events that are not likely to be diminished to zero prevalence and why they are difficult to eradicate.

4. Pick an error in which you were personally involved and do an informal Root Cause Analysis by repeatedly asking "why?" until you get to one or more root causes.

References

1. Gallagher TH, Studdert D, Levinson WN. Disclosing harmful medical errors to patients. *N Engl J Med*, 356(26):2713-9, June 28, 2007.

2. *To Err Is Human: Building a Safer Health System.* Washington, DC: Committee on Quality of Health Care in America, Institute of Medicine, National Academies Press, 2000.

3. Nance J: *Why Hospitals Should Fly: The Ultimate Flight Plan to Patient Safety and Quality Care.* Bozeman, Montana: Second River Healthcare Press, 2008.

4. Gawande, A: *The Checklist Manifesto: How to Get Things Right.* New York, NY: Metropolitan Books-Henry Holt & Co, 2009.

5. Reason J. Human error: models and management. *BMJ*, 320(7237):768-70, 18.

6. Agency for Healthcare Research and Quality http://teamstepps.ahrq.gov/abouttools-materials.htm. Accessed November 2011.

7. The Just Culture Community http://www.justculture.org/algorithm.aspx. Accessed November 2011.

8. Wachter RM. Patient safety at ten: unmistakable progress, troubling gaps. *Health Aff* (Millwood), 29(1):165-73, Jan.-Feb. 2010.

9. Wachter RM. The end of the beginning: patient safety five years after "to err is human." *Health Aff* (Millwood), Suppl Web Exclusives:W4-534-45, July-Dec. 2004.

10. Landrigan CP, Parry GJ, Bones CB, *et al.* Temporal trends in rates of patient harm resulting from medical care *N Engl J Med*, 363(22):2124-34, Nov. 25, 2010.

Chapter 5

The Quality Policy Environment

By David Domann, MS, RPh

Executive Summary

This chapter will address the quality policy environment with respect to the establishment of national quality improvement priorities, the development and endorsement of quality measures for use in public reporting, and incentive programs and policy for health care delivery models. The focus will be on policies emanating from the quality improvement provisions of the Affordable Care Act of 2010 and initiatives carried out by the National Quality Forum and other quality organizations. Many of these policies are important to the physician provider because they are being designed and implemented to enhance quality and efficiency of care for patients.

Learning Objectives

1. Understand the key provisions of the Affordable Care Act and other public and private sector programs that are intended to drive value-based care in the United States.

2. Identify the six priorities of the Department of Health and Human Services National Quality Strategy.

3. Describe the quality measure development and endorsement processes and how these measures will foster provider accountability

4. Describe the accreditation standards for new health care delivery models that will be led by physician providers.

Key Words: National quality priorities, quality measure development and endorsement, quality reporting and incentive programs, quality improvement, value-based care

Introduction

The "Quality Enterprise" in the United States comprises the various stakeholders that are compelled to improve quality and efficiency of health care through a series of activities, including the establishment of a national quality strategy and priorities, the development and testing of quality measures, and the endorsement of these measures and standards through a national consensus standard development process. Stakeholders in the enterprise define the quality measurement that will occur in ambulatory and hospital care, long-term care, and home health. They also support quality measurement and reporting in provider incentive-based quality programs that are designed to improve the value of health care services delivered by physicians and other health care providers. Overall, the stakeholders in the enterprise are focused on promoting value-based care, a concept that links payment directly to the quality of care provided rather than the volume of care.

Figure 1. Relationship among Quality Enterprise Processes in the United States

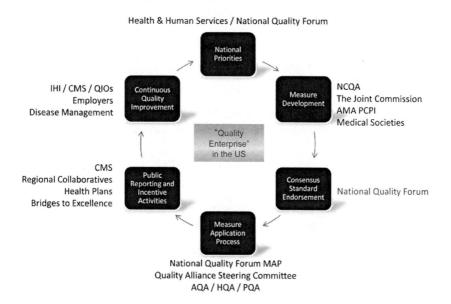

Quality Enterprise Is Focused on Improving Quality and Efficiency of Medical Care

The key processes and their relationships to one another in the enterprise are shown in Figure 1. First, the National Quality Forum (NQF) convenes the National Priorities Partnership[1] to establish national priorities. Next, measure developers, including the National Committee for Quality Assurance (NCQA) and the American Medical Association (AMA) Physician Consortium for Performance

Improvement, develop measures for submission to the Consensus Development Process conducted by NQF. Quality alliances, such as the Hospital Quality Alliance (HQA), have defined quality measure sets for use in various health care settings, while CMS and other private payers have incorporated quality measures developed by members of the enterprise for use in public reporting and in incentive programs. The new NQF-convened Measure Application Partnership is adding more structure to the selection of quality measures for public payer quality reporting and incentive programs. Finally, organizations such as the Institute for Healthcare Improvement (IHI) and the regional Quality Improvement Organizations (QIOs) drive quality improvement initiatives across the U.S. at local and state levels. While many other members play key roles in the enterprise processes, the way in which all stakeholders look to national priorities as a focus for their work is key to these processes.

Over time, the relationship among stakeholders in the enterprise is becoming more aligned in these processes. Participation by physicians in these processes is imperative, but, given the volume of work being taken on in quality measure development and endorsement, it can be a challenge for a physician to keep up with in the course of everyday medical practice.

Recent health policy established through the Affordable Care Act (ACA) of 2010[2] is furthering the push to value-based care through advances in health care delivery and payment models that rely on quality measurement and reporting as a foundation for performance improvement. Many of the quality improvement (QI) provisions depend on leadership from physician providers in implementing more proactive processes that highlight improved care for patients and better management of populations. Increasingly, physician recognition programs are being established to further incentivize and highlight the actions of physician providers who achieve improvements in quality of care. These recognition programs focus on meeting standards for the new health care delivery models (e.g., patient-centered medical home) and on certain structural elements (e.g., use of e-prescribing and health information technology in a meaningful manner) as well as on the management of certain high-value medical conditions. The challenge of changing a medical practice to meet these recognition standards is obvious; however, such change will be of considerable value in advancing improvements in quality of care for patients.

Of great importance to the new public and private sector health policies is the physician provider's engagement in processes to develop and endorse quality measures and standards and in the consensus standard development process that endorses these standards for use in value-based care programs.

The Affordable Care Act of 2010 (ACA)

The ACA[2] includes numerous QI provisions that rely upon physician leadership in establishing new health care delivery models to improve health care service delivery, patient health outcomes, and population health through quality measurement. Specifically, these key provisions are intended to improve health care delivery by establishing patient-centered medical homes and accountable care organizations; advancing new payment models for physicians and health systems, including shared savings programs and episodes of care/bundled payments; and quality performance reporting. Again, while the challenge of keeping up with these changes in health care delivery and payment is recognized, coping with such change is less difficult for physicians working in large medical group practices than for those in private practice.

Health Care Delivery and Payment Models

Accountable Care Organization (ACO)—Shared Savings Program

On March 31, 2011, the Centers for Medicare and Medicaid Services (CMS), proposed new rules under the ACA to help doctors, hospitals, and other health care providers better coordinate care for Medicare patients through ACOs.[3] These entities create incentives for health care providers to work together to manage a population of patients across care settings. Under the proposed rule, an ACO refers to a group of providers and suppliers of services (e.g., hospitals, physicians, and others involved in patient care) that work together to coordinate care for the patients they serve in original Medicare.

As defined in the final rule, the Medicare Shared Savings Program (MSSP) will reward ACOs that lower the growth in health care costs while meeting performance standards on quality of care and putting patients first.[4] If ACOs help save money by getting patients the "right" care at the "right" time, they will share in those savings.

The goal of an ACO is to deliver seamless, high-quality care for Medicare beneficiaries rather than the fragmented care that often results from different providers receiving different, disconnected payments. The ACO would be a patient-centered organization wherein the patient and physician providers are partners in care decisions. The new program is scheduled to begin early in 2012.

Center for Medicare and Medicaid Innovation (CMMI)—Patient-Centered Medical Home (PCMH)

In the CMMI–PCMH demonstration initiated late June of 2010,[5] CMS will participate in multi-payer reform initiatives to make advanced primary care practices more broadly available. This particular program is being conducted in eight states to evaluate the effectiveness of physician providers across the care system who are working in a more integrated manner, while receiving more coordinated payment from Medicare, Medicaid, and private health plans. The demonstration is expected to include more than 1,200 PCMHs serving nearly 1 million Medicare beneficiaries. In this model, physician leadership will be essential to the success of the advanced primary care practice as measured through safety, effectiveness, timeliness, and efficiency of care, as well as improved patient decision making.

Quality Measurement and Reporting

The Physician Compare Web site[6] on Medicare.gov was launched in late 2010 to serve as a health care professional directory. Currently, the site contains information on how to search for physicians who participate in Medicare by specialty etc., and identify those physicians who satisfactorily participated in the Physician Quality Reporting System. By January 2013, physician quality measurement performance information will be posted. This is intended to better inform patients in selecting physicians for their care. This program and Web site align with the Hospital Compare Web site that enables comparison of hospitals based on the results of quality measurement.

Paying Physicians Based on Value Rather than Volume

Beginning January 1, 2015, a new program will tie physician payments to the quality of care they deliver rather than being based on volume of care they provide.[7] Those physicians who provide higher value care will receive higher payments than those with documented lower quality care.

Setting National Quality Priorities and Goals in the United States

National Priorities Partnership

In 2008, the NQF, a private not-profit organization, convened the National Priorities Partnership (NPP), a group of 32 organizations representing various sectors of health care that made a commitment to establishing a set of national priorities and goals.[8] In a national movement to deliver transformative improvements to the nation's health care system, the NPP identified six cross-cutting priority areas that are important across the management of many medical conditions including:

- Patient and family engagement
- Population health
- Safety
- Care coordination
- Palliative and end-of-life care
- Overuse

The priorities and goals established through the NPP contributed to measure development plans by organizations such as the NCQA and the AMA Physician Consortium for Performance Improvement. Both of these organizations develop quality measures for use at either the health plan or the physician reporting level. These priorities also contributed to standards and best practices endorsed by the NQF and provide guidance to its ongoing work in the endorsement of consensus standards.

National Quality Strategy

More recently, the U.S. Department of Health and Human Services (DHHS) released the National Strategy for Quality Improvement in Health Care (National Quality Strategy, March 2011), a provision of the ACA.[9] This was the first effort to create national aims and priorities to guide local, state, and national efforts to improve the quality of health care in the United States.

The National Quality Strategy will promote high-quality health care that is focused on the needs of patients, families, and communities. It is also designed to be an evolving guide for public and private sector efforts to measure and improve health care quality. The strategy is intended to make the system more "user-friendly" for physicians and other health care providers by reducing administrative burdens and fostering collaboration to improve care.

The National Quality Strategy will pursue three broad aims.

1. **Better Care:** Improve overall quality by making health care more patient-centered, reliable, accessible, and safe.

2. **Healthy People and Communities:** Improve the health of the U.S. population by supporting proven interventions to address behavioral, social, and environmental determinants of health in addition to delivering higher quality care.

3. **Affordable Care:** Reduce the cost of high-quality health care for individuals, families, employers, and government.

To help achieve these aims, the strategy also establishes six priorities that will focus efforts by public and private partners (Table 1).

Table 1. Six Priorities Established to Support the Three Aims for the Health Care System

• Making care safer by reducing harm caused in the delivery of care.
• Ensuring that each person and family are engaged as partners in their care.
• Promoting effective communication and coordination of care.
• Promoting the most effective prevention and treatment practices for the leading causes of mortality, starting with cardiovascular disease.
• Working with communities to promote wide use of best practices to enable healthy living.
• Making quality care more affordable for individuals, families, employers, and governments by developing and spreading new health care delivery models.

Source: CMS and the National Priorities Partnership. Publicly available information.

The DHHS asked the NQF to convene the NPP for input on the National Quality Strategy, including guidance on goals, measures for tracking national progress, and strategic opportunities. This work was submitted to DHSS in late 2011.[10]

Quality Measure Development and Endorsement

Because quality measurement has come to play such a critical role in U.S. health care (i.e., performance measurement of physician providers, hospitals, and health plans), it is vital that quality measures be evidence-based with appropriate specification development and testing prior to submitting, endorsing, and implementing them via public and private payer programs. Two important contributors to the development and testing of quality measures for performance measurement are the NCQA and the AMA-convened Physician Consortium for Performance Improvement (AMA PCPI). Both of these organizations are committed to improving patient health and safety through performance measurement.

The NQF also makes a significant contribution to the final phase of measure development through its Consensus Standard Development Process. This organization's new Measure Application Partnership (MAP) will provide input to DHSS on the selection of quality measures for public reporting and performance-based payment programs.[11] Because the MAP is responsible for developing a coordination strategy for clinician performance measurement, physician participation is essential to ensure that appropriate performance measures are considered.

AMA-convened Physician Consortium for Performance Improvement (PCPI)

In recent years, the PCPI has evolved as a key physician-led initiative dedicated to improving patient health and safety through its efforts in developing, testing, and implementing evidence-based performance measures for use at the point of care.[12] Much of PCPI's work has been carried out in collaboration with specialty societies, medical boards, and providers who use measures at the point of care to gain a deeper understanding of the practical use of performance measures. PCPI has been successful in integrating performance measures in certification and licensure programs as well as in public and private payer programs. In fact, the majority of measures used in the CMS Physician Quality Reporting System were developed through PCPI (Table 2).

Overall, PCPI members are committed to:

- Identifying and developing evidence-based clinical performance measures and measurement resources that enhance quality of patient care and foster accountability.

- Promoting the implementation of effective and relevant clinical performance improvement activities.

- Advancing the science of clinical performance measurement and improvement.

Increasingly, the measures created through the PCPI focus on outcomes and processes to determine whether desired goals are achieved and on creating composite measures with a single score for multiple related measures. PCPI also has been on the cutting edge with respect to information technology—e.g., testing the use of performance measures in electronic health record systems.

Table 2. PCPI Measure Sets

• Acute Otitis Externa/ Otitis Media with effusion	• End-stage Renal Disease–Adult	• Oncology
	• End-stage Renal Disease–Pediatric	• Osteoarthritis
• Anesthesiology and Critical Care	• Eye Care	• Osteoporosis
		• Outpatient Parenteral Antimicrobial Therapy
• Asthma	• Gastroesophageal Reflux Disease	• Palliative Care
• Atrial Fibrillation and Atrial Flutter	• Geriatrics	• Pathology
• Care Transitions	• Heart Failure Hematology	• Pediatric Acute Gastroenteritis
• Chronic Kidney Disease	• Hepatitis C	• Perioperative Care
• Chronic Obstructive Pulmonary Disease	• HIV/AIDs	• Prenatal Testing
• Chronic Wound Care	• Hypertension	• Preventive Care and Screening
• Community-acquired Bacterial Pneumonia	• Major Depressive Disorder–Adult	• Prostate Cancer
• Diabetes	• Major Depressive Disorder–Child and Adolescent	• Radiology
• Emergency Medicine		• Rheumatoid Arthritis
• Endoscopy and Polyp Surveillance	• Melanoma	• Stroke and Stroke Rehabilitation
	• Nuclear Medicine	• Substance Use Disorders
	• Obstructive Sleep Apnea	

National Committee for Quality Assurance (NCQA)—HEDIS Measures

The NCQA has been at the forefront of performance measurement at the health plan level for over 20 years.[13] Their measurement set, known as the Healthcare Effectiveness Data Information Set (HEDIS), is a tool used by the majority of U.S. health plans to measure plan performance, to enable comparisons of performance among plans, and to identify general and specific needs for improvement.

HEDIS data are used by a variety of stakeholders: by consumers as they select health plans, by employers who use the results to make improvements in the quality of care they offer employees, and by health plans for participation in the NCQA accreditation process. Published annually for the past 14 years, the NCQA's *State of Healthcare Quality* reports on performance trends based on HEDIS measurement by more than 1,000 health plans in the U.S.[14] The report is widely used for tracking variations in care and for its recommendations on care improvement needs in certain areas. HEDIS measures have been developed to cover a range of important medical conditions and health issues, including the following:

- Asthma Medication Use

- Persistence of Beta-Blocker Treatment after a Heart Attack

- Controlling High Blood Pressure

- Comprehensive Diabetes Care

- Breast Cancer Screening

- Antidepressant Medication Management

- Childhood and Adolescent Immunization Status

- Childhood and Adult Weight/BMI Assessment

Increasingly, organizations such as NCQA are using the priorities established by the NQF-convened NPP to guide the types of cross-cutting measurement types that need to be developed. NCQA follows a rigorous process of measure development that involves identifying appropriate clinical areas to evaluate and types of measures to be developed. In drafting initial measures and specifications, technical subgroups rely on physician providers with expertise in the specific measurement area. Before public comment and final adoption of a measure for the HEDIS set, the measure is tested and vetted with various stakeholders from the standpoint of feasibility, reliability, and validity.

Recently, NCQA has become a leader in evaluating the cost and quality of care simultaneously in its Relative Resource Use (RRU) Program.[15] RRU measures indicate how intensively health plans use physician visits, hospital stays, and other resources to care for members identified as having 1 of 5 chronic diseases: cardiovascular disease, COPD, diabetes, hypertension, and asthma. The RRU Program evaluates the use of resources (i.e., physician visits, hospitals stays) for these conditions alongside HEDIS quality measurement for the same conditions, thus allowing quality and spending to be considered simultaneously. This ability will become even more important as public and private payers evaluate new delivery models of care led by physician providers (e.g., the ACO-Shared Savings program to be implemented by CMS).

National Quality Forum (NQF) Consensus Standard Development Process (CDP)

The NQF was created in 1999 to develop and implement a national strategy for health care quality improvement. Over the years, this not-for-profit organization has grown into an influential consensus-based organization in U.S. health care with a structure that enables private and public sector stakeholders to collaborate on cross-cutting solutions in performance improvement.

The NQF operates under a three-part mission to improve the quality of American health care by:

1. Building consensus on national priorities and goals for performance improvement and working in partnership to achieve them.

2. Endorsing national consensus standards for measuring and publicly reporting on performance.

3. Promoting the attainment of national goals through education and outreach programs.

While measures are developed through many sources, those endorsed by the NQF are increasingly included in public and private payers' performance incentive programs. An NQF endorsement reflects on scientific and evidence-based review, input from the steering committees and working groups throughout the endorsement process, and NQF membership voting on standards.

The Consensus Development Process (CDP) calls for input from, and considers the interests of, stakeholder groups across the health care continuum. Physician expert participation is important in this process to ensure that endorsed quality measures are relevant to medical practice. Importantly, because NQF uses a formal CDP, it meets the definition of a voluntary consensus standards-setting organization as described by the National Technology Transfer and Advancement Act of 1995 and Office of Management and Budget Circular A-119. NQF uses its CDP to evaluate and endorse consensus standards that include; performance measures, best practices, frameworks, and reporting guidelines.[16] The CDP's nine principal steps, sub-steps, and associated specific actions are highlighted in Table 3.[17]

Physician providers can play important roles in the NQF CDP at key points in the process. First, physicians who are members of organizations that are measure stewards or developers can submit measures to the CDP. Second, physicians can serve as members of endorsement project steering committees or working groups, especially those who can provide content expertise and who will broaden the range of viewpoints. Besides serving on committees or workgroups, physicians are included as leaders and members of the Consensus Standards Approval Committee (CSAC) and are influential in making recommendations to the board of directors. Finally, physicians are invited to comment on draft reports during the member and public comment phase and may vote as members of NQF. In summary, physician providers play a prominent and necessary role in the measure development and endorsement processes in the U.S.

Table 3. NQF Consensus Development Process

1. Call for intent to submit candidate standards	Interested measure stewards and developers are invited to notify NQF of their intent to submit measures for endorsement.
2. Call for nominations	Nominations for candidates for steering committees and working groups that will oversee a project. After selection, committee rosters are posted on the NQF Web site to solicit comments on the proposed panel.
3. Call for candidate standards	Developers are allowed to submit a measure or best practice for endorsement through NQF's online submission forms a 30-day period is usually allowed for the submission.
4. Candidate consensus standards review	The expert steering committee conducts a detailed review of the submitted measures using a four-part test to ensure they reflect sound science, will be useful to providers and patients, and will make a difference in improving quality.
5. Member and public comment	Comment is solicited from anyone who wishes to respond to a draft report that outlines the steering committee's assessment of the submitted measures.
6. Member voting	NQF members are able to review the draft report and vote on the endorsement of measures.
7. Consensus standards approval committee decision	The Consensus Standards Approval Committee (CSAC) makes recommendations on endorsement to the Board of Directors based on the merits of the measure and the issues raised during the review process.
8. Board ratification	NQF Board of Directors is asked to ratify the recommendations by the CSAC regarding endorsement.
9. Appeals	A period of time is allowed for anyone to appeal the Board of Directors Decision.

Source: National Quality Forum Website

National Quality Forum Measure Applications Partnership

A new Measures Applications Partnership (MAP)[11] was created in 2010 by the NQF for the purpose of providing input to the DHHS on the selection of performance measures for public reports and performance-based payment programs, as required by the ACA. Specifically, the MAP is charged with 1) providing input to HHS/CMS on the selection of available measures for public reporting and performance-based payment programs, 2) identifying gaps for measure development and endorsement, and 3) encouraging alignment of public and private sector programs across health care settings. To complete this task, a MAP Coordinating Committee was established to provide overall direction to the four working groups identified in Figure 2. Each working group will advise the coordinating committee on measures needed in the hospital environment, for clinicians in ambulatory care, for post-acute care and long term care, and finally for the expanding dual eligibility population. Physician providers have been included on each of these workgroups and on the coordinating committee.

Figure 2. NQF Convened Measure Application Partnership–Organization

Measure Applications Partnership: 2-Tiered Structure

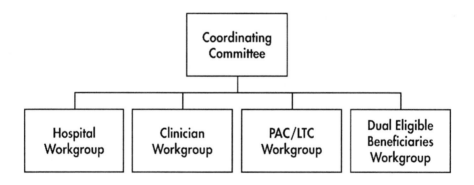

Source: National Quality Forum's Measure Application Partnership

Quality Alliances

The past 10 years has seen the development of a number of alliances devoted to quality measurement and improvement in various care settings. These include the Hospital Quality Alliance (HQA), the Ambulatory Quality Alliance (AQA), the Pharmacy Quality Alliance (PQA), and the Nursing Quality Alliance (NQA) among others. In 2008, the Quality Alliance Steering Committee (QASC)[18] was formed to foster collaboration among existing and emerging sector-specific quality groups as well as leaders among physicians, nurses, hospitals, health insurers, consumers, accrediting agencies, and the public sector. Much of the work of the QASC has been directed at projects such as developing data aggregation methods for quality measurement and establishing models for episodes of care efficiency measurement. All of these alliances offer physician leaders the opportunity to become involved in shaping quality measurement implementation across a variety of settings through participation on steering committees and working groups.

Health Care Delivery and Payment Models

Accreditation Standards for New Delivery Models

As new health care delivery models (e.g., PCMH) evolve, new accreditation standards are being developed to supply the necessary structure for physicians who wish to implement them. The NCQA Physician Practice Connections–Patient Centered Medical Home Program's 2011 standards focus on further promoting patient-centered care, aligning with CMS Meaningful Use requirements and elevating the importance of evaluating patient experience of care.[19]

The NCQA Program for 2011 includes the following six standards that align with core components of primary care:

1. Access and Continuity

2. Identify and Manage Patient Populations

3. Plan and Manage Care

4. Self-care

5. Track and Coordinate Care

6. Performance Measurement and Quality Improvement

Physician participation in such accreditation and recognition programs is expected to result in their achieving financial incentives from public and private payers and recognition as providers of high-quality, patient-centered care. Already, PCMH practices are demonstrating significant improvement in patient and provider experiences and in quality of clinical care.

Incentive Payment and Physician Recognition Programs

Public and private payers are driving value-based care through incentive payment programs that focus on improving outcomes of care versus paying for volume of care. The Physician Quality Reporting Initiative (PQRI) was initiated in the second half of 2007 as a voluntary reporting program offering incentive payments for eligible professionals who satisfactorily report on selected quality measures for services provided to Medicare Part B fee-for-service beneficiaries.[20] In the 2011 program, there are 190 individual measures for claims or registry-based reporting. Changes made to the program under the ACA included authorizing the incentive payments through 2014 and requiring a payment adjustment beginning in 2015 for eligible professionals who do not satisfactorily report data on quality measures in a given reporting year. Because it is now permanent, the program was renamed the Physician Quality Reporting System (PQRS) effective in 2011.

Quality Improvement and Reporting

Under the Quality Improvement Organization (QIO) Program,[21] CMS contracts with a single organization in each state for a three-year cycle referenced as a Scope of Work (SOW). The overall mission of the QIO Program—to improve effectiveness, efficiency, and quality of services for Medicare beneficiaries—is reflected in both completed work and future plans. In the 9th SOW, significant focus was placed on issues related to care transitions. The strategy for the 10th SOW includes two directions to 1) improve individual patient care and safety through reducing health care-acquired conditions by 40 percent and 2) integrate care for populations by improving care transitions that reduce hospital readmission rates by 20 percent. Physicians have played key roles in QIOs as leaders and reviewers.

Physician Provider Engagement in the Quality Enterprise

Of importance for physician providers is the opportunity to inform and shape U.S. policy standards directed at improving the quality of care. These opportunities arise through participation in organizations where measurement development committees and advisory groups exist (e.g., the AMA PCPI) and/or in the consensus standard development process of the NQF.

NQF's unique structure allows private and public sector stakeholders, including physician providers, to work together in the consensus development process to endorse measures and best practices that will lead to solutions to drive continuous quality improvement in the US health care system. The various "Quality Alliances" offer opportunities for engagement of physician leaders, especially in areas where sector-specific quality improvement initiatives are directed.

Conclusion

The quality policy environment has evolved significantly over the past several years through provisions of the ACA that advance new delivery and payment models for physicians and health systems and that expand existing quality measurement and reporting systems. The NQF has played a key role in advancing health care quality policies through the establishment of national priorities that drive members of the Quality Enterprise to develop and endorse quality measures for incentive payment programs for physicians, hospitals, and health plans. The National Quality Strategy, announced in 2011 by DHSS, will further advance the quality improvement direction in the U.S. through three broad aims of better care—health, people, and communities—and driving affordable care. There are ample opportunities for physician provider participation in influencing and shaping policies in health care quality.

Case Study

The NQF convened NPP, whose current 48 members represent a diverse range of stakeholders across health care sectors, is working to bring about improvement in U.S. health care. The NPP first identified a set of national priorities and goals in late 2008 to help focus performance improvement on high-leverage areas, thereby accelerating fundamental change in health care quality. The priorities included: patient and family engagement, improving the health of the population, safety, care coordination, end-of-life care, and overuse.

In late 2010, the NPP was asked by DHSS to offer consultative support on setting national priorities and goals for the DHHS National Quality Strategy that was released early in 2011. This consultation was provided and reflected in a National Quality Strategy that focused on a set of aims and priorities that will promote high-quality health care in which the needs of patients, families, and communities guide the actions of all of those who delivery and pay for care.

In mid-2011, the NPP was asked to recommend goals, measures of success, and strategic imperatives to allow for further implementation of the National Quality Strategy. The role of the NPP in supporting national priorities could not have occurred without broad health care sector stakeholder involvement that included significant physician provider leadership. In fact, Donald Berwick, MD, a pediatrician and former Administrator for the CMS, served as the first co-chair of the NQF-convened NPP.

Study/Discussion Questions

1. Describe how provisions of the Affordable Care Act of 2010 will drive value-based care.

2. What is the three-part AIM referenced in the HHS National Strategy for Quality Improvement in Healthcare?

3. What is the role of the National Quality Forum in endorsing performance standards?

4. How have CMS policies impacted the area of quality improvement?

5. What are the opportunities for physicians to participate in quality reporting and incentive programs?

Suggested Readings and Web Sites

- Report to Congress: National Strategy for Quality Improvement in Healthcare.
- http://www.healthcare.gov/center/reports/quality03212011a.html
- CMS: Roadmap for Implementing Value Driven healthcare in the Traditional Medicare Fee-For-Service Programs. http://www.cms.gov/QualityInitiatives-GenInfo/downloads/VBPRoadmap_OEA_1-16_508.pdf
- NQF Convened National Priorities Partnership. http://www.nationalpriorities-partnership.org/

References

1. National Priorities Partnership. Available at http://www.nationalprioritiespartnership.org/.
2. Affordable Care Act of 2010.
3. Accountable Care Organization / Shared Savings Program. Available at http://www.cms.gov/sharedsavingsprogram/.
4. Final Rule – Medicare Shared Savings Program. Available at http://www.cms.gov/sharedsavingsprogram/.
5. Center for Medicare and Medicaid Innovation—Patient Centered Medical Home. Available at http://www.cms.gov/DemoProjectsEvalRpts/MD/ItemDetail.asp?ItemID=CMS1230016.
6. Physician Compare. Available at https://www.cms.gov/physician-compare-initiative/.
7. Hyatt-Thorpe J, Weiser C. Health Reform GPS: Medicare value-based purchasing programs. Available at http://www.healthreformgps.org/resources/medicare-value-based-purchasing-programs/.
8. National Priorities Partnership. Available at http://www.nationalprioritiespartnership.org/.
9. National Quality Strategy. Available at http://www.healthcare.gov/center/reports/quality03212011a.html.
10. Input to the Secretary of Health and Human Services on Priorities for the National Quality Strategy. National Priorities Partnership convened by the National Quality Forum. Available at www.nationalprioritiespartnership.org.
11. NQF Measure Application Partnership. Available at http://www.qualityforum.org/Setting_Priorities/Partnership/Measure_Applications_Partnership.aspx.
12. AMA Physician Consortium for Performance Improvement. Available at http://www.ama-assn.org/ama/pub/physician-resources/clinical-practice-improvement/clinical-quality/physician-consortium-performance-improvement.page.
13. National Committee for Quality Assurance – HEDIS. Available at http://www.ncqa.org/tabid/59/Default.aspx.
14. NCQA State of Healthcare Quality Report. Available at http://www.ncqa.org/tabid/836/Default.aspx.

15. NCQA Relative Resource Use Program. Available at http://www.ncqa.org/tabid/1231/Default.aspx.

16. NQF Consensus Development Process. Available at http://www.qualityforum.org/Measuring_Performance/Consensus_Development_Process.aspx.

17. NQF Consensus Development Endorsement Process. Available at http://qualityforum.org/Measuring_Performance/Consensus_Development_Process.aspx.

18. Quality Alliance Steering Committee. Available at http://www.healthqualityalliance.org./

19. NCQA Physician Practice Connections: Patient-Centered Medical Home Program 2011. Available at http://www.ncqa.org/tabid/631/default.aspx.

20. Centers for Medicare and Medicaid Services: Physician Quality Reporting System. Available at https://www.cms.gov/PQRS/01_Overview.asp#TopOfPage.

21. Centers for Medicare and Medicaid Services: Quality Improvement Organizations (QIO). Available at http://www.cms.gov/QualityImprovementOrgs/.

Section II.

Measuring Quality:
Application of Quality Measures

Chapter 6

Data Collection: Why Collect Data for Quality Improvement?

By Susan Irene DesHarnais, PhD, MPH

Executive Summary

There are many reasons to collect clinical and administrative data. One important reason is to build databases that are useful for monitoring and improving the quality of the health care that you are providing to your patients. Ideally, these databases will serve your internal data needs as well as providing the information required by external agencies, both voluntary and regulatory.

When deciding what types of data to collect, several possibilities should be considered. It is important to be explicit about what one wishes to measure. Data on patient outcomes, both positive and negative, are certainly needed, but it is essential to risk adjust outcome data to account for differences in patient risk factors at the start of treatment. Process data are also needed in order to understand how to improve care.

Once priorities for quality improvement are defined, the next step is to develop a secure, economical, and usable system that is flexible enough to meet both present and future needs. Ideally, the system should accommodate administrative, regulatory, and billing needs in addition to quality improvement objectives.

The final topic is how to deal with public reporting of data in a positive and constructive manner, so that such reporting offers opportunities for communication, honesty, and the improvement of care.

Learning Objectives

1. Give examples of both positive and negative patient outcomes.
2. Explain why risk adjustment is needed when measuring patient outcomes.

3. Describe two reasons to support transparency when considering public reporting of patient outcomes.

Key Words: Quality, outcomes, processes, data reporting, risk adjustment

Introduction

There are many reasons to collect clinical and administrative data. One important reason is to build databases that are useful for monitoring and improving the quality of the health care that you are providing to your patients. Ideally, these databases will serve your internal data needs as well as providing the information required by external agencies, both voluntary and regulatory.

Data collection for quality improvement should serve multiple purposes, including your own clinical and administrative objectives, and compliance with regulatory and quasi-regulatory agencies.

Internal needs for data collection to improve quality of care

One internal data need is to collect information that allows you to measure the quality of care you are providing your patients. This information should enable you to identify best practices as well as anomalies, both within your practice and in comparison to similar practices. For example, if you can document rates of post-surgical infections of various types for patients who had a certain type of surgery, you can then make informed judgments about whether your infection rates are too high, about as expected, or very low, given the types of patients you are treating. If your rates are significantly higher than they had been (historically) in your practice, you want an "alarm" to go off so that you can take corrective actions. On the other hand, if your rates are much better than expected, it is possible that others could—and should—learn about what you are doing.

Once you have collected information on your clinical events, you should be able to use this information to evaluate and refine your clinical processes and decision-making skills. Processes of care may need to be redesigned to better meet the needs of both the providers and their patients. Process redesigns require reliable data from before and after the changes to determine if the redesigned process is effective in addressing the problem.

Another need for data collection is to assess information and education needs of both clinicians and patients. Physicians cannot assume that they or other clinicians in their organizations really know how to perform all of the tasks and procedures necessary to provide high-quality care. It is necessary to train clinicians and assess and reassess their skills, either through simulated testing or through direct observation of their performance. Without this information, it is impossible to develop well-focused training for clinicians.

Similarly, a physician cannot assume that all of his or her patients with a given chronic disease understand how to manage their disease and deal with its problems and complications. Instead, it is necessary to assess patients' knowledge and verify patients' skills and understanding. One tool for doing this is to develop personal health records (PHR) that engage patients for medication management and self-monitoring. If PHRs are used and evaluated, the patients' needs can be explicitly addressed.

External needs

Multiple organizations either require or ask for data on the quality of care provided by your organization. Because of these demands, it is necessary to collect data on the quality of care for the following reasons:

- To meet requirements for reimbursement incentives, regulatory agencies, licensing, and accreditation.

- To contribute to state and national registries and health information exchanges for benchmarking purposes.

When designing a system for collecting data on quality of care, it is essential to know what types of data these external agencies require, including which classification systems they use for categorizing diseases and complications of treatment. Without addressing these needs, it is virtually impossible to develop an integrated data collection system. One caveat however; it is very unlikely that the various external agencies' requirements will satisfy your own needs for data collection. Clearly, you must define your own data needs for quality monitoring and improvement first, and then develop an integrated data collection system that meets both internal and external requirements.

Outcomes and Processes of Care Measurements

What are outcomes, and why should we measure them?

An outcome can be defined as the condition of the patient following treatment and recovery. We need to monitor the quality of care to determine treatment effectiveness, i.e., to measure the effect the treatment has had on the patient's condition. According to the Office of Technology Assessment (OTA) definition, the whole point of treating the patient is to "increase the probability of outcomes desired by the patient, and reduce the probability of undesired outcomes, given the state of medical knowledge."[1] Thus, we should look at desired (positive) outcomes, as well as undesired (negative) outcomes.

Examples of some desired (positive) outcomes that might be measured

- Better score on a depression scale 3 months after a specific drug treatment.
- Improvement in range of movement of a joint, 1 year following joint replacement.

- Greater time between hospitalizations for acute episodes, for patients with a defined chronic disease.

- Return to work within 60 days from heart surgery.

Note that outcome measurement requires careful specification of the relevant population, measure, and when that measurement is to be taken.

When is it necessary and/or easier to measure adverse outcomes?

Adverse outcomes may be measured for several reasons. Sometimes it is not possible to measure positive outcomes because we do not have any information to follow up on patients' improvements following treatment. For example, a hospital may not be able to link its data system with physical therapy or chemotherapy treatment that occurs in outpatient settings following a patient's discharge, let alone determine longer term patient health status. This may force the hospital to judge quality of care by assessing inpatient records pertaining to adverse outcome avoidance.

Hospital adverse outcomes might include rates of:

- In-hospital mortality for patients receiving a particular surgical procedure.

- Unscheduled readmission to a hospital within three weeks of discharge for diabetic patients.

- Complications of treatment in hospitalized patients, e.g., MRSA, central line infections.

- Urinary tract infections for catheterized patients.

- Complications for diabetic patients where a hospital readmission is required.

Another reason for measuring adverse outcomes is to assist in prioritizing quality improvement projects within a hospital or other type of practice. By monitoring the things that should *not* happen, it is possible to improve processes of care and reduce negative outcomes.

Risk Adjustment

When evaluating providers in terms of quality, it is important to take into account the health outcomes that could reasonably be expected from that provider given the technology available, the severity of the disease treated, and other patient risk factors. Risk adjustment is a method of taking into account the patient's condition when he or she was admitted to a hospital and then using the patient's risk factors to predict a given outcome. Because different hospitals serve patients with different risk factors, it is essential to risk-adjust outcome variables in order to allow for valid comparisons of outcomes across providers.

Risk factors are those *patient* characteristics that are empirically associated, at a statistically significant level, with a higher probability that a specified outcome will occur. The following are some risk factors related to the patient's immediate problem or illness: the reason for admission (principal diagnosis), gender, race, age, comorbid conditions, and whether the patient was transferred from another hospital or nursing home.

Note that comorbidities can be measured in many ways, including:

- Specific comorbidities, e.g., cancer, COPD
- Interactions between comorbidities
- Total number of comorbidities
- Number of body systems with comorbidities

The way that comorbidities are defined and measured affects the risk-adjustment model by producing differences in expected outcomes.

Other risk factors include such things as the patient's social, financial, and economic status—for instance, type of insurance; type of employment; type of residence or homelessness; health literacy, social support system; nutritional habits/status; and use of drugs, alcohol, and tobacco. Information on these variables is not typically available in standard data sets, except for the type of insurance.

How is risk adjustment performed?

In order to measure the effect of provider performance on patient outcomes, we must control (to the extent possible) for risk factors that may affect patient outcomes *Indirect standardization* is an empirical method of computing, for each patient, the probability of a specified outcome, using a large reference population to derive weights for each of that patient's risk factors.

Example of Indirect Standardization

Step 1.

Use logistic regression to construct a preliminary model for a specific condition/outcome combination to enable us to define those variables (risk factors) that are statistically significant. One example might be 30-day post-surgery mortality for a coronary bypass operation. Some candidate predictor variables might be age, gender, race, procedure (e.g., number of vessels bypassed), and presence or absence of five common comorbidities (i.e., those occurring in >1 percent of all cases for this specific condition/outcome combination).

Step 2.

Determine relevant variables to include in the final model by evaluating the relationship of all candidate risk factors to the specified outcome.

Step 3.

Run a final model, with the selected risk factors.

Step 4.

Use the weights derived from the revised logistic regression for each of the predictor variables to compute the predicted score for each person for each outcome of interest.

Using Risk-Adjustment Models to Develop Hospital Performance Reports

Once risk adjustment is complete, it is possible for an oversight organization, health plan, or other entity to develop reports for each hospital, comparing the *predicted* frequencies for each category of adverse event to the *observed* frequencies. Using risk-adjustment models, a predicted probability of each relevant adverse event can be assigned to each case. Then, a comparison can be made of predicted to actual occurrences for a given group of patients. Finally, statistical tests can be performed on the differences between predicted and observed frequencies to determine whether the differences are statistically significant or merely represent random variations. Once this is accomplished, systems profiles can be developed to compare hospitals using these multiple risk-adjusted measures.

How Does Risk Adjustment Differ from Severity Management?

Risk adjustment is an empirical investigation of the relationship of each risk factor to a specified outcome. In contrast, severity measures depend entirely on how one defines severity; for example, what is "severity" for a diabetic? It might be defined as:

- Quality of life
- Independence
- Psychological functioning
- Freedom from pain
- Ability to see things
- Ability to walk
- Results of lab tests
- Days in the hospital per year
- Cost of care per year

Obviously, a given diabetic patient's severity score will vary depending on which of these concepts is used to define severity.

Another problem with severity methods is that they produce a "global" or "summary" severity score for a patient, and that score is used for predicting any and all outcomes. This is not a valid approach. By contrast, a risk score is the empirical relationship of a patient's risk factors to a specified outcome. In risk-adjustment models, risk factors and weights differ for the same patient for different outcomes. Separate models must be used for risk adjustment for each outcome and for each disease/condition.

Interpreting Risk-Adjusted Data

By comparing actual to predicted events for a given hospital, it is possible to compare that hospital's performance with the performance of all hospitals in the population used for the indirect standardization. This can be very useful in identifying priorities for quality improvement. However, one should keep in mind that many of the hospitals used to set the norms could be performing at a less than optimal level of quality. The results are relative to averages, not best practices.

At the individual physician level, outcomes measurements—even with risk adjustment—are often unstable. The number of patients seen by a given physician is often too small for statistically significant findings. Reporting outcomes by physicians may, therefore, be misleading.

Why Measure Processes of Care?

Often it is adequate to measure processes of care, rather than outcomes. It is usually easier to measure processes, and it is appropriate to do so when there is good evidence that certain processes are strongly associated with desired outcomes. For example:

- Percentage of diabetic patients who received eye exams in past 12 months.
- Percentage of women 60-70 years old who received a mammogram in the past 12 months.
- Percentage of pregnant women who received at least six prenatal visits, including one or more in first trimester.
- Percentage of children who received all of the required immunizations during their first two years of life.
- Percentage of women delivering babies during the last six months who received vaginal deliveries rather than C-sections.

At times, processes of care are used to measure problems; for example:

- Percentage of patients with missed appointments.
- Percentage of patients with waiting time beyond acceptable limits.
- Percentage of visits that did not include required assessments or lab tests.

These types of measures are useful if they lead to process improvements. Note that in all of these examples a denominator is needed. The denominator can be defined in various ways. It may be all relevant patients in an insured population, or it may be defined as all patients seen by a given provider or group of providers. The two definitions will produce different results or ratings. For example, in a practice in which half of the identified diabetics do not come in for visits—but all who do show up actually get good care—the ratings on provider process measures will vary from 50 to 100 percent, depending on which denominator is used.

Issues Regarding Data Collection for Quality Improvement

Ensuring privacy and security while meeting HIPAA requirements

It has become evident to most people who use computers—and especially those who use the Internet—that it is very difficult to keep information secure and to keep patient records from falling into the wrong hands. Most health care organizations face possible threats from external sources as well as threats from employees. When collecting data on the quality of care, it is often necessary to abstract patient records or enter data directly through electronic medical records to form an analytical data set. Data on individual patients must be protected by law, and collective data used in reports must be protected to ensure that the quality improvement activities do not compromise the facility's reputation. Thus, protection from unauthorized people outside of the organization is critical.

It is usually necessary to obtain the services of computer security experts or, at the very least, engaging such people to audit the security of the data collection systems and data storage procedures. Such an investment is considered to be worthwhile to ensure that the protected data are actually safe.

It is also necessary to establish security procedures for employees and to train and monitor all employees in protecting data from misuse. Procedures are needed for password protection, who may access which databases, and who may give information to people outside the facility under what circumstances. Procedures are also needed for storing data on laptops or drives that leave the facility. It is also important to ensure that disgruntled employees or those who are terminated do not take or misuse data. The failure to protect patient information could seriously damage efforts to improve quality and safety, as well as result in lawsuits and/or regulatory actions.

Assessing usefulness versus the cost of using different data collection systems

When collecting data for quality improvement, it is important to consider the design of the data collection system to maximize its usefulness while controlling costs. Different types of practices have very different needs when it comes to collecting data to improve quality. Still, some general principles can be applied.

Prioritizing objectives for quality improvement

No single system can meet all present and future objectives. Before choosing a system design for data collection, it is essential to gather all potential users to identify high-priority needs. Clinicians may want to study treatment patterns, while financial experts may want to look at the cost-effectiveness of various practices. Outside organizations will be requesting and/or demanding reports of quality indicators that are very different from those desired by the clinicians. Not all needs can be anticipated in advance, and the system will have to accommodate future needs with minimal disruption.

In addition to involving the end users, the information technology experts should assume an important role in designing a data collection system for quality improvement. The following areas are of special importance:

Understanding the relationship of a proposed data collection system to other existing and/or planned systems

Various computerized systems must be able to "talk to each other". Often, information housed within the billing system is valuable for quality improvement efforts. For example, infection rates and readmission rates can be determined for various subgroups of patients if billing records are coded properly. However, sometimes it is necessary to use the billing system to identify those medical records that need clinical review. The two systems must be linked in order to analyze these records. Information technology staff must understand what linkages are necessary for quality improvement activities and design the systems accordingly.

Priorities inform decisions between "homegrown" vs. "off-the-shelf" systems

There are difficult decisions to make when choosing a system for collecting quality improvement data, and it is important to involve both technical and clinical personnel in making these decisions.

Designing and maintaining a system is never less expensive than purchasing a system off the shelf. The costs in terms of time and personnel invariably will exceed the initial estimate. By the time the system is developed, tested, and installed, expenses are often far greater than buying a system. The question becomes one of modifying existing systems to meet the needs of the organization—a question that must be carefully evaluated by information technology staff. The bottom line: any decision to develop a system internally should be accompanied by a compelling need.

Monitoring the quality of data entered and reports generated by the system

Monitoring the quality and completeness of the data entering the system is no small matter. Standards for coding and abstracting must be specified carefully, and personnel who do this work must be trained and monitored. Periodic checks and retraining to ensure data quality and completeness are essential to producing credible reports.

Public reporting of data

One benefit of reporting heath care-associated infections (HAIs) and other adverse events to the public is a better educated population wherein individuals ask appropriate questions of their physicians (and of other care providers) and use their knowledge to foresee potential problems. The reporting requirement has brought transparency to HAIs and health care quality and safety in general.

When dealing with public reporting systems, it is important to understand that:

- There are multiple reporting systems in use, and the results will differ across reporting.
- Different methods are used, each having certain strengths and weaknesses.

The best approach is one that is honest and transparent (as opposed to a defensive stance). Transparency has helped save lives while providing a forum for defining best practices and the impetus for information sharing across organizations and institutions to improve processes and outcomes of care for all patients.

Conclusion

Well-designed databases can be useful for monitoring and improving the quality of the health care that you provide to your patients. Ideally, these databases serve internal data needs as well as providing the information required by external agencies, both voluntary and regulatory. Several possibilities should be considered when deciding what types of data to collect. Data on patient outcomes, both positive and negative, are important, but outcome data must be risk adjusted to account for differences in patient risk factors at the start of treatment. Process data also are necessary for understanding how to improve care.

Ideally, the system should accommodate administrative, regulatory, and billing needs in addition to quality improvement objectives. Public reporting of data should be approached in a positive and constructive manner. These reports present opportunities for open, honest communication that ultimately leads to improvement in patient care.

Study and Discussion Questions

1. What are the longer term consequences of defensiveness and blaming others when public reporting of patient outcome data reveals specific problems?

2. Should outcome data be linked to payment levels? If so, how should this be done?

3. If you are treating patients who are sicker than average, what is the advantage of using risk adjustment when comparing your patients' outcomes to those of other physicians?

Case Study: Hospital A and Hospital B

You are trying to determine whether you would rather go to Hospital A or Hospital B for a particular type of elective inpatient surgery. You are interested in measuring the outcomes of care for people like you who got the same type of surgery in each of these two hospitals. Assume that you have complete access to billing data and other medical records data for all of the people who had this procedure during the past 18 months at each of these two hospitals. What data would you request? Based on the data, how would you go about analyzing the data to decide which hospital to choose? What outcome measures would you use? Construct a sample table showing how you would do this, inserting your own data.

Suggested Readings and Web Sites

Books

Donabedian, A. *An Introduction to Quality Assurance in Health Care.* New York, NY: Oxford University Press, 2002.

Hubbard, DW. *How to Measure Anything: Finding the Value of Intangibles in Business.* Hoboken, NJ: John Wiley and Sons, 2010.

Iezzoni, LI (ed.). *Risk Adjustment for Measuring Health Care Outcomes.* Ann Arbor, MI: Health Administration Press, 1994.

Lighter, DE. *Advanced Performance Improvement in Health Care: Principles and Methods.* Sudbury, MA: Jones and Bartlett, 2011.

Committee on Quality of Health Care in America, Institute of Medicine, *Crossing the Quality Chasm: A New Health System for the 21st Century.* Washington, DC: National Academies Press, 2001.

Journals

American Journal of Managed Care
American Journal of Medical Quality
Annals of Internal Medicine
Health Affairs
JAMA
Journal of the American Medical Informatics Association
Journal of Healthcare Quality
Medical Care
New England Journal of Medicine

Websites

www.qualitynet.org
www.qualitycheck.org
www.CalHospitalCompare.org
www.hospitalqualityalliance.org

www.qualityforum.org
www.ihi.org
www.healthgrades.com

References

1. Institute of Medicine Committee on Quality of Health Care in America, *Crossing the Quality Chasm: A New Health System for the 21st Century,* Washington, DC: National Academies Press, 2001.

This chapter is based on the extensive research of the author as reflected in the body of published work listed below:

- DesHarnais S, Chesney JD, Wroblewski RT, *et al.* The risk-adjusted mortality index: a new measure of hospital performance. *Medical Care,* 25(12):1129'48, Dec. 1988.

- DesHarnais SI, McMahon LF Jr., Wroblewski RT, Hogan AJ. Measuring hospital performance: the development and validation of risk-adjusted indexes of mortality, readmissions, and complications. *Medical Care,* 28(12):1127:41, Dec. 1990.

- DesHarnais S, McMahon LF Jr, Wroblewski R. Measuring outcomes of hospital care using multiple risk-adjusted indexes. *Health Services Research,* 26(4):425-45, Oct. 1991.

For more information on indirect standardization, please reference the following:
Blumberg, M. S. Risk adjusting health care outcomes: a methodological review. *Medical Care Review,* 43(2):351-93, (Fall 1986).

Chapter 7

Process Improvement Using National Data

By Rick May, MD

Executive Summary

Quality has become *the* new strategic imperative for hospitals and physicians. Over the next 10 years, achieving quality outcomes will be critical to the financial survival of all health care providers in the U.S. Reaching quality Nirvana requires a combination of coherent planning and goal orientation, broad stakeholder engagement, and clear metrics to establish baseline performance and track improvement.

In this chapter we will discuss how to jumpstart your organization's quality journey by using data that are readily available through a variety of national sources.

Learning Objectives

1. Discuss the financial and political factors driving "pay-for-quality" initiatives.

2. Understand the advantages and limitations of using administrative data to evaluate hospital clinical quality.

3. Discuss differences between the three major types of national quality data—public, semi-public, and private—and give examples of each.

4. Conduct a hospital performance "Check-Up" across several major sources of national health care quality data.

5. Know how to turn the "Red Flags" identified during the Check-Up into a series of questions that drive subsequent QI investigations.

Key Words: Health care, Quality, Financing, Pay-For-Quality, Administrative Data, Risk Adjustment, Patient Safety, Mortality, Complication, Readmission, Chart Review, Outcomes

Proper Names: Medicare, Hospital Compare, HealthGrades, *U.S. News & World Report,* ACC-NCDR, STS, Project IMPACT, Thomson Reuters, The Joint Commission, Core Measures, SCIP Measures, Premier, Crimson

Introduction

Quality is *the* strategic imperative.

Depending on your perspective, the U.S. health care system is being reformed, changed, manipulated, or mangled. Whatever verb we choose, titanic forces are stressing the system and moving us toward a new paradigm.

Health care costs are rising unsustainably (Figure 1), but clear-cut solutions to addressing this predicament remain elusive. Clearly, an optimal way to control the nation's health care costs would be to evaluate the services we currently provide to patients and make logical decisions about which services offer the greatest benefit to the largest number of patients. Ineffective treatments, non-evidence-based treatments, and treatments that do not add years of quality life would be scrutinized and, perhaps, not covered by payers—although patients could pay for these treatments out of pocket. But, with the echoes of "death panels" still ringing in their ears, most legislators view even reasonable conversations about limiting services to any constituent group as a highly charged political third rail.

Figure 1.

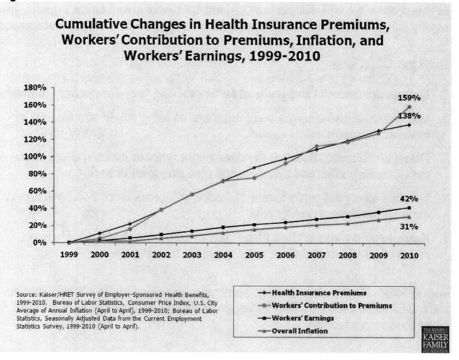

Without a meaningful conversation that might lead us to logical and practical ways of limiting health care expenditures, we are left to choose from more politically palatable but often less effective options. Among these is the seemingly simple but highly complex notion of linking reimbursement for health care services to the quality of those services.

There are a number of reasons why this is not a simple undertaking. We lack a clear definition or consensus around what "quality" in health care really means. Currently, we do not collect enough clinical metrics to monitor even a small percentage of the care being administered on a national level. While consumers are mostly unaware of it now, providing only "quality care" will translate into less care for many patients in certain instances.

Despite these and other shortcomings, this politically appealing solution likely will drive much of health care reform for the next decade. For better or worse, we are entering a new age of "pay-for-quality," "pay-for-performance," or "pay-for-outcomes," and, fortunately, one positive side effect might be to help improve quality. (Figure 2)

Figure 2.

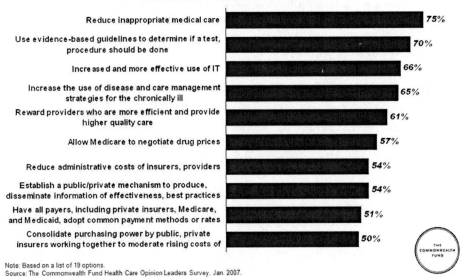

Health Care Opinion Leaders:
Views on Controlling Rising Health Care Costs

"How effective do you think each of these approaches would be
to control rising costs and improve the quality of care?"
Percent saying "extremely/very effective"

Approach	Percent
Reduce inappropriate medical care	75%
Use evidence-based guidelines to determine if a test, procedure should be done	70%
Increased and more effective use of IT	66%
Increase the use of disease and care management strategies for the chronically ill	65%
Reward providers who are more efficient and provide higher quality care	61%
Allow Medicare to negotiate drug prices	57%
Reduce administrative costs of insurers, providers	54%
Establish a public/private mechanism to produce, disseminate information of effectiveness, best practices	54%
Have all payers, including private insurers, Medicare, and Medicaid, adopt common payment methods or rates	51%
Consolidate purchasing power by public, private insurers working together to moderate rising costs of	50%

Note: Based on a list of 19 options.
Source: The Commonwealth Fund Health Care Opinion Leaders Survey, Jan. 2007.

THE COMMONWEALTH FUND

For decades, physicians and hospitals were forced to choose between improving quality and improving financial performance. Because of a natural inclination to keep the lights turned on, many chose the latter. In a new age of pay-for-quality, financial success and ultimate survival will be intimately tied to hospitals' and physicians' ability to provide high-quality patient outcomes and to supply proof of their performance by using appropriate metrics. Pay-for-quality data will force all providers to confront their skills and outcomes more realistically. In a broader sense, pay-for-quality will likely produce a genuine consumer marketplace in health care wherein patients will make purchasing decisions based on whether they are likely to have positive versus adverse outcomes.

The fact that we have arrived at this point should be celebrated by all of us who believe in providing the best possible care for our patients. Now the believers must answer some fundamental but challenging questions:

- How do we understand what quality means?
- How do we know if our organizations are providing it?
- How do we measure it, track it, and benchmark it?
- If we are not providing it consistently, how do we improve?
- How do we educate physicians and staff about it and get them to care about it?
- How do we let patients know that we provide it?

While you may feel that you are adrift in a sea of quality metrics without a paddle, your boat is filled with thousands of other like-minded and like-challenged health care providers, all searching for similar answers. In this chapter, we examine the various types of national quality data that can help you evaluate your organization and explore some relatively simple ways to use these data to drive quality improvement (QI).

Hospitals Drowning in Data

Most hospitals have one or more internal data collection systems. These types of data systems—e.g., Premier, Crimson, Micromedex, Press-Ganey—offer hospitals vast amounts of data at a variety of levels. The big question is: what are hospitals doing with all the data?

In-house clinical reporting systems provide a veritable cornucopia of data, but most of them are never seen or used to drive QI. In a recent conversation with previous employees from two companies that provide clinical data systems to hospitals nationally, I learned a well-kept secret. By polling their clients, these companies found that only 10 percent of hospitals actually use these very expensive data systems on a regular basis. Amazingly, hospitals seem quite aware of this significant underuse.

Data Collection "Driving the Bus"

There are several reasons why all these data are accumulating with little QI to show for the effort. Given the onslaught of national reporting requirements, many hospital quality departments have been reduced to data abstraction shops. Quality directors tell us that they and their staffs spend more than 90 percent of their time collecting data, leaving less than 10 percent of their time and resources to spend on actual QI.

Another reason is that the nurses and physicians with responsibility for implementing the clinical changes necessary for QI do not have time to adequately care for their patients let alone spend extra time reviewing data. Lastly, several studies suggest that much of the data being collected nationally (e.g., Core Measures) do not correlate well, or at all, with patient outcomes, which leads many to question the real value of some of these data.

Taken together, the current allocation of scarce resources, lack of time by health care professionals, and nagging questions about the value of data make using internal data for QI a very challenging and sometimes dicey proposition.

Using Billing Data for Quality Reporting

National data sources, especially those that cover all hospitals and allow for nationwide comparisons, have several limitations. Looking at the evolution of quality reporting in the U.S., it is easy to understand why our current quality systems are often inadequate. Several years ago, researchers began a search for databases that were applicable across most hospitals and physicians in the country for use in producing national health care quality standards. In general, they found that clinical data were rarely being collected in any type of standardized or statistically valid manner, making comparisons between hospitals, or between physicians at the same hospital, difficult if not impossible.

Although most major U.S. industries are on their fifth generation of computer technology, health care electronic information management is in only its first or second iteration. For a majority of individual physicians, in-office electronic health record (EHR) systems are nonexistent or rudimentary. While most hospitals claim to have some type of EHR system, there remains a huge variation in usefulness and utilization, from systems that do little more than help with computerized order entry to those that actually capture physician input. Unfortunately, even the more sophisticated systems often are not used appropriately, and the data captured are often unsuitable for automated extraction of quality metrics.

In the absence of good databases, we have resorted to using the "administrative systems" (i.e., billing systems) that are readily available. Most national quality data available today are based on data collected for the purpose of billing. Although these systems were not designed for clinical data extraction, they provide a data source with consistent formats across essentially all hospitals. Thus, they have become the databases of choice.

Billing Data Advantages

Billing information contains a lot of helpful information related to patient demographics (e.g., age, sex, race), diagnoses, and procedures. While not specifically created to capture clinical information, these systems capture major conditions via the diagnosis codes and events/procedures related to a hospitalized patient's care. Coincidentally, the most important clinical diagnoses and procedures tend to be the ones that pay the most.

Billing Data Limitations

The Medicare inpatient data set (known as MedPAR) exemplifies some of the limitations we face. Medicare makes its information available to a variety of public and private entities nationwide. The cost of buying the data from Medicare is nominal and the technology to upload the data into a variety of database systems for analysis is well within the reach of most relatively computer-savvy organizations.

The challenge comes with the data themselves. First, Medicare publicly reports only the first nine ICD-9 diagnosis codes; therefore, even if a patient is very sick and has 20 or more significant medical conditions, only nine of them will be available for review. Fortunately, these nine conditions will tend to be those that are likely to produce the largest reimbursement and generally will be of the greatest clinical importance. But we are still presented with an incomplete clinical picture.

Next, certain information is challenging to use. In many instances, the patient's age is not reflected accurately—e.g., either not shown at all or stratified into an age range. Because patient race often is recorded inaccurately or unavailable, it cannot be used in any meaningful way to risk-stratify the data. Although physician attribution with respect to procedures is relatively accurate, overall physician attribution is very inaccurate. In general, the record contains a single "physician of record"—usually the admitting physician—and no indication of the other physicians involved in a patient's care. It follows that if a patient is admitted by Dr. Smith, who sees the patient only briefly on the day of admission, we may learn nothing of the 17 other physicians who see the patient during his or her hospital stay. Lastly, Medicare blinds data at a patient level so that multiple encounters for the same patient are disconnected. This makes it impossible to track patients as they move in and out of the system.

These types of databases leave us with:

- A series of disconnected single patient encounters in which we see some, but never all, of the patient's relevant medical conditions.

- Demographic factors of variable accuracy.

- No consistent way of connecting the care the patient received from a majority of care providers.

With only inpatient data available, we see only a small portion of each patient's overall care, usually with no indication of appropriateness of the admission, incomplete past medical history, no information on outpatient medications, inaccurate lists of past procedures, and no indication of what happens to the patient following discharge.

With all of these limitations, why use these types of databases? There are two reasons—one bad and one good. The bad reason is that we lack a better option. The good reason is that, when used correctly, this type of national billing data can yield some fairly powerful results.

Risk Adjustment

Administrative data sets are huge, usually containing tens of millions to hundreds of millions of patient records. Because the risk factors with the highest monetary value for billing also tend to be linked to more clinically relevant diagnoses, many of them are captured in the limited billing data. The combination of a high volume of patients and a system that looks for maximum "badness" among the diagnoses yields rich data for analysis. The risk-adjusted models produced with these data tend to achieve high correlations with outcomes.

Importantly, with proper creation of the logistic regression analyses models and appropriate analysis of hospital data using these models, it is possible to reduce large amounts of hospital data to a series of significant, actionable questions. These are the questions that are critical to using data to drive QI in hospitals.

The Importance of Asking the Right Questions

National quality metrics clearly have limitations but, because they allow us to see a high-level snapshot of hospitals compared to their peers, they provide insight into the areas of opportunity at any given facility.

An analogy

Imagine the vast sea of data as a calm ocean with a clinical treasure somewhere beneath the surface. Given the flat surface and the massive volume of material beneath, it is difficult to know where to begin a search.

Enter the national databases with large data sets running through logistic regression analyses comparing all possible risk factors with outcomes. This regression analysis process creates a computer model with a series of weighted independent variables (risks) on the front end and the likelihood of certain outcomes on the backend. We run our hospital's patient data through the model and, for any select clinical area, we have predicted outcomes expressed as a percentage. We compare our predicted outcomes with our actual outcomes, looking for statistically significant outliers.

Back on the ocean, the flat calm is now punctuated by floating red flags that represent areas of significant variation in the risk-adjusted data. One flag may suggest too many renal complications in knee replacement patients and another may hint that too many stroke patients are aspirating. Each flag represents statistical outliers but do they really represent clinical QI opportunities? Here is where we must take the next step.

Finding Answers

When using national data for QI, it is important to recognize that the red flags generated by models are not answers, but they do represent questions that need to be examined further. The real power of our national data sources lies in generating these questions. Using these national models, we can take huge amounts of data with no clear landmarks and create scores of starting points.

Types of National Data, Data Sources, and Reliability

Table 1 outlines some of the major national databases. Access to the data varies by database. This list is not intended to be comprehensive, but rather to illustrate the types of national data available to support clinical QI.

The major data sources fall into three major buckets: public, semi-public, and private.

- Public: Data available to everyone, generally via the Internet. Although most of the data are now free to patients, in some cases (e.g., MedPAR or state data) the raw data are not very helpful to consumers.

- Semi-Public: Data supplied by public companies and available to almost anyone, usually for a fee. These data are often used by companies to produce business analyses.

- Private: Data created and held by organizations that limit its access to participating hospitals, selected researchers, and sometimes governmental agencies. Generally, these data are not accessible to the public or available for purchase except by participating providers.

Your National Data Check-Up

The multitude of national data sources may at first seem confusing, but it is possible to get a quick snapshot of your hospital or system's performance regarding quality. This quick check up serves two main purposes:

- It will give you a high-level view of how a prospective or current patient sees your facility in terms of quality.

- It should generate a list of Red-Flag areas for further analysis (details outlined in the next section).

Table 1. Comparison of National Databases

Database	Type	Creator/Sponsor	Availability	Comments
Hospital Compare	Public	Medicare	Anyone on the internet.	CMS/HHS-sponsored website with information on more than 5000 hospitals nationwide. Includes information on hospital mortality in several areas, performance on process measures, patient safety scores, etc. Some information is benchmarked and risk-adjusted. www.hospitalcompare.hhs.gov
MedPAR	Public	Medicare	Anyone for a small purchase price.	Audited and standardized data on Medicare inpatient admissions. Made available by Medicare fiscal year (Oct. to Sept.). Blinded to patient and physician. Difficult to use in its raw form, but many organizations perform analyses on the data. https://www.cms.gov/IdentifiableDataFiles /05_ MedicareProviderAnalysisandReviewFile.asp.
State Data (raw)	Public in 19 states, limited in others	Individual States	19 states available to anyone, but the price varies widely.	19 states provide public data (Arizona, California, Colorado, Florida, Iowa, Maine, Maryland, Massachusetts, Nevada, New Jersey, New York Oregon, Pennsylvania, Rhode Island, Texas, Utah, Virginia, Washington, Wisconsin). Formats vary widely as does the timing of the data releases. In some states the data are provided free and in others they are very expensive.
State Data via State websites	Public, Semi-Public, and/or Private	Individual States	Some data available to anyone via the state websites, other data are restricted.	Remarkable variability exists among states. Patients have not demanded a consistent standard across the U.S. Some states have robust websites with lots of free data available. Other states provide no data to help the public evaluate their hospitals' quality.

Table 1. Comparison of National Databases *(continued)*

Database	Type	Creator/Sponsor	Availability	Comments
U.S. News	Public & Semi-Public	*U.S. News and World Report*[1]	Best hospitals ranking information is available to anyone. Other data available for purchase.	Methodology includes ranking most U.S. hospitals in several areas, including reputation, survival (mortality), patient safety, volume, nursing, availability of technology, patient services, etc. Public ratings only list the top performers in several areas, but the website provides some information on all hospitals. http://health.usnews.com/best-hospitals.
HealthGrades[2,3]	Public & Semi-Public	HealthGrades.com	Website provides some free data, other data available for purchase.	Free Website has quality ratings on all non-federal hospitals (5000+) in over 30 clinical areas. HealthGrades is the highest traffic consumer website, with more than 11 million unique patients visiting the site each month. In-depth data available for purchase. www.healthgrades.com.
Thomson Reuters (formerly Solucient)	Public & Semi-Public	Thomson Reuters	Some free, some for purchase.	Annual ratings of health care quality across multiple hospitals and service lines. Much of the information is available free on the Internet. Large data sets and analyses available for purchase. www.thomsonreuters.com.
Joint Commission Quality Check	Public, Semi-Public, and Private	The Joint Commission	Some information available to the public, other information is only available to participating hospitals and select researchers.	The Joint Commission is responsible for inspecting and certifying most U.S. hospitals. Public site notes awards and certifications for each hospital. Much more hospital data recently made available to the public through an improved website. Heavy on mortality, HCAHPS[4], and Core Measures data (from CMS). www.qualitycheck.org/consumer/searchQCR.aspx.

Table 1. Comparison of National Databases *(continued)*

Database	Type	Creator/Sponsor	Availability	Comments
Premier	Private	Premier	Information available to participating hospitals and select researchers.	Collaborative health care alliance among over 2,500 U.S. hospitals. The database has clinical and financial information on more than 130 million patient discharges. www.premierinc.com.
Crimson	Private	The Advisory Board	Information available to participating hospitals.	Participating hospitals collect cost, quality, and utilization data from inpatient, outpatient, and ambulatory care settings. The system provides analyses and benchmarks. www.advisory.com/Technology/Crimson.
Project IMPACT	Private	SCCM — The Society of Critical Care Medicine	To participating hospitals, selected researchers, limited commercial use.	Data on care of ICU patients to track outcomes and costs. Clinical data, chart extracted, collected by participating hospitals. Blinded to patient and physician. www.projectimpacticu.cc.
ACC — National Cardiovascular Data Registry	Private	American College of Cardiology	To participating hospitals, selected researchers, limited commercial use.	Clinical data, chart extracted, collected by participating hospitals. NCDR includes several databases, including cardiac catheterizations, acute coronary syndrome, ICD's, etc. ACC-NCDR is the gold standard for cardiac intervention data. www.ncdr.com.
STS — National Cardiovascular Data Registry	Private	American College of Cardiology	To participating hospitals, selected researchers, limited commercial use.	Clinical data, chart extracted, collected by participating hospitals. STS includes 3 surgery databases, including adult cardiac, general thoracic, and congenital heart surgery. STS is the gold standard for cardiac surgery data. Jan. 2011 STS participating hospitals were allowed the option to display their results publicly. About 250 programs currently show their star ratings. www.sts.org/national-database.

Clinical Areas

When looking at your hospital's clinical quality, it is best to focus on the highest value clinical areas first. In general, the following are the highest value areas for most hospitals in terms of patient volume, financial importance, and clinical opportunity:

- Cardiac medicine: heart failure, acute myocardial infarction, cardiology, interventional cardiology, cardiac catheterization (PCI)
- Cardiac surgery: coronary artery bypass graft, valve replacement
- Pulmonary: chronic obstructive pulmonary disease, pneumonia (community-acquired)
- Critical care: sepsis, pulmonary embolism
- Orthopedic surgery: knee replacement, hip replacement, hip fracture repair
- Spine surgery: spine fusion, disk excision, laminectomy
- Women's health/maternity care: hysterectomy, Caesarean-sections, gynecologic surgery
- Oncology

In addition to specific clinical areas, it is wise to be aware of your national data in the following areas related to outcomes, complications, and patient safety indicators:

- Infections (all, but especially central line and ventilator associated pneumonia)
- Wrong site surgeries
- Decubitus ulcers
- Others (e.g., falls, air emboli, mismatched blood, etc.)

The check-up can be done in any order, but the outline that follows gets the most valuable data first. It is helpful to take notes in a Word® document, cutting-and-pasting data, graphs, and images found during your check-up. As you go through the check-up, note any below average or areas of concern with the "Red Flag" (e.g., a red X or check mark) to make it easy to find for further review later.

Check-Up Steps

To keep it simple, select one or two clinical areas of interest first from the list above when doing the check-up for the first time. Note: Substitute the name of your hospital for "Happy Hospital" used in the examples.

Step 1: Google® Search

Google is critical to how the world sees you, and it is where most of your patients will look to evaluate your hospital. At least 80 percent of health care searches go through Google. About 91 percent of people look at only the first three search results, and about 95 percent never look at anything beyond the first Google page.

Bottom line: don't look much past the first few results since your patients never will.

Search on several variations of the following: "Happy Hospital." "Happy Hospital Quality," "Happy Hospital (insert a clinical area from the above list) Quality," "Happy Hospital Mortality," "Happy Hospital Complications."

For each of these searches, note any quality data that appear: awards, recognitions, etc. Patients are especially interested in graphs and pictures that reflect your quality. Copy and paste a few of these into your notes. Add Red Flags in any areas that look problematic or that appear no better than average if they are important service lines in your hospital.

Step 2: Check HealthGrades®

HealthGrades is searched by over 11 million patients per month, so how your hospital looks in HealthGrades is how most of your patients see you. Great (★★★★★) performance is, of course, fine, and potentially an area to emphasize and build. Average (★★★) performance is acceptable to most patients. Poor (★) performance (generally the bottom 10-12 percent of hospitals nationwide) often leads a patient to look for care elsewhere. Mark any one-star areas and other areas of concern (underperformance) with a Red Flag.

Google "HealthGrades Happy Hospital" and click on the HealthGrades link (it will look something like this: http://www.healthgrades.com/hospital-directory/colorado-co/happy-hospital-hgst3b428d46060034). Check the following tabs and make note of information:

- "Distinctions"
- "Quality and Ratings"
- Clinical area(s) of interest noting Actual and Predicted percentages as well as the star ratings
- "Patient Safety Indicators," noting areas that fall below average

Step 3: Hospital Compare®

Go to www.hospitalcompare.hhs.gov and enter your hospital's zip code or city. We'll do this quick look twice, once for a medical condition (heart failure) and once for a procedure (knee replacement) since the search paths and data are slightly different.

Medical Condition Search

Select "Medical Conditions" and then "Heart Failure" (drop-down box) and then "Find Hospitals." The next screen lists the hospitals in your area. Select your hospital and, if you're curious, select one or two competitor hospitals to see how you compare.

Click on "Compare" and, going through the various tabs, record how your hospital looks, with a focus on the following:

- Process of Care Measures: These reflect performance on Core and SCIP Measures. Mark any areas showing less than 100 percent with a Red Flag.

- Outcomes of Care Measures: 90-95 percent of hospitals are in the "No Different than U.S. National Rate" group. Be very concerned if your hospital is in the "Worse Than U.S. National Rate" in any category.

- Click the 'View Graphs" tab. Unless your actual mortality percentage is substantially lower than the national average, note this as a Red Flag since average performance in the area of heart failure mortality will likely cost you money in the future.

- Click the "View All Measures" tab to access Patient Safety Measures. At the top of the page, three categories are listed: Serious Complications, Deaths for Certain Conditions, and Other Complications and Deaths. Most of this information is not useful in its current form.

  Under the "Hospital Acquired Conditions" section, click on "Get Results for this Hospital." A small box will open with raw numbers that are not benchmarked. Go to "Click here to view the U.S. National Rate for these measures" at the bottom of the box. Scroll down to "Hospital-Acquired Conditions" again for the information you need. Look at the conditions (e.g., pressure sores, falls, air emboli), comparing your hospital to the U.S. National Rate.

  Note how your hospital compares to the national rate. *Mark any area where your occurrence rate is greater than zero with a Red Flag.* Going forward, the occurrence of any of these conditions will hurt your hospital from a financial and ratings standpoint, so you must work toward eliminating them completely. It may not be possible to eliminate all hospital-acquired conditions completely or permanently, but this process is a journey and not a destination.

- Medicare Payment and Volume: These data are collected on an October-September fiscal year basis. The payment information is not benchmarked, but note the total number of medicare heart failure patients treated by adding all three DRGs.

Procedure Search

Now, we'll look at a procedure—knee replacement.

Select "Surgical Procedures" and then, from the drop-down box, select "Neck, Back, Arms & Legs." In the final drop-down box, select "Joint Replacement/ Reattachment" and then "Find Hospitals." From the list of hospitals on the next screen, select your hospital (and any competitors) and click on "Compare."

Again there will be various tabs to choose from. When looking at surgeries, the only areas to focus on are the following:

- Process of Care Measures: These are the Surgical Care Improvement Project (SCIP) measures. Put a Red Flag anywhere that your hospital is not at 100 percent since anything less is becoming unacceptable.

- Medicare Payment and Volume: The data are being collected on a yearly basis (Medicare fiscal year: October to September). Again, the payment information is not useful, but note the total number of Medicare knee replacement patients treated by adding all the DRGs.

Step 4: State Data

Depending on the particular state, you may be able to access state data on your hospital via your state's website. State websites vary considerably in terms of actual existence, data timeliness, and usefulness of the data for QI. Some states merely provide a link to Hospital Compare®. If you find data, note any Red Flag areas.

Step 5: Joint Commission Quality Data Download

- Go to http://www.qualitycheck.org/consumer/searchQCR.aspx or the Joint Commission webpage (www.jointcommission.org). In the upper right corner, open the drop-down box titled "Joint Commission Web Sites" and then click on "Quality Check."

- Enter the name of your hospital and the state and click "Search." Find your hospital and click on the "View Accreditation Quality Report" link.

- When you click on "Download Accreditation PDF Report" in the left column, your hospital's Accreditation Quality Report should appear. This PDF file— about 37 pages long—contains quality information used by The Joint Commission in its evaluation of your hospital. Much of the information comes from CMS, including Core Measures, mortality numbers, and SCIP measures, many of which you will have seen when reviewing your Hospital Compare data.

- Copy pages 3 and 4, the "Summary of Quality Information," for future reference. This outlines your major certifications and quality awards.

- Quickly scan the rest of the report, looking for red minus signs like this ⊖ that denote deficiency areas. Record these in your notes with a Red Flag.

Step 6: U.S. News and World Report

Although these rankings are heavily weighted toward a hospital's reputation and other factors that do not necessarily correlate with quality, there is some useful information on http://health.usnews.com/best-hospitals/rankings. Enter your hospital name, city, and state in the search box on the right side. With the Specialty box on "All," select "Find Hospitals" and find your hospital on the next page.

Click on your hospital for the following details:

- First page, check the overview of your hospital for accuracy.

- Click the 'Rankings" tab for significant data related to quality. Several specialties (e.g., cancer, gynecology, orthopedics) are listed on the left side. Click on each specialty category and record the following few elements that are useful for QI:

  o Reputation with specialists: a measure of how many specialists named your hospital as one of the best in the country for care in this area. While this may help you evaluate your reputation among specialists, it may have little to do with performance on actual objective quality metrics.[5]

  o Survival: a risk-adjusted measure of your hospital's mortality rate in this area. Note that for areas with very low mortality (e.g., orthopedics) the rating is based on a very small number of patients and is not particularly helpful.

  o Patient volume: helpful in comparing with all hospitals nationally.

At this point, you should have several pages of public information related to your hospital's performance in one or two (or more) clinical areas, performance on Core and SCIP Measures and patient safety measures, an overall picture of how the public perceives your hospital, and most importantly, a list of Red Flag areas for further investigation. Again, the Check-Up process will not provide answers, but it will help you reduce a vast amount of information down to a few Red Flag questions.

Beyond Public Data Sources

Once the initial Check-Up using public data is complete, turn to more private data sources such as ACC-NCDR, STS, cancer registries, Premier, Crimson, etc. If any of these are available at your hospital, review them for data to support or refute your preliminary analysis. If you are unfamiliar with these data sources, you may want to speak with your hospital's data system administrator to see what information these databases contain and how to go about getting reports.

Begin by going through your list of Red Flag areas in general terms and seeking additional national data if possible. For example, if your Check-Up of "Hospital Compare" revealed a Red Flag regarding inpatient sepsis at your hospital, it might be helpful to correlate these data with data from the Project IMPACT (critical care) database.

Use all available data sources to get the best possible understanding of the types of patients and the data included in Red Flag areas. You may find it helpful to review the methodology sections of the major national data sites.

Turning Red Flags into Actionable Questions

After identifying and possibly validating Red Flag areas, it is time to turn each flag into a clear, concise, well-defined question. The following are key steps to identifying actionable information for any clinical or patient safety Red Flag.

Step 1: Clearly define the questions prompted by the Red Flags.

For example, a one-star (poor) score in a knee replacement surgery rating on HealthGrades raises questions such as:

- "Is our quality in this area really in the bottom 10 percent of the country?"

- "Is this poor quality "real," or is it the result of coding and documentation issues?"

- "If it is real, what is driving our poor quality?"

- "What can we change to improve our quality?"

Step 2: Clarify Red Flag questions in terms of the data source being used, the time period being measured, and the data metrics that are being gathered.

Also, determine if the data are risk-adjusted. For example, for the HealthGrades one-star in knee replacement[6]:

- Data Source: HealthGrades ratings are based on Medicare inpatient data only.

- Time Period measured: HealthGrades 2012 ratings are based on Medicare fiscal years 2008, 2009, and 2010 (i.e., October 2007 to September 2010).

- Data Metrics: Knee replacement ratings are based on inpatient complications only.

- Risk Adjustment: Data are risk adjusted

Step 3: Use other national data sources to corroborate the Red Flag questions.

For instance, is there a national data source or registry that looks at knee replacement complications? In many areas, there are well-established national data sources that enable further investigation of Red Flag areas.

Step 4: Create internal reports to replicate the data used in the Red Flag areas.

Consider whether your hospital has internal data sources for looking into this area (e.g., Premier, Crimson). For example, many hospital systems can generate internal reports using their own data for knee replacement complications. Involve your information technology department to help address these technical questions.

Step 5: Create the internal report using the same time period and data subset used by the national data source.

For the knee replacement example, we would use national data from Medicare patients (October 2007-September 2010). In most cases, quality issues will affect all patients regardless of insurance status. An internal report that includes all patients will change the volume but, in general, will not change the percentage of deaths or complications significantly.

Step 6: Make sure the ICD-9 codes or DRG's match up with the national data source that raised the Red Flag.

In the preceding HealthGrades example, a one-star in knee replacement is based on inpatient complications. The HealthGrades methodology[6] specifies the ICD-9 procedure codes used (i.e., Principal Procedure: 81.54) and gives a complete list of all the complication ICD-9 codes used to create the rating.

Create your internal report by pulling all knee replacement patients (Principal Procedure: 81.54) with Medicare insurance admitted between October 2007 and September 2010 who had one or more of the complications listed in the HealthGrades methodology. The patients captured in this report—i.e., the same patients and outcomes that raised the Red Flag plus the non-Medicare patients on your hospital's list—can be used to answer the questions we raised in Step 1.

Drilling Down into the Data

Once you have the patient list as described above, you can proceed with the most important steps in the process: Validating the existence of an actual problem, understanding the root causes of the problem, and identifying the steps needed to fix the problem and improve quality.

The following steps can be used to drill down into the data for almost any clinical Red Flag area regardless of how it was identified.

- Clearly identify the population of patients who make up the data set; e.g., all knee replacement patients with one or more complications, CABG patients over 65 who died of sepsis, all patients in the hospital who had a pulmonary embolism after surgery, all heart failure patients who were re-admitted within 30 days.

- Working with your physicians and reviewing the literature, identify five best practices or processes of high-performing hospitals that improve quality in the area under review. These should be care processes that are not already done consistently at your hospital. Completing this important step provides a framework to guide the chart review process. Examples of five best practices:

  o For CABG patients: Risk scoring pre-op, pre-surgery review conference, perfusion scoring intra-op, rapid postoperative extubation, and tight glucose control.

  o For heart failure patients at discharge: Set follow-up appointments prior to discharge, connect patients with an outpatient heart failure nurse, channel all patients through an outpatient heart failure clinic, automatic outpatient nutrition education, scale goes home with the patient for daily weights.

- For patients with a pulmonary embolism after surgery: Start Lovenox pre-op, rapid anti-coagulation post-op, short tourniquet times, bilateral procedures only in low-risk patients, Lovenox bridge if using Coumadin.

- Pull a sufficient sample of charts (20 to 100) from the list of patients in question. Err on the side of more charts—the review will focus solely on identifying common patterns among the patients in question.

- Quickly review each chart to confirm that the problem was not just a coding or documentation error (e.g., the patient really died, was really readmitted in less than 30 days, really qualifies as acute renal failure). You will likely find that more than 90 percent of the problems are real rather than the result of coding or documentation errors.

- Review the charts again, noting how often you did things right. Looking at each patient record, ask, "Of the five best practices that we identified that we should be doing, how many did we provide to this patient?"

- Record all patient information on a spreadsheet, noting any coding problems (Yes or No), the number of your five best practices that were provided to the patient, and (in your judgment) whether the failure to provide these best practices contributed to the bad outcome.

Final Review and Action Plan

Once the chart review is complete, it is time to change something that will actually improve quality. The chart review spreadsheet should reveal some consistent patterns of behaviors that contributed to your suboptimal quality. In most cases, these behaviors will be acts of omission rather than commission; i.e., it was a failure to do the right things consistently that allowed the problems to develop rather than doing the wrong things.

At this point, it becomes important to bring more people into the conversation. Start by sharing the chart review findings with the physician or physicians who were involved in creating the list of five best practices to see if they agree with your evaluation and/or if they have other interpretations. Be prepared to review a few more charts if necessary for validation.

Once consensus is reached in this small group, call a larger meeting to present your findings to a broad range of stakeholders from your hospital. Put together a few slides that outline the following in general terms:

- The national data sources consulted for this round of QI.

- The findings that raised the Red Flag; e.g., a one-star rating on HealthGrades, a red minus on the Joint Commission report.

- The other data sources (if any) used to confirm the issue. Note: Often, we need to pursue QI based on a single data source.

- A quick overview of the internal report created to replicate the national data source and the patient list created using this report.

- A more in-depth review of the five best practices used in the chart review; i.e., who was involved in creating the list, the supporting literature, etc. To save time, be prepared to hand out copies of the relevant articles (or send them out in advance of the meeting, especially to the physicians).

- A high-level overview of the chart review findings. It may be helpful to note at this point in the presentation that only a small percentage of the problems were due to coding and/or documentation errors (if this was indeed the case).

- Note the percentage of patients who received any of the five best practices and the percentage who received all five of them.

- Note how often you felt that the failure to provide the five best practices appeared to contribute to the suboptimal outcome in question.

Based on what they have seen, ask the group what system changes can be made to ensure that future patients in the at-risk group receive the five best practices. Generally, a spirited discussion follows with a focus on implementing consistent best practices in your system.

Your role is twofold: 1) keeping the group focused on agreeing to change something, and 2) avoiding a re-hash of the data. The likelihood is that you have correctly identified a real problem, ruled out coding/documentation errors as a significant factor, and established inconsistent delivery of best practices as the true cause; you have good ideas about how to change your systems to improve your outcomes and fix the Red Flag. Given your diligence to this point, there is little likelihood that your data are significantly incorrect. If at all possible, try to end the meeting with consensus around making at least one change in your system of care.

Going Forward

Hopefully, the process of using national data to drive QI has yielded at least one change in at least one clinical area aimed at improving care and outcomes. Even a small initial change represents the first step on a broad and productive road ahead.

By repeating this process to pursue other Red Flags and/or to look at data from other sources, you will find even more QI directions to follow. Review your list of Red Flags with the other stakeholders at your hospital and ask them what questions to answer next. Prioritize your Red Flags and create a schedule to keep the process moving forward. Don't be surprised if it takes months to years to fully investigate and address the Red Flags that it took a mere few hours to identify. It may help to remember what Atul Gawande wrote in his book *"Better: A Surgeon's Notes on Performance"*:

"Better is possible. It does not take genius. It takes diligence. It takes moral clarity. It takes ingenuity. And above all, it takes a willingness to try."

Epilogue: The Inevitable Pushback

The processes outlined in this chapter almost never evolve smoothly. It would be naïve to assume that all stakeholders at your hospital will automatically believe the data and readily agree to change their practices. Physicians tend to be the most skeptical when presented with new ideas, but nurses, technologists, and other providers may also push back against the data and the process.

The following are the Top 10 most common provider concerns, along with suggested responses:

1. *"Our patients are sicker."* That may be the case but, because national data are risk-adjusted, having sicker patients may actually make us look better in national ratings systems.

2. *"We have aggressive coding, and it picks up more complications."* Aggressive coding generally affects the capture of risk factors more than the identification of complications. This is because most patients generally have several risk factors, some of which are missed, but a smaller number of complications that are rarely missed. Aggressive coding usually improves your risk adjustment more than it increases your complications; thus it often makes you look better rather than worse.

3. *"The data are too old."* It is true that all national data sources use retrospective data. But because hospital systems are so complex, significant changes to those systems usually take years to decades to implement. It follows that problems identified in older data are usually still active.

4. *"The data sets are too small."* The data sets used to create national data analysis models are huge, usually incorporating millions of patient records. This makes for very powerful statistical models that, when applied to somewhat smaller data sets from individual hospitals, still yield very accurate analyses.

5. *"What is the p-value of your data?"* P-values generally are not used in this type of data analysis. With population quality statistics, we commonly use confidence intervals and/or standard deviations from the mean. Generally, one standard deviation from the mean (90 percent CI) is used to create cutoffs for grouping low, average, and high performers.

6. *"Is the difference between me and the best performers statistically significant?"* While the patient numbers for individual physicians may not be large enough to show statistical differences, it is much easier to show statistically valid differences between hospitals. Since most of the variation in quality occurs at the hospital level, it is more relevant to compare performance at that level.

7. *"I think that making these changes to improve quality may decrease my patient volumes and could hurt me financially."* Because Medicare and most major payers are shifting much of their reimbursement to "pay-for-quality" systems, most providers will find that unless they adopt practices to improve quality, they will likely face significant reductions in reimbursement. The worst performers will probably not survive financially.

8. *"There's nothing in this process for me."* Besides the reimbursement issues, most physicians find that system improvements implemented to enhance quality generally make their lives easier. Your patients will die less often, have fewer complications, and be happier. Hopefully those things will make you happier as well.

9. *"This whole process is not about quality; it's just about saving money."* Actually, it's about both. For most inpatient care, it's been shown that improving quality saves money as well. Money drives pay-for-quality, but ultimately this process puts quality front and center as the strategic imperative for hospitals.

10. *"We've tried to make changes before and they always fail."* One of the biggest challenges in QI is to produce lasting change. We face the same challenge with this process. However, never in the history of medicine has delivering quality been so directly tied to hospital and physician financial survival. People will be motivated to make sure it doesn't fail this time.

Conclusion

The unsustainable expansion of health care expenditures is driving fundamental changes in reimbursement policies based on a variety of "pay-for-quality" systems. Health care providers, primarily hospitals and physicians, must fundamentally change the ways in which they evaluate, measure, improve, and demonstrate quality if they wish to survive financially.

Despite their limitations, national databases can help hospitals understand and improve their quality. Using these databases for consistent improvement requires specific knowledge and strategies to be successful.

With a rigorous and consistent approach to reviewing and gathering data from national databases, hospitals can use a wide variety of health care quality data to direct and support their QI journeys.

Study and Discussion Questions

1. What are the demographic and market factors driving the substantial and unsustainable increases in health care spending in the U.S.?

2. Is access to health care a right or a privilege?

3. What are the major cultural and economic characteristics present in hospitals and among physicians who have limited the use of electronic health information systems?

4. How do you define "quality" as it relates to health care? Who should determine the quality metrics that are displayed publicly and that form the basis for payment systems?

5. Should there be different quality standards applied to different patient groups based on socioeconomic status, age, education, or other factors?

Case Studies

Case Study #1: A large suburban hospital performs 2000 knee replacements annually. Based on the acuity of its patients, the hospital is predicted to have a complication rate among its knee replacement patients of six percent. However, the observed complication rate among these patients is 11.5 percent. The cost of these complications to the hospital is estimated to be approximately $1,840,000 annually (2000 patients x 11.5% x $8,000 per complication).

The majority of the complications are "medical" in nature (i.e., related to the patient's overall health status) rather than "technical" (i.e., linked to technique problems during the surgery). Most of the patients who develop complications come through their surgery without problems but develop medical complications between 12 and 72 hours post-operatively.

Current medical literature suggests that all patients presenting for knee replacement should go through a standardized, evidence-based medical evaluation process to identify each patient's unique risk profile. This profile should be used to modify all perioperative order sets to optimize care for each patient.

After implementing this type of program, the hospital experienced a reduction in knee replacement complications down to an actual rate of 1.5 percent.

The cost of implementing the pre-operative evaluation program was approximately $600,000 per year, but the savings to the hospital are approximately $1,600,000 annually, along with substantially better quality. The net savings are $1,000,000 annually.

Suggested Readings and Web Sites

Berwick D. Public performance reports and the will for change. *JAMA*, 288(12):1523-4, Sept. 25, 2002.

Steinberg E. Improving the quality of care—can we practice what we preach? *N Engl J Med,* 348(26):2681-3, June 26, 2003.

Green J et al. In search of America's best hospitals: the promise and reality of quality assessment. *JAMA,* 277(14):1152-5, Apr. 9, 1997.

Schneider E, Epstein A Use of public performance reports: a survey of patients undergoing cardiac surgery. *JAMA*, 279(20):1638-42, May 27, 1998.

Kaiser Family Foundation and Agency for Health Care Research and Quality. National Survey on Consumers' Experiences with Patient Safety and Quality Information. Washington, DC: Kaiser Family Foundation, 2004.

Werner RM, Asch DA. The unintended consequences of publicly reporting quality information. *JAMA*, 293(10): 1239-44, Mar. 9, 2005.

Websites

www.hospitalcompare.hhs.gov
https://www.cms.gov/IdentifiableDataFiles/05_MedicareProviderAnalysisandReviewFile.asp
http://health.usnews.com/best-hospitals
www.healthgrades.com
www.thomsonreuters.com
www.qualitycheck.org/consumer/searchQCR.aspx
www.premierinc.com
www.advisory.com/Technology/Crimson
www.projectimpacticu.cc
www.ncdr.com
www.sts.org/national-database

References

1. Murphy J, *et al.* Methodology: U.S. News and World Report Best Hospitals 2011-12. Pub. RTI International. Version: July19, 2011.

2. Reed, *et al.* HealthGrades Hospital Report Cards Mortality and Complication Outcomes 2012 Methodology. HealthGrades Oct 2011. (Available at www.healthgrades.com/business/img/HospitalReportCardsMortalityComplications2012.pdf).

3. www.healthgrades.com/cms/ratings-and-awards/data-source.aspx- shows the sources and years for all the HealthGrades data.

4. Jha A *et al.* Patients' Perception of Hospital Care in the United States. *N Engl J Med,* 359(13):1921-31, Oct. 30, 2008.

5. Sehgal, A *et al.* The Role of Reputation in U.S. News & World Report's Rankings of the Top 50 American Hospitals. *Ann Intern Med,* 152(8):521-5, 2010.

6. Halasyamani L *et al.*Conflicting Measures of Hospital Quality: Ratings from "Hospital Compare" Versus "Best Hospitals." *Journal of Hospital Medicine*, 2(3):128-34, May 2007. Posted on Medscape.

Section III.

Evaluating Quality: Diverse Dimensions of the Health Care System

Chapter 8

Measuring Quality at the Health Plan Level

By Eric J. Berman, DO, MS, Karen E. Michael, RN, MSN, MBA, and Tina Morton RN, BSN, CCM, CPHQ, CHCQM

Executive Summary

It is increasingly apparent that, without a drastic revision, our current health care system will bankrupt the U.S. While a small percentage of Americans receive their care through truly integrated delivery systems, most of us struggle with an inefficient, disconnected, and misaligned system of health care in which reimbursement is predicated on paying for services and procedures with little emphasis on the coordination, quality, efficiency, and outcomes of those services. Using quality as our "foundation," alignment of incentives for providers and facilities as our "building blocks," and a truly collaborative approach to the management of populations through an effective exchange of information between payers and providers as "mortar," we can build a world-class health care system that provides ready access to the highest quality care at the lowest cost.

Long responsible for administering health care benefits for the vast majority of employer-funded health insurance programs, health plans are increasingly responsible for the administration of government-funded (i.e., Medicare and Medicaid) programs. Health care reform proposals to create health care coverage for currently uninsured Americans will further increase the role of health plans in the delivery of health care services. The foregoing, coupled with the health plan's ability to view health care service information across providers, places the health plan in a central role in health care quality measurement.

Health plans use a variety of standardized metrics to measure and report on quality. The results of health plan quality measures are used to gauge and improve internal performance and drive performance improvement from health care providers. Although challenges exist, advances in information technology and the application of information sharing platforms to health care will greatly expand the health plan's ability to measure quality and use the results.

Learning Objectives

1. Gain an appreciation for the role quality plays in the delivery of health care from the health plan perspective.

2. Understand how health plans measure and use quality information in the delivery of health care.

3. Learn how quality, access, and cost influence the provision of care in the U.S.

Key words:

Health Plan, Pay-for-Performance, Outcomes, Measure, Comparison, Performance

Introduction:

Why do health plans care about quality? Health plans are committed to a culture of quality for three reasons; namely, it ensures that 1) activities are measured, 2) performance is constantly challenged to improve, and 3) the importance of innovation is recognized. As performance levels rise, it becomes progressively more difficult to improve upon previous efforts. This spurs the development of innovative approaches that elevate health plans' capabilities. This, in turn, leads to raising standards so that ever more ambitious goals can be attained. Thus, quality provides the platform for setting standards, measuring progress, and evaluating the effectiveness of health plans' efforts to reach new levels of performance.

From a practical perspective, public and private purchasers (e.g., employers) as well as state and federal regulatory agencies use health plan accreditation standards and quality measures (e.g., the Healthcare Effectiveness Data and Information Set [HEDIS]) to evaluate the performance of health plans and to ensure their commitment to industry standard quality measures. Having such standards also permits comparison of like health plans for consumers of health care service.[1]

Health plans measure quality at the provider and subpopulation level to fuel internal quality improvement (QI) programs. For example, quality measures provide the foundation for most health plan pay-for-performance (P4P) programs, which allow providers to earn additional dollars based on their quality scores. Internal quality metrics are also used to evaluate health plan performance with respect to specific member groups. These subpopulation measures may look at members with a certain chronic condition such as diabetes mellitus or members in a specific demographic segment such as child-bearing females or children under age of two.

Viewed by some in the industry as the "Good Housekeeping Seal of Approval," health plan accreditation is generally a voluntary process conducted by an impartial entity. As health plan accreditation evolved over the past two decades, it has increasingly become a contractual, employer, and consumer expectation.

Accrediting organizations set standards and survey health plans against those standards. New standards are continually developed and existing ones are revised to push health plans to higher levels of performance and promote industry priorities as times change.

A form of quality reporting, accreditation evaluates a health plan's systems, processes, and outcomes against a set of standards and benchmarks. The resulting "report card" serves multiple purposes. For the health plan, it is a means for understanding how it compares to its peers. For competitors and health care purchasers, it provides a mechanism for ranking a plan's quality and value. For governments, purchasers, consumers, boards of directors, funding sources, and potential new business partners, it provides evidence of a plan's commitment to quality.

While accreditation may be a mechanism by which health plans attract members and purchasers, it is primarily an investment in quality. Charges for accreditation vary by accrediting body; however, the true cost of accreditation includes the cost of the application and survey as well as the costs for any systems and processes required to meet the standards.

Accreditation Organizations

Accreditation organizations are usually referred to by their initials. Two organizations provide the majority of accreditation for health plans in the United States.

National Committee for Quality Assurance (NCQA)

A not-for--profit organization created to improve health care quality in the U.S., the NCQA was launched in the late 1970s by the health maintenance organization industry in response to employers' demands for accreditation. Initially, many board seats were held by employers, unions, and consumers. In 1990, NCQA became an independent entity focused on health plan accreditation using a unified set of standards to evaluate core systems and processes as well as the actual health outcomes or results achieved by the plan.

This voluntary accreditation program evaluates the health plan in specific areas such as key dimensions of care, service, and efficiency with the goal of improving care, enhancing service, and reducing cost. The three main components of the final scoring for accreditation include: NCQA standards and guidelines, HEDIS, and the Consumer Assessment of Healthcare Providers and Systems (CAHPS) survey results. NCQA now offers a menu of programs, including accreditation, recognition, certification, and distinction.[2]

Utilization Review Accreditation Commission (URAC)

URAC was founded in 1990 in response to public concerns that there were no uniform standards for utilization review processes. An independent, not-for-profit, nationally recognized accrediting organization, URAC's mission is to promote continuous improvement in the quality and efficiency of health care management through the process of accreditation and education.

URAC's standards include input from practitioners, insurers, and the public. URAC offers a broad range of accreditation programs—from an entire health plan to a single process area such as case management.[3]

Standard Measures of Health Plan Quality

Several standard measures are used to evaluate the quality of services delivered by health plans. The data collection methodology differs by measurement and includes aggregation of administrative data, medical record extraction, and survey.

Health Effectiveness Data Information Set (HEDIS®)

Developed by NCQA, HEDIS is a tool used by more than 90 percent of America's health plans to measure performance on important dimensions of care and service. Altogether, HEDIS consists of 75 measures across 8 domains of care.[1] Because so many plans collect HEDIS data, and because the measures are so specifically defined, HEDIS makes it possible to compare the performance of health plans on an "apples-to-apples" basis.

Health plans use HEDIS results to identify opportunities for improvement. Many health plans report HEDIS data to employers or government funding sources and many use their results to stimulate improvements in their quality of care and service.

Employers, consultants, and consumers use HEDIS data in combination with accreditation information as a basis for selecting the best health plan for their needs.

Consumers benefit from HEDIS data through the *State of Health Care Quality* report, a comprehensive look at the performance of the nation's health care system. HEDIS data are also the centerpiece of most health plan "report cards" that appear in national magazines and local newspapers.

To ensure that HEDIS remains relevant, NCQA has established a *process* to evolve the measurement set each year. NCQA's Committee on Performance Measurement, a broad-based group representing employers, consumers, health plans, and others, debates and decides collectively on the content of HEDIS. This group decides on the HEDIS measures to be included and conducts field tests to determine how measurement is done.

To ensure the validity of HEDIS results, all data are rigorously audited by certified auditors using a process designed by NCQA.[1]

Consumer Assessment of Health Providers and Systems (CAHPS®)

The CAHPS program develops and supports the use of a comprehensive and evolving family of standardized surveys that ask consumer and patients to report on and evaluate their experiences with health care. Surveys topics are those with the greatest importance to consumers, such as the communication skills of providers and the accessibility of services. CAHPS originally stood for the Consumer Assessment of Health Plans Study, but, as the products have evolved beyond health plans, the name has evolved as well to capture the full range of survey products and tools.

The CAHPS program is funded and administered by the U.S. Agency for Healthcare Research and Quality (AHRQ), which works closely with a consortium of public and private organizations. Over the past 10 years, the CAHPS consortium has established a set of principles to guide the development of CAHPS surveys and related tools. These include:

- Identifying and supporting the consumer's or patient's information needs
- Conducting thorough scientific testing
- Ensuring comparability of data
- Maintaining an open development process
- Keeping products in the public domain

Patients and consumers, quality monitors and regulators, purchasers, provider organizations, and health plans use CAHPS survey data to inform their purchasing or contracting decisions and to improve the quality of health care services.[4]

Medicare Health Outcomes Survey (HOS)

In 1998, the Medicare HOS was launched by the Centers for Medicare and Medicaid Services (CMS) in collaboration with NCQA. The first patient-reported outcomes measure to be used in Medicare managed care, the Medicare HOS program goal is to gather valid, reliable, and clinically meaningful health status data in the Medicare Advantage (MA) program for use in QI activities, P4P, program oversight, public reporting, and improving health.

All managed care organizations with MA contracts are required to participate in the Medicare HOS, which is used as part of the effectiveness of care component of the HEDIS data set. In addition to health outcomes measures, the HOS is used to collect the urinary incontinence in older adults, physical activity in older adults, fall risk management, and osteoporosis testing in older women HEDIS measures.[5]

Preventable Quality Indicators (PQIs): Part of a set of Agency for Healthcare Research and Quality (AHRQ) quality indicators developed by investigators at Stanford University and the University of California under a contract with AHRQ, PQIs use hospital inpatient discharge data to assess quality of health care delivery for "ambulatory care-sensitive conditions"; i.e., conditions for which good outpatient care may prevent the need for hospitalization or for which early intervention may prevent complications or more severe disease.

Examples of PQIs abound:

- Patients with diabetes may be hospitalized for diabetic complications if their conditions are not adequately monitored or if they do not receive the necessary patient education for appropriate self-management.

- Patients may be hospitalized for asthma if primary care providers fail to adhere to practice guidelines or to prescribe appropriate treatments.

- Patients with appendicitis who do not have ready access to surgical evaluation may experience delays in receiving needed care, which may result in a life-threatening condition—perforated appendicitis.[6]

Even though PQI indicators are based on hospital inpatient data, they provide insight into the community health care system and services outside the hospital setting. Health plans use PQIs to understand the quality of outpatient care and coordination among the provider groups within their networks. Purchasers use PQIs to rate the health plan's influence on their provider network.

Quality Comparisons

Several mechanisms exist for health plans to compare their quality scores on a national level. These comparisons provide health plans with a mechanism to benchmark their results against comparable organizations.

Quality Compass®: NQCA publishes the Quality Compass, which includes HEDIS results and percentile rankings for all U.S. health plans that submit HEDIS rates. An interactive, web-based tool, the updated Quality Compass is available in the fall of each year.[1]

NCQA Rankings: NCQA ranks the nation's private, Medicare, and Medicaid health insurance plans on the basis their combined HEDIS, CAHPS, and NCQA accreditation standards scores, using a weighted ranking methodology. At present, only managed care organizations (MCOs) are included in the ranking; however, NCQA is working on a method to apply the ranking to preferred provider organizations (PPOs).

NCQA rankings are published in *Consumer Reports* online in early October for commercial health plans and in November of 2010 for Medicare and Medicaid plans. This information was formerly printed in *U.S. News and World Report*.[7]

STAR Ratings: Based on a combination of HEDIS, CAHPS, Medicare HOS, and oversight monitoring metrics, STAR ratings are used by CMS to compare MA health plans. STAR ratings provide an overview of MA health plan performance in five categories[8]:

- Access and Service—how well the health plan provides its members with access to needed care and with good customer service.

- Qualified Providers—health plan activities that ensure each doctor is licensed and trained to practice medicine and that the health plan's members are happy with their doctors.

- Staying Healthy—health plan activities that help people maintain good health and avoid illness.

- Getting Better—health plan activities that help people recover from illness.
- Living with Illness—health plan activities that help people manage chronic illness.

Plans with MCO and health plan accreditation are eligible to receive up to five stars in each of the star rating categories; plans with PPO accreditation are eligible to receive up to three stars in the Access and Service and Qualified Providers categories.

Risk Adjustment and Severity Indexing: Health status risk-adjustment/severity-indexing models were designed as a way to account for illness burden when evaluating health outcomes across a population. Initially used as a tool for gauging hospital payment and for assessing hospital performance, today risk adjustment is commonly used in health plan capitation calculations and in measuring and reporting on health care provider performance.[9]

These models are often used to design programs that provide greater premium dollars to a health plan and/or a greater payment from the health plan to the contracted provider for members identified as higher risk, and lower compensation for members identified as lower risk. Health status risk models can improve the accuracy of capitation development for very large populations in which, hypothetically, the risks are balanced among sicker patients and less-sick patients.[10]

Cost and Quality Comparisons: Several organizations have been exploring the relationship of quality and cost to more accurately enable fair comparisons of health plans, hospitals, physicians, and other health care providers. Episode-based, population-based, and combined approaches are commercially available to evaluate performance. For example, 3M Health Information Systems has analyzed reporting of potentially preventable readmissions (PPR)[11] by several states and recently introduced a methodology for reporting potentially preventable admissions (PPA). This approach has approximately a 70 percent overlap with the AHRQ Ambulatory Care Sensitive Conditions (ACSC),[12] depending on the methodology implemented.

Beginning in 2011 for commercial and Medicare plans, NCQA will utilize a new plan all-cause readmission measure to track hospital readmissions from a post-hospital care perspective. NCQA has also designed an approach using relative resource use (RRU) measures that indicate how intensively health plans use health care resources (e.g., physician visits, hospital stays). Used in tandem with HEDIS quality measures results, RRU measures will make it possible to consider health plans influence on resource use, unit prices and quality.[1, 13] Such approaches allow for objective performance comparisons based on both quality and cost measures.

Paying for Performance (P4P)

Providing payment to improve quality performance is not a new concept. Parents all over the world have entered into P4P arrangements to improve school grades or encourage timely completion of chores. Health plans use P4P arrangements to reward providers for meeting pre-established quality and efficiency targets. Some arrangements include disincentives, wherein a portion of the provider's payment is withheld and released only if the targets are reached. Employers and government agencies that purchase health care insurance are also entering the P4P arena by establishing quality-related incentives for health plans to earn.

With continued growth in medical cost trends, chronic care conditions, health care utilization, and consumer demands, linking provider payments to QI is an alternative to "business as usual"—i.e., straight capitated payment arrangements (which pay for care whether or not the individual gets any services) and fee-for-service arrangements (which pay for every service regardless of the health outcome achieved). P4P incentives are designed to align financial rewards with improved outcomes.[14]

P4P Program Design

There are three key elements to the design of a P4P program: 1) the metrics used to measure quality; 2) the type and amount of reward; and 3) the timing of measurement and reward. Ideally, the program measures should be based on sound clinical principles and, where possible, broadly accepted among program participants. Additionally, the program should not create undue administrative burdens for the participant or the entity administering it. The data needed to calculate performance should be accessible through existing or reasonably enhanced systems. For this reason, metrics based on HEDIS measures are often chosen.

The four basic P4P program designs include bonuses, withholds, adjustable fee schedules, and quality grants.

1. Bonus programs provide participants with additional monies at the end of the measurement period, based on their performance. In general, bonus programs are easier to implement (i.e., contract changes are unnecessary) and more favored by participants (i.e., they represent additional reimbursement).

2. Withhold-based programs involve a portion of the participant's reimbursement being held back and returned if the performance target is met. Withhold programs are less attractive to participants because a portion of their baseline payment is at risk. These programs usually must be written in the participant's contract.[15]

3. Adjustable fee schedule programs provide the participant with a higher reimbursement schedule if quality targets are met. If the participant subsequently falls below the quality threshold, the reimbursement rates drop for the next period.

4. Quality grants are one-time payments by the health plan or the purchaser for a quality project or initiative.[15]

The amount of the reward associated with each P4P program varies from nominal to significant. Although there is no single formula, experts agree that to achieve meaningful results the amount should be sufficient to make it worth the participant's while to change behavior and processes.[15]

The measurement-payout cycle should strike a balance between the administrative work needed to collect and analyze program data and the desire to provide results and rewards in a timely manner. Shorter cycles give the participant frequent feedback to fuel behavior change and provide a closer link between the behavior and the reward. In programs requiring a full year of data collection followed by a three- to six-month period for data analysis, the participant is already six months into the next measurement cycle before receiving any feedback on performance. Despite the time lag, this approach results in more complete data and thus a more accurate reflection of actual performance.

Incentives for Providers

The most prevalent P4P programs are those that provide incentives to physicians for *a combination of provider and member* performance on national quality measures. Most commonly implemented by health plans for their commercial, Medicaid, and Medicare members, physician P4P programs are also offered by some state Medicaid agencies. CMS has several demonstration programs in place that target physician and member performance. Hospital P4P programs are less common. In effect, most hospital programs currently reward the facility for collecting and reporting data.[15,16,17]

Incentives for Health Plans

P4P programs that reward health plans for performance on quality measures exist mainly in the commercial and Medicaid markets. Employer groups offer health plans incentives to improve quality outcomes on their insured employees based on a percentage of premium or a percentage of administrative fees. State Medicaid agencies use the same strategies to incent Medicaid health plans to improve health outcomes for the Medicaid populations they serve. CMS currently collects and publishes quality data on MA health plans and, beginning in 2012, will use those data to determine the per-member-per-month fee paid to the health plan.[18]

Incentives for Members

Another P4P trend is the practice of providing a financial incentive or other reward to individuals for their participation in health and wellness programs. Primarily found in the commercial market, member incentives vary from movie tickets and gym membership discounts to gift cards and bonus payments. The practice of incenting health plan members has not gained as much traction in the Medicaid and Medicare space, where politics limits the use of tax-payer funded dollars.

Does P4P work?

Several studies have looked at the effectiveness of P4P in improving quality and health outcomes. Not surprisingly, the experience is mixed.[19,20,21,22] Some evidence supports improvement in quality and reduction of costs as a result of P4P, and an equal amount of evidence shows no traceable impact.[19,20] Some reports identify unintended consequences of P4P programs, including the avoidance of high-risk patients whose outcomes may negatively impact quality scores.[20] The wide variation in program design and paucity of rigorous evaluation make it difficult to link P4P programs with changes in provider performance.[21]

Future of Health Plan Quality

Several trends and external factors will influence the evolution of quality at the health plan level.

Data Exchange

Probably the strongest future influence will be the increasing availability of and access to health care data. The federal government has recognized the importance of expanding access and improving the quality of health care data for the purpose of research on comparative effectiveness and the need for investment in data infrastructure.[23]

Access to high-quality data is critical to innovation, QI, and increased efficiency in health care. The federal government has signaled that expanding access to and improving the quality of health care data for the purpose of research is a priority. In its report to Congress, the Federal Coordinating Council for Comparative Effectiveness Research emphasized the need for investment in data infrastructure and access to support comparative effectiveness research.[24] The Office of the National Coordinator for Health Information Technology included the promotion of a nationwide health information technology infrastructure to facilitate health and clinical research as part of its mission. The importance of data access was also underscored by the American College of Physicians' position paper, *Achieving a High-Performance Health Care System.*[25]

Developed in response to President Obama's Open Government Directive,[23] the April 2010 release of the Department of Health and Human Services' open government strategy was a major step forward in expanding health data access.

Health Information Exchanges (HIEs) allow providers to share data electronically across different information systems without losing the meaning of the information. Functioning HIEs provide health care workers and consumers with access to clinical data to facilitate the provision of safe, timely, efficient, and effective health care services. HIEs also enable health plans and other entities to analyze health care outcomes at the population level. The recent influx of federal dollars for health information technology has greatly increased interest in establishing HIEs.[26]

The challenges associated with implementing HIEs are numerous. A central issue is governance and responsibility for the data sets exchanged through the service. Who is responsible for the accuracy of the information? Who ensures that data errors are corrected? Who controls access to the data? Another problematic element is liability. Is a practitioner responsible for every piece of information (e.g., abnormal lab result) available through the HIE?

Another very basic hurdle for HIEs is the health system's relative inability to deliver information from multiple sources in a usable format. Currently, data elements as simple as an ICD.9 diagnosis code on a claim record may be stored on one system as a three-character-decimal point-two character field and in another system as a character field with no decimal point. One system may recognize leading zeroes, while another does not.

Once the barriers are overcome, HIEs will be invaluable to health plans, providers, and members alike. Access to HIE data will improve the health plan's ability to analyze population-based data, measure outcomes related to QI activities, and structure/design future quality initiatives. Access to a complete set of current health care data on a member will enhance the clinical care provider's ability to deliver appropriate, high-quality care that will, in turn, improve member outcomes. By reducing unnecessary and duplicative studies and medications that may translate into avoidable initial admissions or readmissions, HIEs stand to benefit the entire health care system.

Integration of Behavioral Health, Physical Health and Pharmacy: Another bump on the road to data sharing is the inability to integrate and share certain physical health, behavioral health, and pharmacy data across provider types. Federal HIPAA regulations permit the sharing of protected health information (PHI) for the purpose of treatment and health care operations, which include most health plan quality initiatives. Many states, however, have laws specific to the ability to share what is sometimes referred to as "extra-sensitive PHI," i.e., PHI related to behavioral health conditions and HIV.[27] In general, these regulations prevent health plans from sharing information pertaining to these conditions among providers.

The practical applications of these regulations are vast. For example, a health plan's quality program may allow network clinicians and emergency rooms to access a list of a member's medications filled through the plan's pharmacy benefit. Regulations requiring that extra-sensitive PHI and medications related to behavioral health and HIV be redacted from the list severely limit the usefulness of the information.

HIPAA 5010 and ICD.10: The planned implementation of HIPAA 5010 transactions and the introduction of ICD.10 diagnosis codes will further impact the ability of health plans to leverage data for quality initiatives. Developed by the World Health Organization, the ICD.10 diagnostic coding system is used almost everywhere in the world except the U.S. With more than 64,000 codes, the ICD.10 code set tracks more diagnoses at greater levels of specificity than the ICD.9 system currently used in the U.S. ICD.10 codes contain three to seven characters with several number/letter combinations, compared to the three- to five-character ICD.9 system, which only uses letters as an option for the first character.[28]

Although many believe the specificity afforded by the ICD.10 system will greatly enhance the level of reporting and accuracy of reimbursement,[29] the need to track and report data using the same coding scheme as the rest of the world is the main impetus behind HIPAA 5010 requirements. The current schedule called for health care organizations to be prepared to perform HIPAA 5010-compliant electronic health care transactions on January 1, 2012. The transition to ICD.10 codes for Medicare claim submission is planned for 2013 and other payers are expected to follow suit.

Implementing the system changes necessary to accomplish these transitions will create multiple challenges. Health plan information systems will need to remediate diagnosis fields and prepare to accept and integrate data using both formats during the cross-over. Complex crosswalks will be needed to allow the health plans to pull data for comparison over different time periods. For example, the code set to identify members who received a hip replacement due to a fracture will be different dramatically from pre- to post-ICD.10 implementation.

Increasing Transparency

Another trend with implications for the future of health plan quality is the move toward increased transparency. Purchasers and consumers are insisting on full disclosure of cost and quality metrics to enable them to make informed choices about the health care services they receive.

Initiatives are under way at the state and federal level to promote transparency. The federal government launched www.healthcare.gov to provide access to quality comparisons for hospital, home health, nursing home, and dialysis providers. Users of the site can also search for and compare health insurance options.[30] Some states (e.g., Wisconsin) have introduced their own laws mandating disclosure of price and quality information.[31]

Despite this push, experts agree that there are limitations to consumers' ability to use the information to guide their health care decisions. Price alone is not a barometer of quality. Current quality information is inadequate at best and is often unavailable or not accessed during the decision-making process. Additionally, most health care decisions are made during emergency or highly emotional situations. Increased transparency, alone, will not promote value-based decisions by health care consumers; however, the push for increased transparency will continue into the future.[32]

Evolving Communication Channels

Changes in how we communicate with each other will have a profound impact on the design of future health plan quality initiatives. Communication is becoming ever more mobile, with an emphasis on short exchanges and immediate gratification. Health plans that traditionally have promoted quality-related health care behaviors through mail and telephone must begin to transition to electronic communication channels such as email, text-messaging and mobile-device applications.

Text Messaging

Clearly the communication channel of choice for the younger generation, text messaging is the most widely used mobile phone service.[33] As mobile phones surpass land lines for personal use, texting is likely to become the primary mechanism for communication.

Using text messages to promote quality initiatives poses some challenges. First and foremost, the health plan's information system needs a mechanism to distinguish between mobile phone numbers and land lines. For maximum impact, the content needs to be contained in a single message, limiting the text to 160 characters.

Additionally, a health plan must walk the tightrope of PHI disclosure. PHI may be included in telephone and mail communications because mechanisms exist to validate the recipient. Because there is no such mechanism for text messages, a health plan must either convince a member to sign up to receive text messages related to his or her health care or create generic messages without a link between the recipient and a specific health condition.

On the plus side, text messages tend to be cheaper than telephone outreach or mailed communications. And, unlike automated phone calls and letters, receivers of texts rarely ignore the message.

Email

Growing in popularity, email is an inexpensive alternative to phone and mail communication as well as a "green" approach to communicating larger amounts of information. The two main challenges to email as a communication channel for quality initiatives are access to email addresses and Internet security. Historically, health plans' information systems have not captured member email addresses in a usable field. Since email messages sent out over the public Internet are not considered secure enough to transmit PHI, health plans need to establish secure email behind a health plan fire wall.

An "App for That"

Mobile applications will be the next frontier in health care quality.[34] The emergence of the mobile health or "mHealth" field was jump started by provisions in two pieces of federal legislation; 1) the broadband plan requirements in the American Recovery and Reinvestment Act (ARRA), and 2) the planned addition of 45 million currently uninsured Americans to the health care system under the Patient Protection and Affordable Care Act. ARRA requires the Federal Communications Commission (FCC) to create a national broadband plan that will create jobs and businesses and improve health care. Adding this stimulus to an industry that desperately needs to embrace automation to survive amidst the shortage of primary care providers and an impending tidal wave of uninsured will spark innovative uses for mobile health applications.[35]

Mobile devices are already the communication tool of choice for the under 40 set, with a significant presence in older age groups as well. For demographic subgroups with high transiency (e.g., Medicaid benficiaries), mobile devices are often the only means of communication. Sixty-four percent of physicians already use a smartphone device, and that number is projected to reach 81 percent in 2012.[36] Applications that help people manage their diabetes, monitor respiratory flows for asthma, retrieve health histories ,and connect patients and providers are emerging daily. Health plans may benefit from these innovations by linking to applications that address the needs of their at-risk populations.

Performance-Based Contracting

Directly tied to the value-based purchasing movement, performance-based contracts seek to align cost efficiency and quality parameters into an arrangement that benefits both the payer and the provider. More sophisticated than traditional P4P programs, performance-based contracts contain a blend of quality outcome measures, utilization expectations, and cost thresholds. In return for greater latitude in service delivery, the provider agrees to meet the contract parameters. If the parameters are not met, the provider's reimbursement level drops for the next measurement cycle.

A lighter version of the financial risk arrangements prevalent in health care in the 1990s, performance-based contracting is seen by some as a path forward toward provider-based accountable care organizations (ACOs).[37,38] For health plans, performance-based contracts are a mechanism to balance cost and quality while exploring their role in the emerging ACO frontier.

Making Every Member Contact Count

A key element of success for any business is the ability to sell products and services *in addition* to the item originally sought by the customer. Combining this approach with data-fed algorithms produces the Jiffy Lube experience. Jiffy Lube has figured out how to *make every contact count*. When a customer brings a car to Jiffy Lube for an oil change, Jiffy Lube associates access their information system, compare the car's previous service history with the manufacturer's recommendations, and present the customer with a list of additional services that are appropriate for the car. These optional services can be completed in about the same time as the originally planned oil change, and therefore create no additional inconvenience to the customer.[39] Health plans must engage a similar approach to make the most out of every contact with their members.

Closing Gaps in Care

Health plans have rich data sets on the services and diagnoses of their members. One mechanism for making every member contact count is to turn those data sets into actionable information. Just as the Jiffy Lube attendant is presented with the evidence-based needs for the car, the physician should be prompted with a list of incomplete recommended health care services at the time he or she accesses the patient's record. Health plan information can be put into the hands of the provider at the point of service in one of two ways: feeding data directly to the physician's electronic medical record (EMR) or providing information to the office staff during an online eligibility check.

Improving Quality of Care for Chronic Conditions

Diabetes, heart disease, hypertension, asthma, chronic obstructive pulmonary disease, and serious mental illness, as well as combinations of these conditions, are some of the more common chronic conditions that drive health care costs. The following statistics are sobering;

- 45 percent of the U.S. population (120 million people) have one chronic medical condition.[40]
- 50 percent of these individuals (60 million people) have multiple chronic conditions.[40]
- 83 percent of Medicare beneficiaries have one or more chronic medical conditions.[41]
- 23 percent of Medicare beneficiaries have five or more chronic medical conditions.[41]
- By 2015;
  - An estimated 150 million Americans will have at least one chronic medical condition.[40]
  - Health care spending is expected to reach $4.0 trillion and amount to 20 percent of the GDP.[42]

For decades, payers, providers, federal and state governments, public health efforts, and others have attempted to control the impact of chronic conditions and the other drivers of rising health care cost. Several studies have demonstrated the need to completely redesign processes for transitions of care to improve quality and reduce inherent costs.[43-47] Studies also have demonstrated that, for coordination of care to be effective, *care coordinators must interact in person with the patients* and *collaborate closely with patients' physicians* to reasonably improve outcomes.[48-51]

Rebalancing the Specialist Spend

As health plans seek more resources to fund their quality initiatives, one opportunity may be to reduce the percentage of the health care dollar that goes to specialty care. For decades, specialty physicians have seen their fees climb steadily while primary care physicians have seen only modest increases in some areas and decreases in others.

Payment rates and lifetime earning potential are a significant factor for medical students deciding between primary care and higher paying specialty care.[52] By some calculations, specialists earn twice what a primary care physician does, often with a less demanding schedule.[53] The looming shortage of primary care physicians threatens access to primary care at a time when the importance of primary care is being heralded as the backbone of preventive care and an avenue to lower health care costs.[54,55] It is no fluke that the other industrialized countries studied in comparison to the U.S. all spend far less (per capita and GDP) on health care, outperform us on quality, emphasize primary care, and use specialist care more judiciously.[56]

Recent federal legislation addresses payment issues through proposed increases to primary care payment rates for Medicare beneficiaries and provisions that will raise Medicaid payment rates to the Medicare level.[53,57] Since changes must be budget neutral, many expect the additional primary care dollars to come from fees currently paid to specialists. Challenged to follow suit, health plan payment changes may tie primary care increases to quality measures and use shared accountability contracts or capitation to control specialty costs.[58]

Several of these suggestions have been addressed through health care reform under the Affordable Care Act[59] or a realignment of financial incentives to promote coordinated care. Some examples include; the patient-centered medical home, bundled payments, ACOs, and reductions in Medicare inpatient payments to hospitals with higher than expected readmission rates beginning in 2013.

The Access, Cost/Efficiency, Quality Equation

The role of MCOs, whether they be health plans, integrated delivery systems, or other entities, is to provide their members with reliable access to high-quality care at the most cost-effective price point. Although conceptually simple, discerning and maintaining an optimal balance between access to the appropriate type and level of care that provides consistently high-quality outcomes at an acceptable cost is a highly complex exercise. This will become obvious as we explore the core characteristics of each component.

The criteria for "access to care" is generally set by state regulations requiring a minimum number of providers in a given specialty to be available to a member within a set distance from his or her residence. These criteria may vary by state, population density in different geographic regions, and availability of highly specialized providers or facilities (e.g., pediatric neuro-ophthalmology, medical genetics, or regional children's hospitals). Other factors influencing access to care include a provider's after hours availability and whether open scheduling is offered by the practice. Although the latter is not a regulatory requirement, both can be patient satisfiers and assist in reducing inappropriate ER visits.

The "cost/efficiency" component of the equation is driven by the combination of unit cost or the amount paid for a service and utilization or the frequency with which that service is utilized.   Depending on the product (i.e., Medicare, commercial [e.g., Indemnity, PPO, HMO], or Medicaid), the services needed, availability of those services, market share, region of the country, cost, and/or efficiency may vary considerably even within a single federal program as reported in the Dartmouth Atlas of Health Care for Medicare.[60]

Financial outcome measures consisting of the unit cost and utilization rate are frequently measured by medical cost trend or medical loss or medical cost ratios. These calculations are generally available at the book of business, product, facility, practice, or individual provider level. Because age, gender, and medical conditions factor into financial outcomes, several methods are used to adjust for the severity of illness within given populations. The addition of risk adjustment/ severity indexing improves the accuracy of comparative performance.[61]

Efficiency calculations are further affected by contracting issues and capacity. A primary care provider (PCP) who is part of a large university contract is expected by that arrangement to refer to specialists within that system. The PCP and his or her department may be penalized if the hospital and/or specialist contract is not cost-effective. Likewise, the most efficient orthopedic provider in a given network might be a solo practitioner who manages his or her own post-operative joint replacement anticoagulation and whose patients receive outpatient rehabilitation rather than a university practice that admits all joint replacement patients to an acute rehabilitation facility for management of post-operative needs. Despite the solo practitioner's superior efficiency, his capacity to manage referrals for the network is limited. However, his superior performance on quality and efficiency may command higher reimbursement through performance-based contracting.

Given the broad acceptance of standard quality measures for comparing performance on quality measures, quality is uniquely positioned to drive the agenda on reforming our health care system. Quality also provides the impetus for a culture that never settles for the status quo. It presses us to strive for continuous improvement across clinical, administrative, and customer service measures to deliver safe, caring, efficient, customer-focused, outcome-driven care. When coupled with efficiency, the intersection of quality and efficiency becomes the barometer for assessing our progress in pursuit of this more effective and equitable approach to health care.

An important goal for health plans is to redesign their traditional reimbursement models to permit plans, providers, and hospital systems to align their incentives around key measures of quality and efficiency. This will enable health plans to promote true partnerships in the management of populations. In such a collaborative environment, there will be greater potential for consistent, sustainable improvement in quality, efficiency, and access. This, in turn, will deliver services safely, responsibly, and affordably.

Case Study[51]

Introduction

Mercy Health System, a member of Catholic Health East, serves southeastern Pennsylvania and Philadelphia through four acute care hospitals, community and home care services, and affiliated physician practices. The system is one of two corporate parents of Keystone Mercy Health Plan (KMHP), a Medicaid MCO serving more than 300,000 Medicaid recipients in the greater Philadelphia region. In 2008, the organizations launched a pilot project to improve the quality and efficiency of care and services delivered to their shared population. The initiative targeted three components of the system: 1) to make the primary care practice a medical home for patients, 2) to ensure that transitions from hospital to community reconnected the patients with their medical homes, and 3) to leverage community resources to create a community health team to supplement the efforts of the provider and payer.

Methods

Embedding a Care Coordinator in a Primary Care Practice: Beginning in November 2008, a care coordinator—a social worker certified in case management—began working one day per week. The position, funded by KMHP, gradually expanded to five days per week. In addition to addressing social barriers to care (e.g., transportation and public utilities issues), the coordinator received specialized training to coach patients in medication adherence and other aspects of self-care. Using the health plan's data, she provided the practice with a more complete picture of each patient seen (e.g., whether prescriptions were filled, whether the patient had any recent hospital or emergency department admissions, whether care was rendered by other providers).

Removing Barriers to Care: Key to the success of the on-site coordinator was her ability to identify and close gaps in care. By comparing combined patient data with algorithms representing recommended care, we identified a 45- year-old woman needing a mammogram, a diabetic who missed his yearly retinal exam, and an asthmatic child who filled a prescription for a rescue inhaler but not a controller and was behind on his immunizations.

Care coordinators at KMHP were made aware of clinical information generally not available to them (e.g., spirometer results, x-ray reports on a member with chronic obstructive pulmonary disease). NaviNet—Keystone Mercy's provider portal used by Mercy Health System caregivers to verify eligibility and make referrals—was programmed to note care gaps in patient summaries and to generate a pop-up alert when eligibility checks were run.

The physical presence of an on-site coordinator positively impacted the outcomes. Viewed as a member of the clinical team as well as a health plan liaison, she gained a level of rapport with members that is not possible from phone conversations. More importantly, she was able to influence members and engage them as active participants in the management of their health.

Transition from Hospital to Ambulatory Care. Beginning in May 2009, KMHP provided a full-time registered nurse at Mercy Fitzgerald Hospital to manage transitions of care for members. Her focus was to educate members and reduce unnecessary emergency department visits by addressing non-medical barriers to care, assisting with housing, making referrals to food pantries, and arranging for skills training. Importantly, she reconnected members with their medical homes by making follow-up appointments with their PCPs or specialists and forwarding discharge instructions. She also enlisted the support of the plan's case managers to coordinate these services as needed.

Leveraging Community Resources. Relationships with community partners, such as The Enterprise Center Community Development Corporation in West Philadelphia, were enhanced by providing the existing outreach team with additional training. Outreach team members visit Keystone Mercy members who live in their zip codes following a hospital discharge. The meetings include discussions regarding doctor follow-up; medications; assessing the member's comfort level with self-care; and, if needed, reconnection of the member to the care management team at KMHP. Community outreach also is enlisted when a member cannot be reached by phone.

Results

179 KMHP members who received enhanced care coordination at the primary care practice at Mercy Fitzgerald hospital were tracked. From 2008 to 2009, the hospital admission rate per 1000 members per year dropped 17 percent and the average length of stay fell 37 percent for a 48 percent decrease in inpatient days per 1,000 members. Hospital days per admission declined from 4.3 days to 2.7 days. The 30-day readmission rate for this high-risk group fell from 30 percent before the pilot began to 7 percent afterward. In contrast, the 30-day readmission rate for members not managed in the pilot program was 16 percent in 2008 and 13 percent in 2009. Despite the drop in total hospitalizations, the hospital benefited because the members engaged in the pilot program were more likely to choose that hospital when they required acute care.

When asked by the transition care coordinator why they chose to visit the emergency department at Mercy Fitzgerald, 36 percent reported coming because they didn't know what else to do. Another 20 percent said they came because their PCP was unavailable. Statistical analysis of the emergency department diagnostic codes for these patients, employing a methodology developed by New York Presbyterian Hospital, suggests that more than half of these visits were for non-emergent care and might have been prevented with proper ambulatory management.

Conclusion

Health plans are uniquely positioned to lead the transformation of the U.S. health care system by leveraging their comprehensive data, population management perspective, and ability to appropriately align incentives to compensate for measureable improvements in quality and cost outcomes. Such change, however, will require that health plans, providers, and plan members engage in a collaborative effort to improve the health of entire populations. Plans will contribute the information and analysis to determine which interventions yield the desired results. Providers will utilize this information to improve their efficiency, drive quality, and share in the rewards of these efforts. Members will be incentivized to opt for healthier behaviors that improve health and reduce the overall cost of care or be required to bear increasing financial responsibility for their choices. It is only by redesigning our system to deliver improved quality at a lower cost and sharing the dividends of these collaborative efforts that we will be able to join our rightful place along side of the rest of the industrialized world in solving the health care challenges of the future.

References

1. *What is HEDIS?* National Committee for Quality Assurance. http://www.ncqa.org/tabid/187/default.aspx. Accessed 3/14/2011.

2. *Accreditation.* National Committee for Quality Assurance. http://www.ncqa.org/tabid/66/Default.aspx. Accessed 3/14/2011.

3. *General Questions about URAC Accreditation.* URAC. http://www.urac.org/healthcare/accreditation/. Accessed 3/14/2011.

4. *CAHPS Overview.* Agency for Healthcare Research and Quality. http://www.cahps.ahrq.gov/About-CAHPS.aspx. Updated 12/15/2008. Accessed 3/14/2011.

5. *Health Outcomes Survey (HOS) Overview.* Centers for Medicare and Medicaid Services. https://www.cms.gov/hos/. Accessed 3/14/2011.

6. *Prevention Quality Indicators.* Agency for Healthcare Quality Research. http://www.qualityindicators.ahrq.gov/modules/pqi_overview.aspx. Accessed 3/14/11.

7. *Health Insurance Plan Rankings.* National Committee for Quality Assurance. http://www.ncqa.org/tabid/506/Default.aspx. Accessed 3/14/2011.

8. The Kaiser Family Foundation. *What's in the Stars? Quality Ratings of Medicare Advantage Plans, 2010.* December, 2009. http://www.kff.org/medicare/upload/8025.pdf. Accessed 3/14/2011.

9. Haislmaier E. *State Health Care Reform: A Brief Guide to Risk Adjustment in Consumer-Driven Health Insurance Markets*, Washington, DC: The Heritage Foundation, July 28, 2008.

10. *Disease Management: A New Paradigm for Managed Care. February 2, 2010.* Hospitals and Doctors. http://hospitals-doctors.com/lenyeg/archive/a9.html. Accessed 3/14/2011.

11. Goldfield NI, McCullough EC, Hughes JS, *et al.* Identifying Potentially Preventable Readmissions. *Health Care Financing Review* 30(1):75-91, Fall 2008.

12. Agency for Healthcare Research and Quality. *Refinement of the HCUP Quality Indicators.* Rockville, MD: U.S. Department of Health and Human Services. http://www.ahrq.gov/clinic/epcsums/hcuptab2.htm. Accessed 3/14/2011.

13. The State of Health Care Quality 2010. National Committee for Quality Assurance. http://www.ncqa.org/tabid/836/Default.aspx. Accessed 3/14/2011.

14. Baker G, Haughton J, Mongroo P. Pay for Performance Incentive Programs in Healthcare: Market Dynamics and Business Process. The Leapfrog Group. 2003. http://www.leapfroggroup.org/media/file/Leapfrog-Pay_for_Performance_Briefing.pdf. Accessed 2/9/11.

15. *Medicaid Pay for Performance Programs Slow to Gain Traction.* 2007. University HealthSystem Consortium. http://www.naph.org/Publications/medicaidpayforperformanceprogramsslowtogaintraction.aspx?FT=.pdf. Accessed 2/9/2011.

16. Felt-Lisk S, Gimm G, Peterson S. Making P4P Work in Medicaid. *Health Affairs*, 26(4):516-27, July-Aug. 2007.

17. Campion F X. Medicare's P4P Program Aims to Improve Care. *Managed Healthcare Executive*, March 1, 2009.

18. Appleby J. Administration Unexpectedly Expands Bonus Payments for Medicare Advantage Plans. *Kaiser Health News*, Nov. 16, 2010. http://www.kaiserhealthnews.org/Stories/2010/November/16/Medicare-Advantage-bonuses.aspx. Accessed 3/14/2011.

19. *Pay for Performance*. Mathematica. December 2008. http://www.mass.gov/eohhs/docs/dhcfp/pc/2009-02-13-pay-for-performance-c3.pdf. Accessed 3/14/2011.

20. Rosenthal MB, Frank RG. What is the Empirical Basis for Paying for Quality in Health Care? *Medical Care Research and Review*, 63(2):135-57, Apr. 2006.

21. Felt-Lisk S, Fleming C, Natzke B, Shapiro R. Using Payment Incentives to Improve Care for the Chronically Ill in Medicare: First-Year Implementation of the Medicare Care Management Performance Demonstration (MCMP). Princeton, NJ: Mathematica Policy Research, Inc., March 4, 2009.

22. Tanenbaum SJ. Pay for Performance in Medicare: Evidentiary Irony and the Politics of Value. *Journal of Health Politics, Policy and Law*, 34(5):717-46 , Oct. 2009.

23. Conway PH, VanLare JM. Improving Access to Health Care Data—The Open Government Strategy. *JAMA*, 304(9):1007-8, Sept. 1, 2010.

24. Federal Coordinating Council for Comparative Effectiveness Research. *Report to the President and Congress*. Washington, DC: U.S. Department of Health and Human Services, June 2009. http://www.hhs.gov/recovery/programs/cer/cerannualrpt.pdf. Accessed 3/1/2011.

25. "Achieving a High-Performance Health Care System with Universal Access: What the United States Can Learn from Other Countries." Position Paper, American College of Physicians. *Ann Int Med*, 148(1):55-75. http://www.annals.org/content/148/1/55.full.

26. *Health Care IT Market for Continued Growth over Next Five Years: Compass Intelligence.* June 16, 2010. http://www.news-medical.net/news/20100616/Health-Care-IT-market-set-for-continued-growth-over-next-five-years-Compass-Intelligence.aspx. Accessed 2/13/2011.

27. Gordon EL. Release of Behavioral Health, Developmental Disabilities, HIV, and Substance Abuse Information: Guidelines for Legal Compliance. Matthew Bender & Company, Inc. 2000. http://www.google.com/url?q=http://www.uhlaw.com/files/Publication/f3d6d48a-aa2b-4ed5-980e-0185eabe5f28/Presentation/PublicationAttachment/84aa8b23-8689-4b96-8dae-05e65f2316f5/Lynn%2520Gordon%2520Health%2520Care%2520Law%2520Monthly.pdf&sa=U&ei=Ccl_Tez-2F6uF0QGbz_T1CA&ved=0CBgQFjAD&usg=AFQjCNElWCBA14ny-BljN0-Z63J6WWNdTw. Accessed 3/14/2011.

28. American Medical Association. Preparing for the ICD-10 Code Set: October 1, 2013 Compliance Date. June 2, 2010. http://www.ama-assn.org/ama1/pub/upload/mm/399/icd10-icd9-differences-fact-sheet.pdf. Accessed 3/14/2011.

29. *Exploring the Benefits of ICD-10*. ICD-10 Taskforce Bulletin. July 2010.Health Information Communication Alliance. http://www.nchica.org/hipaaresources/ICD-10/JulyBulletin.pdf. Accessed 3/14/2011.

30. Montalbano E. White House Launches Healthcare Transparency Site. *Information Week*, July 1, 2010. http://www.informationweek.com/news/government/policy/showArticle.jhtml?articleID=225702091. Accessed 2/12/2011.

31. Dolan M. Wisconsin's health care transparency law comes into effect. January 7, 2011. http://blogs.ipro.org/abouthealthtransparency/2011/01/07/wisconsins-health-care-transparency-law-comes-into-effect/. Accessed 2/12/2011.

32. Collins SR, Davis K. Transparency in Health Care: The Time Has Come. The Commonwealth Fund, March 15, 2006. Accessed 2/12/2011.

33. *Facts and Figures: Mobile Text Messaging Usage in the U.S.* August 5, 2009. Mosio: Mobile Reference + Text Messaging. http://www.textalibrarian.com/mobileref/facts-and-figures-mobile-usage-and-text-messaging-in-the-u-s/. Accessed 3/14/2011.

34. Dolan B. *Google Health: The Future of Healthcare Is Mobile.* May 8, 2009. http://mobihealthnews.com/2155/google-health-the-future-of-healthcare-is-mobile/. Accessed 2/13/2011.

35. Kleinberg K. *Mobile Healthcare: Applications, Vendors and Adoption.* Gartner Healthcare. 2002. http://www.himss.org/content/files/proceedings/2003/Sessions/session102_slides.pdf. Accessed 2/22/2011.

36. *The Future of Wireless in Healthcare – Powering the Applications for 21st Century Care.* Healthcare IT News. November 2010. http://www.healthcareitnews.com/sites/healthcareitnews.com/files/resource-media/pdf/sprint_full_report_12.08.10.pdf . Accessed 2/13/2011.

37. Florian M. Provider payment reform: An accountable care approach to alignment of health care goals and incentives. *Health Watch*, 64:52-4, September 2010.. http://www.soa.org/library/newsletters/health-watch-newsletter/2010/september/hsn-2010-iss64-florian.pdf. Accessed February 20, 2011.

38. Draper DA, Gold MR. Provider Risk Sharing in Medicaid Managed Care Plans. *Health Affairs,* 22(3):159-67, May-June 2003.

39. Porritt C. *The Basics of Business–A Top-Down Approach to Succeeding in Business.* 4th ed. Porritt Publishing, 2006, pp. 7-9.

40. Wu S, Green A. *Projection of chronic illness prevalence and cost inflation.* Santa Monica, CA: RAND Health, October 2000.

41. Anderson GF. Medicare and chronic conditions. *NEJM*, 353(3):305-9, July 21, 2005.

42. Centers for Medicare & Medicaid Services. Office of the Actuary, National Health Statistics Group. *National health expenditures aggregate, per capita, percent distribution and annual percent change by source of funds: calendar years 1960-2005.* http://www.cms.gov/NationalHealthExpendData/downloads/tables.pdf. Accessed 3/14/2011.

43. Naylor M, Brooten D, Jones R, *et al.* Comprehensive discharge planning for the hospitalized elderly: a randomized clinical trial. *Ann Intern Med*, 120(12):999-1006, June 15, 1994.

44. Naylor M, Brooten D, Campbell, R, *et al.* Comprehensive discharge planning and home follow-up of hospitalized elders: a randomized clinical trial. *JAMA*, 281(7):613-20 Feb. 17, 1999;.

45. Naylor M, Brooten DA, Campbell, RL, *et al.* Transitional care of older adults hospitalized with heart failure: a randomized, controlled trial. *J Am Geriatr Soc*, 52(5):675-684, May 2004.

46. Coleman E, Parry C, Chalmers S, Min S. The Care Transitions Intervention: Results of a randomized controlled trial. *Arch Intern Med*, 166(17):1822-8, Sept. 25, 2006.

47. Jack BW, Chetty VK, Anthony D, *et al*. A reengineered hospital discharge program to decrease rehospitalization: a randomized trial. *Ann Intern Med*, 150(3):178-87, Feb 3, 2009.

48. Peikes D, Chen A, Schore J, Brown R. Effects of care coordination on hospitalization, quality of care, and health care expenditures among Medicare beneficiaries: 15 randomized trials. *JAMA*, 301(6):603-18, Feb. 11, 2009.

49. Sochalski J, Jaarsma T, Krumholz HM, *et al*. What works in chronic care management: the case of heart failure. *Health Affairs,* (Millwood). 28(1):179-189, Jan.-Feb. 2009.

50. Ayanian, JZ. The elusive quest for quality and cost savings in the Medicare program. *JAMA*, 301(6):668-70, Feb. 11, 2009.

51. Bielaszka-KuVernay C. Improving the coordination of care for Medicaid beneficiaries in Pennsylvania. *Health Affairs,* 30(3):426-30, Mar. 2011.

52. Hauer KE, Durning SN, Kernan WJ; *et al*. Factors associated with medical students' career choices regarding internal medicine. *JAMA*, 300(10):1154-4, Sept. 10, 2008. http://jama.ama-assn.org/content/300/10/1154.full. Accessed February 20, 2011.

53. The Hastings Center. Narrowing the Pay Gap between Primary Care Physicians and Specialists. *Health Care Cost Monitor,* October 16, 2009. http://healthcarecostmonitor.thehastingscenter.org/wesleyboyd/narrowing-the-pay-gap-between-primary-care-physicians-and-specialists. Accessed February 20, 2011.

54. US Department of Health & Human Services. Fact Sheet: Creating Jobs and Increasing the Number of Primary Care Providers. http://www.healthreform.gov/newsroom/primarycareworkforce.html. Accessed February 20, 2011.

55. Seward ZM. Doctor shortage hurts a coverage-for-all plan. *Wall Street Journal,* July 25, 2007:B1. http://online.wsj.com/article/SB118532549004277031.html#. Accessed February 20, 2011.

56. "Achieving a High-Performance Health Care System with Universal Access: What the United States Can Learn from Other Countries," Position Paper, American College of Physicians. *Ann Int Med*, 148(1):55-75, Jan. 1, 2008. http://www.annals.org/content/148/1/55.full. Accessed 3/14/2011.

57. Arvantes J. CMS proposes rule to increase primary care payments. American Academy of Family Physicians, July 8, 2009. http://www.aafp.org/online/en/home/publications/news/news-now/government-medicine/20090708cms-cpt-rule.html. Accessed February 20, 2011.

58. DeMuro PR. Paying specialists and subspecialists on a capitated base. *Healthcare Financial Management,* July 1995. http://findarticles.com/p/articles/mi_m3257/is_n7_v49/ai_17383082/?tag=content;col1. Accessed February 20, 2011.

59. The Affordable Care Act: A Timeline. HealthCare.gov. http://www.healthcare.gov/law/timeline/index.html. Accessed 3/14/2011.

60. Fisher E, Goodman D, Skinner J, Bronner K. Health Care Spending, Quality and Outcomes. The Dartmouth Institute for Health Policy & Clinical Practice, February 27, 2009. http://www.dartmouthatlas.org/downloads/reports/Spending_Brief_022709.pdf. Accessed 3/14/2011.

61. Winkelman R, Mehmud S. A comparative analysis of claims-based tools for Health Risk Assessment. Society of Actuaries, April 20, 2007 http://www.soa.org/files/pdf/risk-assessmentc.pdf. Accessed 3/14/2011.

Chapter 9

Measuring Quality of Inpatient Care

By Adrianne Seiler, MD and Evan M. Benjamin, MD, FACP

Executive Summary

Measuring and improving inpatient quality is a complex endeavor requiring expertise from diverse stakeholders: from patients and the community to health care providers, hospital boards, and a multitude of public and private organizations. To be successful, we must first define quality and then select and execute the appropriate measurements to ensure safe and effective care that is free from harm. Providing high-quality inpatient care requires that the right data be collected, publicly reported, and acted upon in order to achieve the daunting but rewarding goal of improving hospital-based quality and safety.

Learning Objectives

1. Understand the methodologies for defining quality.
2. List the common quality indicators for hospitals and describe how they are measured.
3. Understand how safe care is identified and measured.
4. Discuss the implications for future remodeling of quality improvement efforts and the health care system.

Key Words: Harm, Hospital-Acquired Conditions, Inpatient Quality Indicators, Never Events, Patient Safety Indicators, Sentinel Events

Introduction

Although about 30 percent of personal health care expenditures in the United States go toward hospital care,[1] evidence suggests that there is a great deal of variation in the quality and outcomes of inpatient care. For this reason, a great deal of hard work and research has been focused on measuring and improving the quality of inpatient care in recent years.

To understand how the quality of inpatient care is measured, we must first understand what is meant by "quality" as it applies to the inpatient realm. Next, we will explore how and why we measure quality care and where the data come from. It will become evident that quality isn't just the practice of evidence-based care, but also the avoidance of harm. Many measures of inpatient health care quality, including measures documenting the patient experience, are being developed and utilized every day by organizations such as the National Quality Forum (NQF), The Joint Commission (JC), the Centers for Medicare and Medicaid (CMS), and the Leapfrog Group. Understanding the foundation of inpatient quality data will allow us to explore the potential uses of this valuable information for patient, providers, and payers.

Finally, we will discuss issues in quality measurement such as public reporting and future directions in health care redesign. We hope that this chapter will give the reader a good foundation for understanding how and why we measure and report on inpatient quality as well as some of the difficulties that confront us now and in the future.

Community Expectations in Defining Quality

Over the past 10 years, our eyes have finally opened and there is general agreement that the health care community must be held accountable for closing the enormous gap between the health care we should be getting and the health care we actually receive—the so called "quality chasm" discussed in the 2001 report by the Institute of Medicine (IOM). By now, we all are familiar with the IOM's landmark report, *To Err Is Human*, citing that between 44,000 and 98,000 deaths due to medical errors occur in hospitals every year.[2]

Clearly, patients, families, and communities all know that something must change. So, what does the consumer, or the community, perceive as "high-quality health care"? High quality means excellent clinical care delivered in a safe, effective, and compassionate manner. It's the care we all feel we deserve. The IOM defines the six aims of high-quality health care—i.e., care that is safe, effective, patient-centered, timely, efficient, and equitable[3]—and hospitals must be accountable to their communities for providing care that satisfies each of these domains.

Framework of Inpatient Quality Measurement

Analysis of the IOM's framework for high-quality care enables us to understand why we measure what we do in terms of inpatient quality metrics. It is true that existing quality measures address some of the IOM's domains more extensively than others, but this framework provides a good basis for understanding the nuts and bolts of inpatient quality measurement. Overall, the majority of measures assess effectiveness and safety; a handful of measures inspect timeliness and patient centeredness; and a few measures address the efficiency and equity of care.[4]

Effectiveness and Safety

Safe care is care that protects the patient from being harmed by what is intended to help them; for instance, metrics for catheter-related blood stream infections and wrong site surgeries. Effective care is care based on scientific knowledge that is delivered only to those patients who might benefit and not to those who will not likely benefit. Measures of effective care track the avoidance of underuse and misuse errors through metrics such as beta-blockers after myocardial infarction (MI) and appropriate antibiotic selection for community-acquired pneumonia.

Patient-Centeredness and Timeliness

Patient-centered care means providing respectful care that is responsive to individual patient preferences, needs, and values and allows these principles to guide all clinical decisions.[5] We are becoming more adept at measuring patient-centeredness mainly through the *Hospital Consumer Assessment of Healthcare Providers and Systems* survey (HCAHPS), the first national, standardized, publicly reported survey of patients' perspectives of hospital care. It contains 27 questions pertaining to recently discharged patients' hospital stays.[6] Next, timely care is care that reduces waits and potentially harmful delays for those who give and receive care. Examples of timely care metrics include door-to-balloon time for cardiac catheterization procedures in acute ST-elevation MIs and time to preoperative antibiotics.

Efficiency and Equity

Efficient care is defined as the avoidance of waste, including equipment, supplies, personnel, ideas, and energy. Hospitals are becoming more adept at measuring efficiency by using "lean" methodologies such as tracking emergencydepartment throughput times and aligning staffing requirements to patient volume trends. Finally, equitable care allows for no variance in quality due to personal characteristics such as gender, ethnicity, geographic location, or socioeconomic status. We currently struggle with this metric, relying on data such as access to care and regional utilization of resources by patient characteristic or location to ensure equitable care provisions. The Dartmouth Atlas of Health Care is an exceptional resource for measuring and tracking care variations across geographic regions.[5]

Quality Indicators

Now that we understand the meaning and relevance of quality metrics, we are ready to delve a little deeper into the specific quality indicators we measure in the hospital setting. A quality indicator is a measure that assesses a particular health care process or outcome. Among their multitude of functions, quality indicators serve to "document the quality of care; make comparisons (benchmarking) over time between places (e.g., hospitals); make judgments and set priorities (e.g., choosing a hospital or surgery); support accountability, regulation, and accreditation; support quality improvement (QI); and support patient choice of providers."[7] Because defining quality is complex and multidimensional, understanding quality requires many different measures.

A pioneer of QI science, Donabedian defined quality in terms of structure, process, and outcome measures,[8] a framework that can be applied in the hospital setting (Table 9-1). Structural measures relate to characteristics of the health system that can affect its ability to provide high-quality care. Structural measures include hospital teaching status, patient volume, proportion of specialists, and access to specific technologies (i.e., magnetic resonance imaging, cardiac catheterization).

Table 1. Examples of Inpatient Quality Indicators by Measure Type

Structure

- Access to MRI
- Presence of Stroke Unit
- Access to PCI (angioplasty lab)
- ICU Nursing to Patient Ratio

Process

- % eligible Pts with stroke receiving t-PA
- % Pts receiving pneumococcal assessment/vaccination
- % pts getting smoking cessation counseling

Outcome

- Mortality
- % Avoidable Readmissions
- % CLA-BSI

Conversely, process indicators evaluate what was done during an episode of care to reach the ultimate outcome. Process measures constitute the majority of inpatient quality metrics and include such things as the proportion of eligible stroke patients given the clot-busting drug t-PA, appropriate venous thromboembolism prophylaxis, and the proportion of heart failure patients given discharge instructions.[7] In fact, most metrics in the JC/CMS Core Measure Set are process measures, the use of which is supported by scientific evidence showing that these specific medications or procedures produce better outcomes (Table 2). Each core measure is a "bundle" of evidence-based treatments, all of which must be completed for outcome improvement. For example, if a patient with an MI is given an aspirin and a beta-blocker on arrival but is never prescribed a beta-blocker at discharge, the patient will not fully benefit from the "Acute Myocardial Infarction Bundle" and patient outcomes may suffer. Table 2 shows examples of some initial quality process measures used by regulatory agencies. Additional bundles exist for the Surgical Care Improvement Project (SCIP), venous thromboembolism (VTE), and stroke.

Table 2. Examples of CMS/JC Hospital Core Measure Bundles

Acute Myocaridal Infarction	Community-Acquired Pneumonia	Heart Failure
• Aspirin on arrival • Aspirin prescribed at discharge • ACEI or ARB or LSVD • Adult smoking counseling • Beta Blocker at arrival • Beta Blocker at discharge • Time to thrombolytics within 30 min • Time to PCI within 120 minutes • Inpatient mortality	• Oxygenation assessment • Pneumococcal screening/vaccination • Adult smoking counseling • % of patients receiving 1st dose of antibiotic within 240 minutes	• Discharge instructions • LVF assessment • ACEI or ARB or LSVD • Adult smoking counseling

Source: Data from publicly available information

Last but not least, there are outcome measures that describe the effects of care on the health status of patients and populations; for example, metrics such as mortality, hospital-acquired infections (e.g., catheter-related blood stream infection), and hospital readmission rates.[7]

Sources of Inpatient Quality Data

Inpatient quality data are derived from sources that range from large billing and other administrative databases to clinical data from chart reviews to voluntary and prompted error-reporting systems. The largest reservoir of inpatient quality data comes from two sources: the administrative data source (MSDRGs), and chart-abstracted clinical processes of care (CMS core measures). Additional resources may also include third-party payers. Administrative data include acute and 30-day mortality and complication rates such as hospital-acquired conditions (HAC) and Patient Safety Indicators (PSI) as well as readmissions data. HACs and PSI's were developed for the purpose of using administrative data to track the quality of inpatient care.

Developed by the Agency for Healthcare Research and Quality (AHRQ), the PSIs are administrative data-based indicators that identify potential inhospital patient safety events with a special focus on preventable harm.[10] In contrast, CMS's core measures (e.g., the percentage of patients admitted with an MI who receive aspirin on arrival and the percentage of surgery patients who receive DVT prophylaxis) are driven by chart-extracted clinical data.

Each data source has its strengths and limitations. Although using administrative data is a fast and efficient way to access data, the data lack clinical context and may have validity issues. Risk-adjustment methods that are sufficiently robust for comparability purposes have not been established.[11] Administrative data can be used to provide directional information for QI though they lack the ability to track predefined quality metrics.

In comparison, there is a large reservoir of useful information in clinical data—e.g., data extracted from manual chart reviews. Unfortunately, the benefit of providing data with clinical context is offset by the high cost and labor intensity of data extraction. Together, all of these data sources provide a robust source of clinical indicators that lay the foundation for QI initiatives. See Figure 1 for an illustration of public reporting data flow.

Figure 1: Public Reporting Data Flow

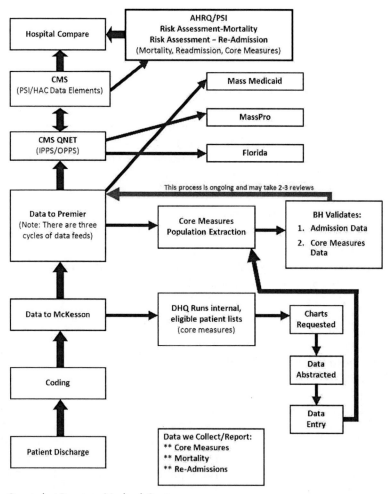

Source: Created at Baystate Medical Center

Measuring Safe Care

With a better understanding of how quality of care is measured, we will focus on how we measure and ensure safe care. Safe care can be viewed from a variety of angles. We can compare risk-adjusted mortality rates for a given diagnosis across hospitals; however, we must keep in mind that mortality rates are only one piece of the puzzle. They do not answer the all-important question of why mortality rates differ. Without knowing this, improvement cannot occur.

To find the answer, hospitals must also focus on harm. The precept of "Do No Harm" or "nonmaleficence" is taught to all physicians in medical school and serves as the foundation of shared medical ethics among all care providers. Providing safe care is one of the hallmarks in measuring inpatient quality. The Institute for Healthcare Improvement (IHI) defines harm as "unintended physical injury resulting from, or contributed to by, medical care (including the absence of medical treatment) that requires additional monitoring, treatment, or hospitalization, or that results in death."[12] Such injury is considered harm whether it resulted from a medical error, whether or not it was preventable, or whether or not it occurred within a hospital. According to the IHI, about 30-35 percent of current hospital admissions are found to have adverse events. This translates to about 90 adverse events per 1,000 patient days, or 40 adverse events per 100 admissions.[13]

Today, hospitals seek to recognize, report, and prevent these episodes of harm. Widely accepted definitions of harm have been developed by a variety of organizations, including the AHRQ PSIs and the predefined HACs created as part of CMS's Inpatient Prospective Payment System (IPPS) 2009 Final Rule. HACs came about after the Deficit Reduction Act of 2005 required the Secretary of Health and Human Services to identify conditions that are "high cost or high volume or both, result in the assignment of a case to a diagnosis-related group (DRG) that has a higher payment when present as a secondary diagnosis, and could reasonably have been prevented through the application of evidence-based guidelines." Under a new provision, hospitals will no longer be paid for services associated with 10 categories of HACs if and when they occur during a hospitalization (Table 3, page 146).[14]

Harm and error data are obtained from error-reporting systems that may be linked to a hospital's electronic medical record and/or based on a voluntary error-reporting system within the institution. An error-reporting system is a structured system that allows everyone involved in a patient's care to report any actual or potential errors or harm that occur during care. The power of the system is that it focuses on system issues rather than personal blame. Error-reporting systems concentrate on "the what, why, and when" of an error instead of the "who." In addition, the IHI has developed a Global Trigger tool to detect harm that occurs in hospitals. The trigger tool is a structured chart review process that, when used on randomly selected charts, helps to identify trends in harm that hospitals can use for internal QI. This will be discussed in more depth later in this chapter.

Table 3. Hospital-Acquired Conditions (HACs)

- Foreign Object Retained after Surgery
- Air Embolism
- Blood Incompatibility
- Stage III and IV Pressure Ulcers
- Falls and Trauma
  - Fractures
  - Dislocations
  - Intracranial Injuries
  - Crushing Injuries
  - Burns
  - Electric Shock
- Manifestations of Poor Glycemic Control
  - Diabetic Ketoacidosis
  - Nonketotic Hyperosmolar Coma
  - Hypoglycemic Coma
  - Secondary Diabetes with Ketoacidosis
  - Secondary Diabetes with Hyperosmolarity

- Catheter-Associated Urinary Tract Infection
- Vascular Catheter-Associated Infection
- Surgical Site Infection Following:
  - Coronary Artery Bypass Graft - Mediastinitis
  - Bariatric Surgery
    - Laparoscopic Gastric Bypass
    - Gastroenterostomy
    - Laparoscopic Gastric Restrictive Surgery
  - Orthopedic Procedures
    - Spine
    - Neck
    - Shoulder
    - Elbow
- Deep Vein Thrombosis/Pulmonary Embolism
  - Total Knee Replacement
  - Hip Replacement

From: CMS at http://www.cms.gov/HospitalAcqCond/06_Hospital-Acquired_Conditions.asp

A discussion of harm would not be complete without addressing surgical complications. Postoperative infection and surgical complications are a major cause of patient injury, mortality, and health care cost. An estimated 2.6 percent of nearly 30 million operations are complicated by surgical site infections each year. Infection is estimated to increase a hospital stay by an average of 7 days and add over $3,000 in charges.[15] Safety and harm in surgical practices were addressed by the Surgical Care Improvement Project, known as SCIP. SCIP is a CMS-sponsored project in collaboration with 34 national partners, including the American Hospital Association (AHA), Centers for Disease Control and Prevention (CDC), IHI, and the JC. The project encompasses a bundle of measures involving: surgical site infection prevention, venous thromboembolism prophylaxis, and mitigating adverse cardiac events, with the ultimate goal of reducing surgical complications nationally by 25 percent.[16]

Given their preventability and the harm they cause, hospital-acquired infections (HAIs) have been closely scrutinized in recent years. The CDC estimates that 100,000 people die each year due to HAIs, with associated hospital costs reaching up to $45 billion each year. Specifically, the CDC reports that patients develop more than 250,000 central line-associated bloodstream infections (CLABSIs) and more than 290,000 surgical site infections (SSIs) each year while hospitalized.[17]

In addition to the aforementioned SSIs and CLABSIs, the major HAIs include catheter-associated urinary tract infections (CA-UTIs) and ventilator-associated pneumonias (VAPs). The majority of these are part of the larger set of HACs discussed earlier in the chapter.[18] New HAI reporting regulations have been adopted by the Department of Health & Human Services (HHS) under the MIPPS. Also, health reform legislation includes a requirement that HAIs be included in the pay for performance program.

Beginning in January 2011, hospitals are required to report rates of CLABSI in the intensive care unit (ICU) and the neonatal ICU to the CDC. These rates will become publicly available on the Hospital Compare web site. At first, Medicare payments will be made to hospitals for simply reporting infection rates. After the first year, payments will be linked to meeting infection rate standards. Similarly, hospitals will be required to begin reporting on SSIs in 2012.[17]

Sentinel Events

Further addressing inpatient safety and harm is the JC, an independent, not-for-profit organization that accredits more than 19,000 health care organizations in the United States. This certifying agency is nationally recognized as a symbol of quality, safety, and efficacy in health care.[19] The JC's 2011 Hospital National Patient Safety Goals include positively identifying patients, using medications correctly, improving staff communication, identifying patient safety risks, and preventing infections and mistakes in surgery.[20] Moreover, the JC has developed a framework for "Sentinel Events" that is widely accepted and has been utilized in all accredited hospitals since 1995. Specifically, a "Sentinel Event" is defined as "an unexpected occurrence involving death or serious physical or psychological injury, or the risk thereof. Serious injury includes loss of limb or function for which an event reoccurrence would carry a risk of a serious adverse outcome." The events are "sentinel" because they indicate an immediate need for system-wide investigation and response. It is important to note that the terms "sentinel event" and "medical error" are not interchangeable. Simply put, not all sentinel events are due to an error and not all errors result in sentinel events.[21]

In addition to the predefined sentinel events (Table 4, page 148), the JC requires each accredited organization to define its own sentinel events and to create systems to monitor and detect these events. Thus, accredited hospitals are expected to identify and respond appropriately to all sentinel events through a timely, thorough, and credible root cause analysis that looks at causal factors with a focus on systems and processes rather than individual performance.

Table 4. Examples of Joint Commission Reviewable Sentinel Events

Any patient death, paralysis, coma, or other major permanent loss of function associated with a medication error.

A patient commits suicide within 72 hours of being discharged from a hospital setting that provides staffed around-the-clock care.

Any elopement, that is, unauthorized departure, of a patient from an around-the-clock care setting resulting in a temporally related death (suicide, accidental death, or homicide) or major permanent loss of function.

A hospital operates on the wrong side of the patient's body.

Any intrapartum (related to the birth process) maternal death.

Any perinatal death unrelated to a congenital condition in an infant having a birthweight greater than 2,500 grams.

A patient is abducted from the hospital where he or she receives care, treatment, or services.

Assault, homicide, or other crime resulting in patient death or major permanent loss of function.

A patient fall that results in death or major permanent loss of function as a direct result of the injuries sustained in the fall.

Hemolytic transfusion reaction involving major blood group incompatibilities.

A foreign body, such as a sponge or forceps, that was left in a patient after surgery.

From Joint Commission Table 1 accessed from: www.jointcommission.org/assets/1/6/2011_CAMH_SE.pdf

The all-too-prevalent medical culture of individual "shame and blame" has been abolished and replaced with one that recognizes errors as a byproduct of bad systems and processes, not bad people. After event identification, action plans are formulated to implement and monitor improvements to decrease the likelihood of future event reoccurrences. Although each accredited hospital is encouraged (but not required) to report any sentinel event to the JC, the Commission may become aware of an event by alternate methods, such as through patient, family, the media, or employee communication.

If the JC becomes aware of a reportable sentinel event, the hospital is expected to prepare a root cause analysis and action plan within 45 calendar days of the event. The JC tracks events in a database to ensure that events are adequately analyzed, undesirable trends are recognized, and resolution plans are implemented.[21]

Leapfrog Measures

The Leapfrog Group recommends that, in addition to a root cause analysis, organizations report and disclose the error, apologize to the patient, and waive all costs associated with the event.[22] The Leapfrog Group is a voluntary conglomeration of large health care purchasers who have banded together to leverage the group's purchasing power in order to "trigger giant leaps forward in the safety, quality, and affordability of health care by supporting informed health care decisions by those who use and pay for health care and promoting high-value health care through incentives and rewards." The group promotes improvements in the safety, quality, and affordability of health care in a variety of ways. Key Leapfrog measures for quality and safety include use of computerized physician order entry (CPOE), ICU staffing, outcomes in key clinical high-risk areas such as mortality rates for MI, CABG, aortic abdominal aneurysm repair, and compliance with key patient safety best practices. [23]

"Never Events"

Finally in regards to harm, the NQF devised a list of "Never Events." The idea was first introduced in 2001 by former NQF CEO Ken Kizer, MD, in response to particularly appalling medical errors that should never occur—e.g., wrong site surgeries. Once created, the list was expanded to "signify adverse events that are unambiguous (clearly identifiable and measurable), serious (resulting in death or significant disability), and usually preventable." The list is organized into six categories: surgical, product or devices, patient protection, care management, environmental, and criminal.

The original 2002 NQF "Never Event" list was revised in 2006 and will be again in 2012. It now includes 28 discrete occurrences, examples of which can be seen in Table 5, page 150. The NQF's never events are also considered sentinel events by the JC, thus reporting regulations are similar. Furthermore, in August 2007, CMS announced it would no longer pay for additional costs associated with many preventable errors, including never events. Individual states and private insurers have followed suit. Furthermore, never events are now publicly reported to both improve care quality and increase accountability. [22]

Initiatives to Reduce Harm

A discussion about harm would not be complete without mentioning the IHI's leadership role in reducing harm. IHI's work with its "100,000 Lives Campaign" grew exponentially into the "5 Million Lives Campaign." These campaigns guided over 4,000 hospitals and facilities in reducing harm and improving safety by implementing the campaign's 12 interventions—interventions aimed at avoiding over 5 million incidents of medical harm over a two-year period. The interventions focused on reducing MRSA infection, surgical complications, and medication errors; preventing pressure ulcers, CHF readmissions, and high-alert medication errors; and engaging governing boards on the importance of QI.[24]

Table 5. Examples of NQF "Never Events"

Surgical Events
- Surgery performed on the wrong body part
- Surgery performed on the wrong patient
- Wrong surgical procedure performed on a patient
- Unintended retention of a foreign object in a patient after surgery or other procedure

Product or device events
- Patient death or serious disability associated with the use of contaminated drugs, devices, or biologics provided by the health care facility

Patient protection events
- Infant discharged to the wrong person
- Patient death or serious disability associated with patient elopement (disappearance)

Care management events
- Patient death or serious disability associated with a medication error (e.g., errors involving the wrong drug, wrong dose, wrong patient, wrong time, wrong rate, wrong preparation, or wrong route of administration)
- Patient death or serious disability associated with a hemolytic reaction due to the administration of ABO/HLA-incompatible blood or blood products

Environmental events
- Patient death or serious disability associated with an electric shock or electrical cardioversion while being cared for in a health care facility
- Any incident in which a line designated for oxygen or other gas to be delivered to a patient contains the wrong gas or is contaminated by toxic substances

Criminal events
- Any instance of care ordered by or provided by someone impersonating a physician, nurse, pharmacist, or other licensed health care provider
- Abduction of a patient of any age

From: Agency for Healthcare Research and Quality. Accessed from: http://psnet.ahrq.gov/primer.aspx?primerID=3).

IHI's Global Trigger Tool (GTT) is at the forefront of harm recognition and reduction. Traditional efforts to detect adverse events focus primarily on voluntary error-reporting systems and error tracking. However, researchers find that only 10-20 percent of errors are ever reported and, of those, 90-95 percent do not cause harm to patients. For this reason, the IHI developed the GTT to identify and measure adverse events (AE). The tool functions by conducting a systematic retrospective review of patient records using pre-defined triggers to identify possible

AEs.[13] At least 10 times more serious events have been identified and confirmed by using the GTT than by using voluntary reporting or PSIs alone. Shockingly, the GTT found that AEs occurred in one-third of all hospital admissions.[25] It appears that a combination of voluntary reporting, PSIs, and tools such as the GTT will lead to overall improvements in the safety of our health care system.

Public Reporting

We wouldn't have gotten very far in improving U.S. health care quality and safety without public reporting. In fact, public reporting and the subsequent comparison of quality data are as important as the measurement itself. Because health care performance transparency is critical to the optimal functioning of the health care system, the Hospital Inpatient Quality Reporting (Hospital IQR) program was mandated as part of the Medicare Prescription Drug, Improvement, and Modernization Act (MMA) of 2003. The MMA Act authorized CMS to pay hospitals that report designated quality measures a higher annual update to their payment rates to incentivize quality and safety reporting.[26]

Public reporting gets "more bang for its buck" than favorable payment rates. That is, hospitals not only receive a financial incentive to report the quality of their services, but CMS also uses much of the hospital-reporting data to help consumers make more informed decisions about their health care. Via a consumer-oriented website, patients and their families can find care recommendations for an adult being treated for a surgery, heart attack, heart failure, and pneumonia, as well as patient experience data captured by HCAHPS.[6,27] In this way, public reporting of hospital data improves the nation's health literacy and allows each patient to make his or her own informed decision before purchasing health care.

The aforementioned data can be found on the Hospital Compare website at: www.hospitalcompare.hhs.gov. The website was formed by CMS in collaboration with the Hospital Quality Alliance (HQA) in an effort to support informed consumer decisions and to improve the quality of inpatient care in the U.S.[27] In addition to the initial set of process measures, Hospital Compare recently added outcome measures, including rates of risk-adjusted mortality and 30-day readmission for patients hospitalized with acute MI, pneumonia, and heart failure.[28] Other entities also contribute to enhancing health care transparency—e.g., the Leapfrog Group's Hospital Survey, first launched in 2001.[29]

Conclusion

Improving the quality of inpatient care is only one piece of the U.S. health care jigsaw puzzle. Even so, it is a strategic piece that will permit many others to fall into their rightful locations. Through the efforts of CMS, AHRQ, NQF, AHA, IHI, the JC, the Leapfrog Group, and a host of other alphabet-soup initialism, we have laid the initial groundwork for improving the quality and safety of hospital-based health care. Nonetheless, much work remains. How we proceed from here remains a subject of a great debate, but forward thinking will likely be the key to success.

An example of such forward thinking is the Partnership for Patients, developed collaboratively by CMS and the AHA. This public-private partnership's goal is to reduce inpatient harm by 40 percent and decrease readmissions by 20 percent in three years starting in October 2011 by "bringing together leaders of major hospitals, employers, physicians, nurses, and patient advocates along with state and federal governments in a shared effort to make hospital care safer, more reliable, and less costly." Forward thinking has allowed allocation of resources to help engaged hospitals achieve these important goals. Because achieving these goals may save up to $35 billion across the health care system and reduce Medicare costs by $50 billion over the next 10 years, it becomes a "win" for everyone. Such "out of the box" thinking can redirect us on the path toward a sustainable health care system.[30]

Realistic forward thinking reveals that, in many areas, the necessary foundations for improvement have yet to be discovered. Dr. Michael Porter declares the need to define "value" in health care as the real means to improvement. He defines true health care value in terms of the patient, as health outcomes achieved per dollar spent. Within this framework, we are compelled to question what "value" is in the context of health care, and how will we define and measure it. Unfortunately, but all too evidently, much of today's quality reporting does not fit Porter's framework. To achieve the IOM's six aims, we must question and redesign our system down to the level of its very infrastructure.[31] Achieving true patient-centered value will require research, discussion, pilot testing novel structures and strategies (e.g., bundled payments, value-based purchasing initiatives), and new models of collaboration. The quality of inpatient health has come a long way, but a long and bumpy road still lies ahead.

Study and Discussion Questions

1. Describe the framework for inpatient quality measurement.

2. What are some of the common inpatient quality measures, including structural, process, and outcome measures?

3. Describe, compare, and contrast the various sources of inpatient quality data.

4. How do hospitals measure "harm"? Can you think of any novel ways to improve upon "harm" measurement?

5. Why is public reporting important? What are some barriers to public reporting and how can they be overcome?

Case Study: Congestive Heart Failure Performance

Standardized—or "core"—performance measures, also called "Hospital Quality Measures," are integral to improving the quality of care provided to hospital patients. BFMC began collecting data on CHF in 2002. Performance for 2003 is shown on page 153.

2003 Congestive Heart Failure Performance

	2003 Q4	2003 Q3	2003 Q2	2003 Q1
Heart Failure	%	%	%	%
DC instruction	60	59.1	17.4	38.1
LVF assessment	100	96.7	100	100
ACEI for LVSD	77.8	81.8	83.3	87.5
Adult Smoking Cessation	25	0	0	0

In the fall of 2003, BFMC senior leadership and its physician partners were assigned to lead strategies in each area. The strategies focused on collecting, tracking, and acting on clinical quality and safety data in the measured areas, consistent with regional and national quality benchmarks. Developed in 2004, a new core measure dashboard enabled measures to be shared internally with the hospital's key clinical departments, the Performance Improvement Council, the Strategic Planning Team, the Medical-Executive Committee, and BH quality colleagues. The goal was to be in the top 10 percent percent of all hospitals reporting the CHF measures.

When left as a responsibility of the clinicians providing care on inpatient units, performance on smoking cessation counseling had been poor. Key issues included the lack of a defined process to provide the needed education to smokers and the lack of clear accountability as to who was responsible for assessing the patient's smoking history, providing the education, and documenting the process in the medical record.

Implementation of an EMR facilitated a method for assessing all patients admitted to the hospital as a routine part of the nursing assessment. If the patient met the requirements for smoking cessation counseling, the EMR created a "task" for the respiratory therapist to provide education and offer the patient the "Quitworks" program (a Massachusetts state-funded program). The respiratory therapist documented the intervention in the EMR.

By creating a structure wherein the assessment was to be completed, and assigning accountability for smoking cessation counseling to the respiratory therapist, the process change improved the completion of the smoking cessation counseling. However, results remained inconsistent (see 2005 data below).

	2005 Q4	2005 Q3	2005 Q2	2005 Q1
Heart Failure	%	%	%	%
Adult Smoking Cessation	71.4	100	66.7	0

You are a member of the Board of Trustees Performance Improvement Committee

1. Are you satisfied with the results and approach presented?

2. What additional information do you want in order to fulfill your responsibilities for overseeing quality on this committee?

3. What recommendations or next steps would you recommend to management?

Suggested Websites and Readings

Agency for Healthcare Research and Quality. Patient Safety Primers: Never Events. http://psnet.ahrq.gov/primer.aspx?primerID=3. Accessed November 2011.

The Joint Commission. Sentinel Events. Accessed from: http://www.jointcommission.org/assets/1/6/2011_CAMH_SE.pdf

Porter, M. What Is Value in Health Care? *NEJM* 363(26):2477-81, Dec. 23,2010.

The Dartmouth Atlas Website — http://www.dartmouthatlas.org/

CMS Website — www.cms.gov

www.healthcare.gov

www.hospitalcompare.hhs.gov.

Institute for Healthcare Improvement Website — www.ihi.org

References

1. Table 2 National Health Expenditure Amounts, and Annual Percent Change by Type of Expenditure: Selected Calendar Years 1998-2014. http://www.cms.hhs.gov/NationalHealthExpendData/downloads/nheprojections2004-2014.pdf. Accessed November 2011.

2. Kohn L, Corrigan J, Donaldson M, eds., *To Err Is Human: Building a Safer Health System*. Washington, DC: National Academies Press, 1999.

3. Institute of Medicine, *Crossing the Quality Chasm: A New Health System for the 21st Century*. Washington, DC: National Academies Press, 2001.

4. Institute of Medicine. *Performance Measurement: Accelerating Improvement*. Washington, DC: National Academies Press, 2005.

5. Agency for Healthcare Research and Quality. The Six Domains of Healthcare Quality. https://www.talkingquality.ahrq.gov/content/create/sixdomains.aspx. Accessed November 2011.

6. Centers for Medicare and Medicaid Services. HCAPHS: Patients' Perspectives of Care Survey. https://www.cms.gov/HospitalQualityInits/30_HospitalHCAHPS.asp. Accessed November 2011.

7. Mainz, J. Defining and classifying clinical indicators for quality improvement. *International Journal for Quality in Health Care,* 15(6):523-30, Dec. 2003

8. Donabedian A: The quality of care. How can it be assessed? *JAMA,* 260(12):1743-8, Sept. 23-30, 1988.

9. Joint Commission Core Measure set. http://www.jointcommission.org/core_measure_set/. Accessed November 2011.

10. Rivard P, Elwy R, Loveland S, *et al.* Chapter 1: Applying Patient Safety Indicators (PSIs) Across Health Care Systems: Achieving Data Comparability. From Henriksen K, Battles JB, Marks ES, et al., editors. *Advances in Patient Safety: From Research to Implementation.* Volume 2: Concepts and Methodology. Washington, DC: AHRQ, 2005.

11. Rothberg, M, Morsi, E, Benjamin, *et al.* Choosing the Best Hospital: The Limitations of Public Quality Reporting. *Health Affairs,* 27(60;1680-7, Nov-Dec. 2008.

12. Institute for Healthcare Improvement. www.ihi.org

13. Griffin FA, Resar RK. *IHI Global Trigger Tool for Measuring Adverse Events (Second Edition).* IHI Innovation Series white paper. Cambridge, MA: Institute for Healthcare Improvement; 2009.

14. Centers for Medicare and Medicaid Services. Hospital Acquired Conditions. http://www.cms.gov/HospitalAcqCond/06_Hospital-Acquired_Conditions.asp. Accessed November 2011.

15. New Mexico Medical Review Association. Surgical Care. http://www.nmmra.org/providers/hospitals_scip.php. Accessed November 2011.

16. Premier. Surgical Care Improvement Project. http://www.premierinc.com/safety/topics/scip/.Accessed November 2011.

17. New HHS Regulations Require Public Reporting of Certain Hospital Infections. http://www.safepatientproject.org/2010/08/new_hhs_regulations_require_na.html. Accessed November 2011

18. IPPS FY 2009 Final Rule HAC Fact Sheet. https://www.cms.gov/apps/media/press/factsheet.asp. Accessed on September 6, 2011.

19. The Joint Commission. http://www.jointcommission.org/about_us/about_the_joint_commission_main.aspx. Accessed November 2011.

20. The Joint Commission. Hospital 2011: National Patient Safety Goals. http://www.jointcommission.org/hap_2011_npsgs/. Accessed November 2011.

21. The Joint Commission. Sentinel Events. http://www.jointcommission.org/assets/1/6/2011_CAMH_SE.pdf. Accessed November 2011.

22. Agency for Healthcare Research and Quality. Patient Safety Primers: Never Events. http://psnet.ahrq.gov/primer.aspx?primerID=3. Accessed November 2011.

23. The Leapfrog Group. http://www.leapfroggroup.org/about_us. Accessed November 2011.

24. The Institute for Healthcare Improvement. 5 Million Lives Campaign. http://www.ihi.org/offerings/Initiatives/PastStrategicInitiatives/5MillionLivesCampaign/Pages/default.aspx. Accessed November 2011

25. Classen D, Resar R, Griffin F, Federico F, Frankel T, Kimmel N, Whittington J, Frankel A, Seger A, James B. 'Global Trigger Tool' Shows That Adverse Events in Hospitals May Be Ten Times Greater Than Previously Measured. *Health Aff,* 30(4:581-9, Apr 2011.

26. Hospital Inpatient Quality Reporting. Centers for Medicare and Medicaid Services. https://www.cms.gov/HospitalQualityInits/08_HospitalRHQDAPU.asp. Accessed November 2011.

27. Hospital Compare. Centers for Medicare and Medicaid Services. https://www.cms.gov/HospitalQualityInits/11_HospitalCompare.asp#TopOfPage. Accessed November 2011.

28. Calculation of 30-Day Risk-Standardized Mortality Rates and Rates of Readmission. Outcome of Care Measure. US Department of Health and Human Services. http://www.hospitalcompare.hhs.gov/staticpages/for-professionals/ooc/calculation-of-30-day-risk.aspx. Accessed November 2011.

29. The Leapfrog Group. Leapfrog Hospital Survey. Accessed from: http://www.leapfroggroup.org/for_hospitals/leapfrog_hospital_survey_copy. Accessed November 2011.

30. Healthcare.gov. Partnership for Patients: Better Care, Lower Costs. http://www.healthcare.gov/center/programs/partnership. Accessed November 2011

31. Porter M. What is value in health care? *NEJM*, 363(26):2477-81, Dec. 23, 2010.

Chapter 10

Measuring Quality of Long-Term Care

By Richard G. Stefanacci, DO, MGH, MBA, AGSF, CMD

Executive Summary

Prompted by concerns regarding the quality of care in nursing homes, the Institute of Medicine (IOM) issued a report focused on improving the quality of care. On the basis of this report, Congress enacted the landmark Omnibus Budget Reconciliation Act of 1987 (OBRA), which raised quality-of-care standards and strengthened federal and state oversight of nursing homes participating in Medicare and Medicaid. As a result, attention has been shifting from regulation to culture change within nursing to achieve improved outcomes.

Improvements in quality are promoted through public reporting by the Centers for Medicare and Medicaid Services (CMS) *Nursing Home Compare* website as well as the *Nursing Home Value-based Purchasing Demonstration* (NHVPD). In addition there is a move to care for nursing home eligible seniors in the community. *Home and Community-Based Services* (HCBS) provides states with greater flexibility to expand HCBS benefits and financial eligibility through a Medicaid state plan amendment that replaces the more restrictive waiver process.

Special needs plans (SNPs) have been introduced to provide all the benefits available under Medicare with added flexibility to increase the scope of services and provide payment incentives to care for nursing home residents in a more efficient and effective manner.

While the OBRA regulations, NHVPD and SNPs are all important steps in the ongoing effort to improve care for long-term care (LTC) facility residents, the focus must broaden beyond mere regulation, reporting, and financial realignment. The goal must be to transform the culture in order to provide the resources necessary for delivering high-quality care to the LTC resident.

Learning Objectives

1. List the critical IOM report and legislation that led to many of the quality improvement initiatives in nursing homes.

2. Explain how the movement toward patient-centered care is being implemented through Home and Community-based Services (HCBS).

3. Describe the Nursing Home Value-based Purchasing Demonstration.

4. Explain how financial incentives are being utilized to provide more efficient and effective care through models like Special Needs Plans (SNPs)

Key Words: Skilled Nursing Facility (SNF), Institute of Medicine Report: Improving the Quality of Care in Nursing Homes, Omnibus Budget Reconciliation Act of 1987 (OBRA), Balanced Budget Act of 1997 (BBA 97), Balanced Budget Refinement Act of 1999, Affordable Care Act of 2010, Home and Community-based Services (HCBS), National Demonstration Project on Culture Change, Minimum Data Set (MDS), State Operations Manual (SOM), Nursing Home Quality Initiative, Nursing Home Value-based Purchasing Demonstration, Special Needs Plans (SNP), Eden Alternative, Wellspring Model

Introduction

The current focus on quality in nursing homes was spurred by a general perception that quality was lacking. Often highlighted by the media in public scandals, nursing facility care in the 1980s was characterized by the prevalent use of physical restraints, inappropriate use of psychotropic medication, overuse of urinary catheters, and the consequences of these conditions—pressure ulcers, weight loss, and behavioral problems.

Because of widespread poor quality of care in nursing facilities, Congress asked the IOM to study how to improve the quality of care in the nation's Medicaid and Medicare certified nursing facilities. In its 1986 report, *Improving the Quality of Care in Nursing Homes,* the IOM expert panel recommended:

- A stronger federal role in improving quality

- Revisions in performance standards and in the inspection/survey process

- Better training of staff

- Improved assessment of resident needs

- A dynamic and improved regulatory process

LTC Legislation and Regulation: A Historical Perspective

As a result of this report, Congress subsequently enacted the landmark Omnibus Budget Reconciliation Act of 1987 (OBRA), which raised quality-of-care standards and strengthened federal and state oversight of nursing homes participating in Medicare and Medicaid.

With the passage of OBRA 1987, surveyors of nursing facilities shifted their focus from the nursing facility to resident outcomes. The quality of life and the quality of care of each resident became the two basic areas of review. Under quality of life, the concept of the living environment maintaining or improving the residents' well-being became the major focus. In addition to physical and mental health, well-being includes the resident's functional status, self-esteem, relationships, appearance, as well as their social and spiritual needs.

The changes that OBRA brought to the care of residents in nursing facilities are noteworthy. Among the most important provisions listed below are a number of "resident rights":

- Emphasis on resident quality of life as well as the quality of care

- A resident assessment process leading to development of an individualized care plan

- New expectations that each resident's ability to walk, bathe, and perform other activities of daily living will be maintained or improved unless an underlying medical conditions precludes it

- The right to be free of unnecessary and inappropriate physical and chemical restraints

- The right to choose a personal physician and to access their medical records

- The right to organize and participate in a resident or family council

- The right to return to the nursing facility after a hospital stay or have an overnight visit with family and friends

- The right to safely maintain personal funds with the nursing facility

- The right to remain in the nursing facility unless non-payment, dangerous resident behavior, or a significant change in the resident's medical condition occurs

- Prohibitions on asking family members to pay for Medicare and Medicaid services

- Uniform certification standards for Medicare and Medicaid homes

- 75 hours of training for paraprofessional staff

- New opportunities for residents with mental retardation or mental illness to access services inside and outside the nursing facility

- New penalties for certified nursing facilities that fail to meet minimum federal standards

As a result of OBRA, state surveyors no longer spend their time exclusively interviewing staff or reviewing facility records. Conversations with residents and families and observations of dining and medication administration are now important survey elements. OBRA has changed the care and lives of residents of nursing facilities across the United States for the better; for instance, significant improvements in the comprehensiveness of care planning have occurred, anti-psychotic drug use has declined by 28-36 percent, and physical restraints have been reduced by 40 percent.

Since OBRA 87, new regulations have been continuously introduced in hopes of raising the bar for quality of care for nursing home residents. The Balanced Budget Act of 1997 (BBA 97) mandated the establishment of case mix-adjusted prospective payment systems for various Medicare post acute care services, including nursing facility and home health services. The BBA 97 also moved nursing facility services into a prospective payment system (PPS), a change that had the unintended consequence of bankrupting many nursing homes. With a substantial number of nursing homes falling into bankruptcy, the Balanced Budget Refinement Act of 1999 temporarily increased the federal per diem nursing home rate by 20 percent.

The most recent report from the IOM on LTC quality came in 2001. In its report on "Improving the Quality of Long-Term Care" that year, the IOM identified three complementary approaches that are generally used for ensuring quality of care and life in LTC: 1) standards set and enforced by government and accrediting agencies and incentives for quality improvement through Medicare and Medicaid and other payers, 2) consumer information, choice, and market competition, and 3) organizational and professional commitment to quality improvement.[1]

The IOM identified several principles that it believes will help shape efforts to protect and improve the quality of LTC.

1. LTC should be consumer-centered rather than solely provider-centered.

2. A system of consumer-centered LTCs should be structured to serve people with diverse characteristics and preferences.

3. Reliable and current information about the options available and the quality of care provided should be easily accessible to allow people to make informed choices about LTC.

4. Access to appropriate LTC services is both a quality of care and a quality of life issue.

5. Measures of the quality of LTC should incorporate its many dimensions, especially quality of life.

6. Providers should be held accountable for their performance in providing high-quality LTC, including the outcomes of care that they are able to affect.

7. A motivated, capable, and sufficient work force is critical to high-quality LTC.

8. Improving the quality of LTC requires sustained government commitment to develop and implement fair, effective regulatory and financing policies.

9. Improving quality of care must be an ongoing objective.

It is interesting to note the evolution of the IOM's position from its initial report, which focuses on setting standards of care, to its current report, which focuses on quality of care. This has set the stage for a quality of care approach that is increasingly resident-centered.

Despite the impact of OBRA, nursing home quality continues be a common and serious concern. Many facilities continue to operate with serious deficiencies because the inspection system either fails to detect violations or because detection does not guarantee prompt correction. In a 2005 investigation, the Government Accountability Office (GAO) found inconsistencies in how state surveyors were conducting their nursing home inspections and questioned whether surveyors understood the serious deficiencies they found.[2] A follow-up study in March 2007 indicated that CMS enforcement policies allow some nursing homes with the worst compliance histories to escape immediate sanctions designed to punish them for putting residents at risk.[3] In light of these findings, it should come as no surprise that the national LTC ombudsman reporting system for the Administration on Aging received almost a quarter of a million consumer complaints over a 12-month period.[4]

Historically, LTC has been synonymous with nursing homes. It has long been recognized that the nursing home was a place providing care both to residents with needs requiring short stays and to those with more chronic conditions requiring longer, if not permanent, care.[5]

Impact of Health Reform Implementation

With the passage of the Affordable Care Act of 2010 (ACA), a trend toward moving LTC beyond the walls of the nursing home is gaining momentum. In recent years, there has been a rise in assisted living facilities and in other LTC settings as possible alternatives to nursing homes for individuals requiring long-term care.[6] At the same time, the need for post acute care in nursing homes, requiring shorter stays, has grown.[7]

Home and Community-Based Services (HCBS) is the driving force behind the current movement toward caring for individuals needing nursing home level of care outside of the nursing home. State Plan Option (ACA Section 2402) allows states the flexibility to expand HCBS benefits and financial eligibility through a Medicaid state plan amendment instead of the more restrictive waiver process. Furthermore, the Community First Choice Option (ACA Section 2401) allows states to provide HCBS attendant supports and services through a state plan amendment and receive a six percentage point increase in the Federal Medicaid

Assistance Percentages (federal matching funds) for those services. Money Follows the Person Demonstration (ACA Section 2403) extends to 2016 the Money Follows the Person (MFP) rebalancing demonstration created through the Deficit Reduction Act of 2005.

In contrast to more traditional approaches, the push for high-quality outcomes is oriented more toward changing the culture than heavy-handed regulatory oversight. For example:

- ACA Section 61111 sets aside Federal Civil Money Penalty (CMP) funds, which currently are deposited to the US Treasury, to provide a stable funding stream for resident-centered care.

- ACA Section 6107 describes a GAO study on the Five Star Quality Rating System for nursing homes, the purpose of which is to determine how the system is being implemented, identify problems, and suggest improvements.

- ACA Section 6114 includes the "National Demonstration Project on Culture Change" for the development of best practices in skilled nursing facilities and nursing facilities that are involved in the culture change movement, including the development of resources for facilities to find and access funding in order to undertake culture change.

The movement toward resident-centered care is at the root of all aspects of nursing home care as well. This is borne out by recent changes in the Minimum Data Set (MDS). MDS assessments must be completed on admission to a nursing facilty and updated quarterly, annually, and when there is a significant change (wo rsened or improved) in a patient's condition. These assessments include areas such as tasks of daily living (ADLs), mobility, cognition, continence, mood, behaviors, nutritional status, vision and communication, recreational activities, psychosocial well-being, pain, and falls and injuries. Information from the MDS is utilized to drive care planning, to provide quality measurements, and as a basis for payment.

Government Regulation, Oversight & Reporting

Surveys and Public Reports

Federal regulators delegate oversight of LTC facilities to the states via the State Operations Manual (SOM), which sets forth survey investigative protocols and interpretive guidelines to provide guidance to state surveyors. In addition to clarifying and explaining the intent of the federal regulations, these protocols and guidelines direct the surveyor's attention when preparing for the survey, conducting the survey, and evaluating the survey findings. The survey is conducted to determine whether a facility is in compliance with state and/or federal regulations. A citation of non-compliance is issued if deficiencies (i.e., violations of the state and/or federal regulations) are noted and supported by surveyor observations of the nursing facilities' staff performance and care practices. (Table 1, page 163)

Table 1. Sample Deficiencies Report

Deficiencies			
Severity	**Score**		
	Isolated	**Pattern**	**Widespread**
No actual harm with potential for minimal harm	A	B	C
No actual harm with potential for more than minimal harm that is not immediate jeopardy	D	E	F
Actual harm that is not immediate jeopardy	G	H	I
Immediate jeopardy to resident health or safety	J	K	L

From CMS - State Operations Manual, Chapter 7 - Survey and Enforcement Process for Skilled Nursing Facilities and Nursing Facilities, (Rev. 63, 09-10-10), Page 93

The survey results are used not only by the state and facility but also as one of several measures making up CMS's public posting of quality indicators for every nursing facility, also known as "report cards."[4]

Nursing Home Quality Initiative

In a number of ways, the Department of Health and Human Services' (DHHS') *Nursing Home Quality Initiative* has become an integral part of a national effort to improve nursing facility care. CMS started with board quality initiatives that focused in part on the care needs of frail elders who reside in nursing facilities. As CMS developed more structured provider-based programs, the subsequent *Nursing Home Quality Initiative* responded by expanding and refining its measures to improve resident outcomes and care effectiveness (e.g., reducing the occurrence of pressure ulcers and avoiding potentially preventable hospital admissions).

Public quality data reporting is meant to guide consumers in choosing a high-quality provider while motivating deficient providers to improve their quality scores. To date, the availability of quality data has had little impact on LTC occupancy rates, either in favor of high-performing facilities or against those with deficiencies.[8] The reasons for this lack of impact include:

- Efforts to disseminate quality information in a form that consumers can actually understand have been inadequate. A study suggests that few consumers are using or are even aware of these Web sites.[9]

- The quality data currently being disseminated for consumer use may not be accurate.[10]

A critical element in the *Nursing Home Quality Initiative* is CMS's posting of 10 quality indicators for every nursing home.[11] The CMS quality initiative redirects focus from processes of care to the clinical care needs of frail elderly patients— evidence of the shift toward the resident and away from the institution. Although fairly well received, these nursing home report cards have limited value because they fail to adjust for differences in risk among LTC facilities.[12]

Medicare Five-Star Rating

Using a five-star rating system (Table 2), CMS/Medicare assigns an overall rating to nursing homes along with separate ratings on three types of performance measures:

1. Health inspections—based on number, scope, and severity of deficiencies during the three most recent annual state inspection surveys and substantial findings from the last 36 months of complaint investigations.

2. Staffing—based on RN, LPN, and nurse aide hours per resident day in addition to information on staff turnover and tenure and discussions of how staffing patterns affect quality and consideration of different staffing demands for different levels of care.

3. Quality measures

Table 2. Medicare Nursing Home Compare Web Page

Facility Name and General Information	Overall Ratings	Quality Measures	Health Inspections	Staffing	Program Participation	Total Number of Certified Beds	Type of Ownership	Continuing Care Retirement Community
	what is this?	what is this?	what is this?	what is this?				What is this?
Basic Spring 5255 East Main Street Fairfax, VA 22081 (555) 555-0555 Located in a hospital Resident & Family Councils: Both	★★★★★ 5 Stars	★★★★ 4 Stars	★★★★★ 5 Stars	★★★★ 4 Stars	Medicare and Medicaid	100	For-Profit Corporation	Yes
Lakefront View 2455 West Pecos Road Fairfax, VA 22081 (555) 555-0988 Resident & Family Councils: Both	★★★★ 4 Stars	★★★★ 4 Stars	★★★ 3 Stars	★★★★ 4 Stars	Medicare and Medicaid	95	Non-Profit Corporation	Yes
Glencrest Gardens 2012 West Southern Ave Fairfax, VA 22031 (555) 555-9800 Resident & Family Councils: Both	★★★ 3 Stars	★★★ 3 Stars	★★★ 3 Stars	★★★ 3 Stars	Medicare and Medicaid	89	Non-Profit Corporation	No
Holton Mills 2750 Lee Highway Fairfax, VA 22031 (555) 555-0988 Resident & Family Councils: Resident	★★ 2 Stars	★★ 2 Stars	★★ 2 Stars	★ 1 Star	Medicare	69	For-Profit Corporation	No

Source: Screen shot of CMS Nursing Home Compare Web Page
http://www.medicare.gov/NHCompare/Include/DataSection/Questions/SearchCriteriaNEW.asp?version=default&
browser=IE%7C8%7CWindows+7&language=English&defaultstatus=0&pagelist=Home&CookiesEnabledStatus=True

One study found no associations between staffing levels and quality indicators. Another study found the presence of a certified medical director to be an independent predictor of quality in U.S. nursing homes.[13] The combined findings of staffing studies indicated that a supportive practice environment was associated with better quality outcomes.[14]

Under the health care reform law, the GAO is required to conduct a study of the Five-Star System. Within two years of enactment, a report must be submitted to Congress detailing the results of the study along with any recommendations for legislation or administrative action. The measuring and reporting of nursing home quality measures will likely continue to evolve and change based on public demand and political initiatives.

Nursing Home Compare

The health care reform law requires that additional information be posted on CMS's *Nursing Home Compare* web site (www.medicare.gov/nhcompare) within one year of the law's enactment. CMS also must review the accuracy, clarity of presentation, timeliness, and comprehensiveness of information reported on *Nursing Home Compare* and develop a process to review the content and to make necessary revisions in consultation with state LTC ombudsman programs, consumer advocacy groups, provider stakeholder groups, and others.

To improve the timeliness of the web site's information, states must provide inspection information simultaneously to CMS and the affected facilities. In turn, CMS must update the information on Nursing Home Compare at least quarterly.

The *Nursing Home Compare* web site must be modified to include a consumer rights page that explains facility-specific information, includes tips on choosing a nursing facility, and describes state-specific services available through the LTC ombudsman program.

Under its 2007 Action Plan,[6] CMS is now focusing on nursing facility quality improvement through:

- Refining the Web-based report card at *"Nursing Home Compare"*
- Expanding the certification and survey process
- Establishing a pilot demonstration project on pay-for-performance under the term *"Value-Based Purchasing"*

Nursing Home Value-Based Purchasing Demonstration

Combining portions of the *Medicare Five-Star Rating* program with new financial incentives results in a newer CMS quality initiative, the *Nursing Home Value-Based Purchasing (NHVBP)* demonstration project. NHVBP is expected to result in cost savings for Medicare through reductions in hospitalizations and subsequent skilled nursing facility stays.

NHVBP is a type of pay-for-performance initiative in which CMS will offer financial incentives to free-standing and hospital-based nursing homes in Arizona, New York, and Wisconsin in exchange for meeting certain qualityof care conditions. Points will be awarded in four domains—staffing, appropriate hospitalizations, MDS outcomes, and survey deficiencies (Table 3, page 167). Within each state, nursing homes that score in the top 20 percent and are in the top 20 percent with improved scores will be eligible for a portion of the state's savings pool. The problem is that if a nursing facility performs well without associated cost savings performance, incentive payments will not be made.[7]

Obviously, CMS has moved over time from simple regulation to public reporting and now toward the use of financial incentives to promote improvement in quality in LTC.

Beyond Regulation and Reporting

Insights into the likely direction of LTC quality improvement can be gained by examining results of a recent national survey of 2,577 LTC providers, policymakers, public officials, and consumer advocates (response rate 38.5 to 51.5 percent) regarding policies, regulations, and quality demonstrates the thoughts from LTC key stakeholders with regard to payment and regulations.

• 53.3 percent believe payment incentives are effective.

• 47.7 percent believe higher staffing requirements are needed.

• 46.9 percent believe increased payment rates are needed.

• 43.4 percent want more technical assistance.

• 43.5 percent want more aggressive regulatory enforcement.

Despite Medicare's focus on reporting quality to the public, increased availability of consumer report cards was ranked least effective in improving quality by 32.7 percent of those polled. Consumers (41 percent) and public officials (44 percent) expressed greater belief in their efficacy than did providers (24.2 percent) and policy experts (21.5 percent). Compared with policymakers and providers, consumers ranked increased staffing requirements and more aggressive regulatory efforts higher (76.2 and 70.5 percent, respectively). Providers ranked increased staffing (32.3 percent) and regulatory enforcement (29.6 percent) lower, and increased payments higher (64.6 percent).[15]

Finally, 67.7 percent of respondents felt strongly that greater regulation is needed for assisted living, specifically application of regulatory and quality initiatives currently used for nursing homes. Respondents ranked support for quality initiatives in assisted living as follows: 56.1 percent support implementation of quality improvement efforts, 43.8 percent support collection of resident assessment data, and 41.6 percent want to see resident surveys regarding care received.[15] These survey findings indicate that quality in LTC is multidimensional and includes clinical information, quality of life, and patient and caregiver satisfaction.

Table 3. Nursing Home Value-Based Purchasing (NHVBP) Demonstration

Quality Domains (% of total score)	Measures
Staffing (30%)	• RNs, director of nursing hours per resident day • Total licensed nursing hours per resident day • Certified nurse aide hours per resident day • Nursing staff turnover rate
Appropriate Hospitalizations (30%)	• Separate measures for short and long stays • Based on hospitalization rates for potentially avoidable hospitalizations, risk adjusted using covariates of Medicare claims and MDS
MDS Outcomes (20%)	Chronic care residents: • Percentage of residents whose need for help with daily activities increases • Percentage of residents whose ability to move in and around their rooms worsens • Percentage of high-risk residents who have pressure ulcers • Percentage of residents who have had a catheter left in their bladder • Percentage of residents who were physically restrained Post acute care residents: • Percentage of residents with improving level of ADL functioning • Percentage of residents who improve status on mid-loss ADL functions • Percentage of residents experiencing failure to improve bladder incontinence
Survey Deficiencies (20%)	• Citation for substandard quality of care or actual harm: ineligible for performance payment • Score values assigned according to scope and severity of survey deficiencies

Source: http://www.cms.gov/DemoProjectsEvalRpts/downloads/NHP4P_FactSheet.pdf

Payment Reform

Nursing Facilities and Medicare: A "Navigation" Guide

While regulation and reporting have been applied to improve quality, there is a growing movement toward utilizing financial incentives as a means to improve the quality of care for LTC residents. To appreciate the significance of these financial incentives, some background knowledge into the current "quit payment system" is vital.

Within most nursing facilities, residents typically receive either skilled or non-skilled nursing care. Skilled care (i.e., care delivered when a resident requires more intensive nursing and rehabilitation services) is available to Medicare beneficiaries following a hospitalization under Medicare Part A. Non-skilled (i.e., general nursing facility care) is typically paid for privately or by state Medicaid programs. (Table 4)

Table 4. Skilled Versus Non-Skilled Nursing Facility Care

	Eligibility	Room & Board	Physician Services	Medication
Skilled	For Medicare beneficiaries requiring skilled nursing care following a 3-day acute hospitalization.	Part A	Part B	Part A
General Nursing Care (Non-skilled)	ADL/IADL needs	Medicaid / LTC insurance / Private Payment	Part B	Part D
			Part C	

Source: Based on the information from CMS including that available in the Medicare & You Handbook   http://www.medicare.gov/Publications/Pubs/pdf/10050.pdf

Medicare beneficiaries who need short-term skilled care (nursing or rehabilitation services) following a hospital stay require at least three days of hospitalization. Hospital observation days cannot help a Medicare beneficiary qualify for covered services in a skilled nursing facility (SNF). The Medicare SNF benefit pays facilities a pre-determined daily rate for each day of care up to 100 days. The prospective payment system (PPS) rates are determined through Resource Utilization Groups (RUGs). Residents are assigned to one of 53 RUGs based on resident characteristics and expected service use (e.g., skilled nursing, rehabilitation). After the first two weeks of a skilled facility stay, Medicare Part A no longer covers 80 percent of the cost. This presents a financial difficulty for many elderly persons.

Also known as Medical Insurance, Medicare Part B covers practitioner (e.g., physicians, physicians' assistants, and nurse practitioners) and rehabilitation services (e.g., occupational therapy, physical therapy, speech therapy) for non-skilled residents. Medicare Part B also covers vaccines such as influenza and pneumococcal pneumonia.

Medicare is expanding programs for beneficiaries in- and outside of the traditional nursing facility. Under Medicare Part C (i.e., Medicare Advantage), managed care organizations are responsible for providing all the benefits available under Medicare Part A, B, and D. In 1987, United Healthcare launched the Evercare program, which utilizes NPs within nursing facilities to provide timely care, thereby reducing emergency department evaluations and hospital admissions and increasing preventive care. The Evercare program also provides skilled level services at nursing facilities without Medicare's three days of hospitalization requirement.

More recently, the Medicare Modernization Act allowed continuing development of these types of programs as well as a broader range of options under Medicare Advantage (MA) and Special Needs Plans (SNP). SNPs are authorized to focus on one of three distinct patients groups: residents of nursing homes, dually eligible seniors (those who are entitled to Medicare Part A and/or Part B *and* are eligible for some form of Medicaid benefit), or those suffering from multiple chronic illnesses. The SNFs receive financial incentives to provide care that improves health outcomes and prevents hospitalizations.

Medicare Part D, the prescription drug benefit that took effect on January 1, 2006, moved drug coverage from Medicaid to Medicare for those individuals with both Medicare and Medicaid (Dual Eligibles). Residents enrolled in Medicaid receive Medicare Part D medications without copayments or premiums. While Medicaid no longer pays for Part D covered medications for the dually eligible, Medicaid does cover non-Part D medications such as benzodiazepines. Medicaid also covers the daily cost of nursing facility room and board for non-skilled stays.

All state Medicaid programs have two eligibility requirements that regulate which beneficiaries may obtain Medicaid financial support for their nursing facility stays; 1) financial eligibility and 2) medical eligibility. With respect to medical eligibility, each state adopts its own procedures and criteria set, because CMS grants medical necessity determinations to the states. Medicaid is the principle payer for nursing home care, responsible for room and board as well as most medical services.[15] Medicaid reimbursement is critical, in that improvements in clinical quality have been demonstrated to increase as a result of higher Medicaid payments.[16]

Unfortunately, current payment systems do not include incentives for nursing homes to care for residents within the facility rather than sending them to the hospital. In effect, the nursing staff can either 1) complete an assessment, provide the information to the attending physician, obtain diagnostic tests as ordered, and manage the resident during the shift, or 2) simply call the attending, state "the resident does not look good," and recommend that the resident be sent to the hospital. Given the choices, it is easy to see why the nurse often opts for the hospital emergency department.

From the attending physician's perspective, sending the resident to the emergency department for assessment and any future management translates into decreased liability. And, for attending physicians who follow their hospitalized patients, it can mean increased visit revenue for acute care management.

For the nursing home administrator, a resident being transferred to the hospital signifies decreased liability as well as increased revenue when that resident returns under the Medicare Part A subacute stay.

One can easily see that the current incentives, or lack thereof, do nothing to encourage the nursing home to raise its clinical services to a level at which they might care for urgently ill residents on site, thus avoiding hospitalizations.

The cost of failing to provide appropriate urgent care to NH residents is significant and likely to grow. Beyond the overall increased health care costs related to paying for acute hospitalization rather than ongoing care in the nursing home setting, there are indirect costs such as the emotional trauma to the resident and family due to a transition in care and the well-established adverse effects and iatrogenic complications of hospitalization. A recent study from the Kaiser Family Foundation asserts that a 25 percent reduction in hospitalizations among Medicare residents in long term care facilities could have yielded a savings of $2.1 billion last year alone.[17]

Fortunately, efforts are under way to correct this problem. The alignment of incentives is a cornerstone of Special Needs Plans (SNP).[18] SNPs are Medicare Advantage plans that, rather than serving all Medicare beneficiaries in a geographic region, can focus on one of three unique groups of beneficiaries; those suffering from a specific chronic illness such as Alzheimer's Disease, those having both Medicare and Medicaid, and nursing home residents. United Healthcare's Evercare focuses on nursing home residents as a specific population served by a Medicare managed care plan.

With responsibility for Medicare Parts A, B, and D and the freedom to operate more efficiently than Medicare, the Evercare program offers unique services. For instance, the Evercare program increases the availability of primary care services by having a dedicated NP available in the nursing home. This level of availability increases the likelihood that an acute change in condition can be assessed directly on-site by a member of the primary care team rather than over the phone by an attending physician who may not be fully aware of the resident's current status and needs. Beyond increased PCP services, Evercare can provide immediate skilled services without the Medicare-required three-day hospitalization (i.e., allowing residents who need intravenous hydration and medications to receive these when needed in the nursing home setting).

Quality of care can be affected, for better or worse, during the transition of care from one setting to another. When residents transition from the LTC facility to another setting, they are at high risk for the adverse effects of prescribing or transcription errors. Overlooked appointments, diagnoses, or laboratory tests as well as missed or duplicated medications are just a few of the potential errors that can lead to poor outcomes.

Seamless transitions from the hospital to home, skilled nursing care, or home health care will reduce these errors. Selected Quality Improvement Organizations (QIOs) under contract with CMS are trying to improve care coordination; promote seamless transitions; and reduce re-hospitalizations. Medicare is striving to improve transitions by encouraging provider investments in health information technology as well as anticipating a "bundled" payment system that would financially tie hospitals and nursing facilities together for an episode of resident care. Medicare is also encouraging the development of systems that will hold hospitals financially accountable for poor outcomes during transitions of care in a system that will have interdisciplinary teams to work on ensuring improved transitions.

Future Challenges and Direction

Even the approaches discussed may not be enough to overcome the challenges facing nursing homes today. These challenges include:

- Workforce shortages coupled with increasing demand
- Continued inadequacy of public financing
- The need for increasing application of technology
- Process-oriented (vs. outcome-based) regulations
- An increasingly litigious environment

In meeting these challenges, nursing homes are likely to face additional regulatory changes, new financial models, and delivery models increasingly focused on resident-centered care. Beyond these approaches, there is a movement focused on transforming the culture within LTC.

The following are the three principal transformative models aimed at improving the quality of care in LTC:

The Eden Alternative is an international not-for-profit organization whose vision is to eliminate loneliness, helplessness, and boredom by improving the lives of elders and their care partners and transforming the communities in which they live and work. *The Eden Alternative's* principle-based philosophy empowers care partners to transform institutional approaches to care into the creation of a community where life for elders is worth living.

The Green House Model, developed by Dr. William Thomas after The Eden Alternative, creates a small intentional community for a group of elders and staff. A radical departure from traditional skilled nursing homes and assisted living facilities, *The Green House* model alters facility size, interior design, staffing patterns, and methods of delivering skilled professional services. Its primary purpose is to serve as a place where elders can receive assistance and support with activities of daily living and clinical care, without the assistance and care becoming the focus of their existence. *The Green House* model is intended to de-institutionalize LTC by eliminating large nursing facilities and creating habilitative, social settings.

The Wellspring Model for improving quality of care in nursing homes was pioneered in 1994 by an alliance of 11 not-for-profit providers in Wisconsin. *Wellspring* seeks to enhance the well-being of residents by improving the quality of care, increasing staff skill levels, and reducing employee turnover. The model includes:

- Clinical training modules,

- Interdisciplinary teams whose members attend trainings and create and implement interventions to improve the quality of care for residents within the facility,

- A *Wellspring* Coordinator at each facility to guide the teams through the implementation process, and

- A *Wellspring* Nursing Consultant who serves as an advisor, educator, and consultant.

CMS's Quality Improvement Organizations are equipped to assist with this transformation. CMS contracts with 53 QIOs—one in each state and territory—to work with consumers, physicians, nursing homes, and other entities to refine care delivery systems and investigate complaints of poor quality care. In their 8th scope of work (SOW), QIOs are focused on several initiatives in nursing homes. These initiatives include decreased restraint use; improved management of chronic pain; improvement in high-risk pressure ulcers; and advancement in excellence in care.

In 2008, QIOs began work on the 9th SOW, a major theme of which is care transitions to reduce hospital readmissions. QIOs are using an Internet-based standardized assessment instrument, the Continuing Assessment Record and Evaluation (CARE). QIOs will likely continue to be a resource for LTC providers in their quest for improvements in the quality of care.

To date, the results have been impressive. Some nursing homes have accomplished cultural change, e.g., less staff absenteeism and lower staff turnover, fewer resident behavioral problems, lower use of psychoactive medications, decreased incidence of pressure ulcers and contractures, and fewer complaints.[19] Clearly, for continued improvement in LTC the focus must broaden beyond regulation, reporting, and financial realignment. Cultural transformation will be essential to provide the resources necessary for delivering comprehensive high-quality care to the LTC resident.

Study and Discussion Questions (Answers on page 174)

1. In its 1986 report, *Improving the Quality of Care in Nursing Homes*, the IOM expert panel recommended all of the following except:

    A. A stronger federal role in improving quality

    B. Revisions in performance standards, and the inspection—i.e., survey process

C. Improved staff training

D. Reducing requirement around assessment of resident needs

E. A dynamic and improved regulatory process.

2. Name the pivotal legislation that came out of the Institute of Medicine Report: *Improving the Quality of Care in Nursing Homes* that has been key in raising quality-of-care standards and strengthening federal and state oversight of nursing homes.

A. Omnibus Budget Reconciliation Act of 1987 (OBRA)

B. Balanced Budget Act of 1997 (BBA 97)

C. Balanced Budget Refinement Act of 1999

D. Affordable Care Act of 2010

E. Home and Community-Based Services (HCBS)

3. Name the regulation responsible for the current movement in caring for nursing home level of care individuals outside the nursing home that provides states with new flexibility to expand benefits and financial eligibility through a Medicaid state plan amendment instead of the more restrictive waiver process.

A. Omnibus Budget Reconciliation Act of 1987 (OBRA)

B. Balanced Budget Act of 1997 (BBA 97)

C. Balanced Budget Refinement Act of 1999

D. Affordable Care Act of 2010

E. Home and Community-Based Services (HCBS)

4. The "value-based purchasing" concept embedded in the Nursing Home Value-Based Purchasing Demonstration is expected to result in cost savings for Medicare through reductions in hospitalizations and subsequent skilled nursing facility stays.

A. True

B. False

5. Following a minimum 3-day inpatient hospitalization, the subacute nursing home stay is paid for by:

A. Medicare Part A

B. Medicare Part B

C. Medicare Part D

D. Medicaid

6. A Special Needs Plan that provides services to nursing home residents is covered through which program:

A. Medicare Part A

B. Medicare Part B

C. Medicare Part C

D. Medicare Part D

E. Medicaid

Answers: 1 (D), 2 (A), 3 (E), 4 (False), 5 (A), 6 (C).

Case Study

Evercare is one of several SNPs that operate within nursing homes. SNPs are *Medicare Advantage* plans that provide all the benefits available under Medicare but with additional flexibility that permits them to broaden the scope of services and provide payment incentives to care for nursing home residents in a more efficient and effective manner.

Discuss how the traditional Medicare benefit provides disincentives for efficient and effective care for nursing home residents and how, by contrast, a SNP can provide positive incentives.

Suggested Readings

Institute of Medicine Report: *Improving the Quality of Care in Nursing Homes*

MedPac Report on Nursing Homes available at http://www.medpac.gov/publications%5 Ccongressional_reports%5CMar04_Ch3C.pdf

Kaiser Family Foundation Report on Nursing Homes available at http://www.kff.org/ medicaid/longtermcare.cfm

SCAN Foundation Research & Reports on LTC available at http://www.thescanfoundation.org/

References

1. Institute of Medicine. *Improving the Quality of Long-Term Care.* Washington, DC: National Academies Press, 2001.

2. US Government Accountability Office. Despite Increased Oversight, Challenges Remain in Ensuring High-Quality Care and Resident Safety (GAO-06-117). Washington, DC: US Government Accountability Office, 2005.

3. US Government Accountability Office. Nursing Homes: Efforts to Strengthen Federal Enforcement Have Not Deterred Some Homes from Repeated Harming Residents (GAO-07-241). Washington, DC: US Government Accountability Office, 2007.

4. Administration on Aging. National Ombudsman Reporting System Data Tables, 2005.

5. Reschovsky JD. The demand for post-acute and chronic care in nursing homes. *Medical Care,* 36(4);475-90. April 1998.

6. McCormick JC, Chulis GS. Growth in residential alternatives to nursing homes 2001. *Health Care Finance Review,* 24(4):143-50, Summer 2003.

7. Cromwell J, Donoghue S. Gilman BH. Expansion of Medicare's definition of post-acute transfers. *Health Care Finance Review,* 24(2):95-113, Winter 2002.

8. Shugarman LR, Garland R. *Nursing Home Selection: How Do Consumers Choose?* Volume II: *Findings from the Website Content Review.* Santa Monica, CA: RAND Corporation, 2006.

9. Stevenson DG. Is a Public Reporting Approach Appropriate for Nursing Home Care?" *Journal of Health Politics, Policy and Law,* 31(4):773-810, Aug. 2006.

10. Minority Staff, Special Investigations Decision, Committee on Government Reform, US House of Representatives. HHS "Nursing Home Compare" Website Has Major Flaws. Report prepared for Rep. Henry A. Waxman and Sen. Charles E. Grassley, February 21, 2002.

11. Nursing Home Compare. Medicare: The official U.S. government site for people with Medicare website Available at http://www.medicare.gov/NHCCompare/home.asp.

12. Mukamel DB, Glance LG, Li Y, *et al.* Does risk adjustment of the CMS quality measures for nursing homes matter? *Med Care,* 46(5):532-41, May 2008.

13. Rowland FN, Cowles M, Dickstein C, Katz PR. Impact of Medical Director Certification on Nursing Home Quality of Care. *JAMDA,* 10(6):431-5, July 2009.

14. Flynn L, Liang Y, Dickson GL, Aiken LH. Effects of Nursing Practice Environments on Quality Outcomes in Nursing Homes. *JAGS,* 58(12)2401-6, Dec. 2010.

15. Miller EA, Mor V, Clark M. Reforming long term care in the United States: findings from a national survey of specialists. *The Gerontologist,* 50(2):238-252, Apr. 2010.

16. Grabowski DC, Feng Z, Intrator O, *et al,* Medicaid nursing home payment and the role of provider taxes. *Med Care Res Rev,* 65(4):514-27, Aug. 2008.

17. Mor V, Gruneir A, Feng Z, *et al.* The effect of state policies on nursing home resident outcomes. *JAGS,* 53(1):3-9, Jan. 2011.

18. Jacobson G, Neuman T, Damico A. *Medicare Spending and Use of Medical Service for Beneficiaries in Nursing Homes and Other Long Term Care Facilities: A Potential for Achieving Medicare Savings and Improving the Quality of Care.* The Henry J. Kaiser Family Foundation, October 2010. http://www.kff.org/medicare/upload/8109.pdf. Accessed Dec. 6, 2010.

19. Centers for Medicare and Medicaid Services. Special Needs Plan—Fact Sheets & Data Summary. www.cms.hhs.gov/SpecialNeedsPlans/Downloads/FSNPFACT.pdf. Accessed July 22, 2010.

20. Lopez RP, Amella EJ, Strumpf NE, *et al*. The Influence of nursing home culture on the use of feeding tubes. *Arch Intern Med*, 170(1):83-8,Jan. 11, 2010.

Chapter 11

Measuring Quality in Ambulatory Care

By Bettina Berman, RN, CPHQ, CNOR
and Valerie P. Pracilio, MPH, CPPS

Executive Summary

To a great extent, quality measurement has been an inpatient phenomenon, and hospitals have invested substantial resources to meet regulatory and compliance requirements. As national efforts have shifted to controlling costs and advancing quality of care, the ambulatory setting has become a target for improvement.[1] Ambulatory care is complex and fragmented with a broad clinical scope that includes prevention, counseling, and chronic disease management.[2] A high utilizer of health care services, the typical Medicare beneficiary visits seven physicians in four practice settings annually.[3,4] Those with chronic conditions visit 10 physicians across seven practices.[4] Patients are responsible for navigating between clinics, laboratories, and radiology suites, as well as between their providers. How well patients and providers work together to coordinate all aspects of ambulatory care affects the overall value of patient care.

National priorities aimed at improving care quality, coordination, and cost control offer hope. The patient-centered medical home and the accountable care organization models, outgrowths of the Patient Protection and Affordable Care Act (ACA), are beginning to increase accountability for ambulatory providers to achieve quality goals. Progress toward these goals is aided by performance measures such as the Physician Quality Reporting System (PQRS). But all of these strategies hinge on an organizational commitment to achieving value (a function of quality and cost) by implementing the processes necessary to comply with new standards.

Learning Objectives

1. Recognize the quality challenges in the ambulatory setting.
2. Understand the strategies that can be used to increase value in ambulatory care.
3. Introduce and describe the various components of quality measurement.
4. Increase provider awareness of new models for delivery of care.

Key Words: Accountable Care Organization (ACO), Accreditation, Affordable Care Act (ACA), Ambulatory Care, Chronic Disease, Patient-Centered Medical Home (PCMH), Pay-for- Performance, Physician Quality Reporting System (PQRS), Prevention, Quality, Quality Measures

Introduction

Some describe the U.S. health care system as the best in the world; the technology is advanced, the tools are cutting edge, and the providers are well-trained. Even with these characteristics, 1.2 billion visits[3] to health care institutions in a given year lead to 6.3 million injuries.[5] Despite the efforts of many well-intentioned people, the system, or lack thereof, is at the heart of most challenges we currently face. This was first made apparent by the Institute of Medicine in 1999 with the publication of *To Err Is Human*,[6] a report that led health care leaders to seek a better understanding of the magnitude of the problem and its underlying causes, thus defining the field of quality and safety improvement.

To date, most health care quality improvement (QI) efforts have focused on the hospital inpatient setting. Relatively little consideration has been given to the ambulatory environment where patients receive more than half of their care.[7] The greatest opportunities to improve coordination, and increase value, exist in the ambulatory environment.

The Ambulatory Setting

Ambulatory care encompasses a range of health services that can be provided on an outpatient basis and that do not require an overnight stay. The health professionals who practice in ambulatory settings—physicians, nurses, nurse practitioners, physicians' assistants, and pharmacists, among others—diagnose, observe, treat, and provide rehabilitation and preventive services that are essential to achieve high-quality patient outcomes.

Ambulatory providers are expected to serve as care coordinators. With chronic disease ranked as the number one cause of death, disability, and increasing health care costs, care coordination remains a formidable challenge.[3,8] Chronic disease management is among the many issues physicians address during ambulatory visits. Coordination of care relies on the combined efforts of all health professionals to share information and work together with the patient to meet her or his health care needs. With almost 45 percent of the U.S. population suffering from at least one chronic condition, there is an imminent need to improve efficiency and effectiveness of health care delivery.[8]

The ambulatory environment is the place where patients most frequently interact with health care professionals and receive preventive, observational, and rehabilitative care. With the recent implementation of the patient-centered medical homes (PCMH) model, the primary care setting has become a gateway for all health care services. In theory, patients who receive the majority of their care in the ambulatory setting (i.e., patients who have repeated interactions with the same provider or provider group over time) may have better outcomes, because continuity creates more opportunities for monitoring chronic conditions.

It is also important to note the patient's role in care management and in information exchange. Partnerships between patients and providers are powerful tools in delivering safe and effective care—two key aims for achieving better health care that will be described later.[9]

Ambulatory Quality

Quality is "the degree to which health services for individuals and populations increase the likelihood of desired health outcomes and are consistent with current professional knowledge."[6] Since the IOM published its report using this definition, a number of measurement systems have been developed to assess quality of care. Clinical guidelines, a product of collective evidence-based knowledge, have been established by professional societies. Despite this progress, there is a significant need to identify mechanisms to further improve ambulatory care, where the volume of care delivery far exceeds that of the inpatient environment.[7]

Care delivered in the ambulatory environment addresses three primary purposes; prevention, management, and treatment. U.S. statistics show that slightly more than half of recommended preventive care (54.5 percent) and chronic care (56 percent) is actually received.[7] Facilitating the continuity of relationships between patients and their ambulatory providers is a tool that could have lasting effects on all aspects of patient care.[7] While progress has been made in terms of availability of information to make decisions and guide strategies in the ambulatory environment, there is still significant work to be done.

Prevention

The U.S. health care system is under considerable pressure to increase its efficiency. Due to the significant proportion of the population affected, a full 75 percent of health care spending is on chronic illness. One strategy for increasing efficiency is to focus on the two types of prevention: clinical preventive services and community preventive services. Clinical prevention involves screening, immunizations, and counseling by health care professionals whereas community prevention is focused on policies and programs aimed at the population level.[10] For the purposes of this chapter, "prevention" refers to clinical quality of care delivered in ambulatory settings.

The benefits of prevention can be measured in terms of productivity and cost-effectiveness. Administratively, prevention produces value for the organization; clinically, prevention saves lives. Increasing the use of five recommended preventive services (daily dose of aspirin, smoking cessation counseling, colorectal cancer screening, flu immunization, and breast cancer screening) to 90 percent would save more than 100,000 American lives each year.[8] Released in June 2011, the first National Prevention Strategy recognizes that preventing disease will improve the nation's health.[11] The strategy outlines a number of actionable recommendations, including educating patients about the benefits of preventive services and team-based approaches to sharing information that providers can use to address patient needs.[11]

Management

The ambulatory environment is where most conditions are diagnosed and managed. Screening to assess disease control, monitoring medication lists, counseling, and education all take place in this setting. Regular follow-up care and disease management education rely on the combined efforts of the provider and the patient. Current quality initiatives focus on incentivizing providers who meet certain quality goals, but patient adherence is the component that offers the greatest opportunity. While patient adherence is difficult to measure and often relies on capturing information from multiple systems, we know that patients are more likely to take action when counseled to do so by their physicians. Provider recommendations are integral to both prevention and disease management.

Treatment

Providing health care to an aging population is one of the greatest challenges our health system faces. One out of every two Americans suffers from at least one chronic disease (e.g., heart disease, cancer, and stroke), and beneficiaries with chronic conditions spend 99 percent of Medicare dollars.[10] Factors that contribute to the prevalence of chronic disease include obesity and smoking. Each of these has behavioral components that could be affected by provider counseling in the ambulatory setting.[3] Almost a quarter of Americans are prescribed three or more drugs, some of which are used to manage these conditions and require close monitoring.[3] Numerous policy debates have highlighted these issues, which remain a growing concern. In order to increase efficiency, better value must be achieved by balancing quality and cost. The ambulatory environment is the ideal place to start.

Institute of Medicine's Six Quality Aims

The IOM's second landmark report described the "chasm" between the quality of the current U.S. health care system and one that is founded on quality. To narrow the chasm and move toward improved quality, the IOM outlined six characteristics of a good quality health care system: safe, effective, patient-centered, timely, efficient, and equitable.[12] These characteristics are explained in detail in Chapter 2. Each of the six characteristics has a place in the ambulatory environment.

Through provider-patient partnerships, health care professionals gain an understanding of patients' needs and preferences, both of which are essential for patient-centered care. The provider-patient relationship is a tool by which providers can deliver safe care using evidence-based strategies. Efficiency and timeliness are operational elements at the organizational level. Addressing these aims requires collaboration between providers and administrative professionals in order to recognize and address elements that affect value and patient experience. In the ambulatory environment, this may require development of practice policies related to testing procedures and information exchange with other institutions, as well as metrics to identify when a coordination is improving.

The Quality Measure Development Process

The rising cost of care has increased the urgency to measure quality of care and hold institutions and providers accountable for performance.[13] Measuring quality of care requires development of metrics, which are often derived from evidence-based clinical guidelines that provide diagnostic or therapeutic guidance for providers.[14] Quality measures, while predicated on the same body of evidence, represent standards of care—either a diagnostic or therapeutic action—that the provider *must* perform in order to meet the measurement criteria. Instances in which the provider achieves the measure objective are expressed in the numerator. The population of those for whom the action should be taken according to the measure specifications is reflected in the denominator.

The Centers for Medicare and Medicaid Services (CMS) promotes the use of quality measures through the Physician Quality Reporting System (PQRS) program, and the National Committee for Quality Assurance (NCQA) utilizes the Healthcare Effectiveness Data and Information Set (HEDIS) measures to rank health plan performance. The benefit of validation by organizations such as CMS and NCQA is that they are able to expedite incorporation of new evidence into clinical practice through these measurement programs.[14]

Quality measures follow a three-component framework (structure-process-outcome), originally identified by Avedis Donabedian, for assessing quality of care.[15]

- *Structure* refers to the health care setting where care is provided. Structural measures can include assessments of electronic medical records (EMRs), patient registries, staff expertise, and organizational structure.

- *Process* measures focus on the actions involved in care delivery, taking both the environment and key players into account. Medication management, blood pressure screenings, preventive testing, and compliance with evidence-based guidelines are all examples of process measures.[6]

- *Outcomes* measures are indications of health as a direct result of the care provided. Health outcomes can be divided into intermediate or proximal, and long-term or distal.[15] Examples of proximal outcomes for patients with diabetes are control of glycemic or lipid levels. Distal outcomes include events such as lower extremity amputation, kidney disease, or mortality.[16]

Composite measures that combine results of several quality measures to provide a comprehensive assessment of an episode of care and measures that assess patient experience are becoming more common strategies to evaluate outcomes.[17] (Table 1, page 182)

Table 1. Ambulatory Quality Measure Examples

Structural Measures

Measure Definition	Measure Description
Health Information Technology (HIT): Adoption/Use of Electronic Health Records (EHR)	Documents whether provider has adopted and is using health information technology. To report this measure, the eligible professional must have adopted and be using a certified Physician Quality Reporting system qualified or other acceptable EHR system.
Adoption/Use of Medication Electronic Prescribing Measure	Documents whether the eligible professional has adopted a qualified electronic prescribing (eRx) system and the extent of use in the ambulatory setting.

Process Measures

Measure Definition	Measure Description
Oral antiplatelet therapy prescribed for patients with coronary artery disease (CAD)	Percentage of patients aged 18 years and older with a diagnosis of CAD who were prescribed oral antiplatelet therapy.
Screening or therapy for osteoporosis for women aged 65 years and older	Percentage of female patients aged 65 years and older who have a dual-energy X-ray absorptiometry (DXA) measurement ordered or performed at least once since age 60 or pharmacologic therapy prescribed within 12 months.
Documentation of current medications in the medical record	Percentage of patients aged 18 years and older with a list of current medications documented by the provider.

Outcomes Measures

Measure Definition	Measure Description
Diabetes Mellitus: Hemoglobin A1c poor control in diabetes mellitus	Percentage of patients aged 18 through 75 years with diabetes mellitus who had most recent hemoglobin A1c greater than 9%.
Diabetes Mellitus: Low-density lipoprotein (LDL-C) control in diabetes mellitus	Percentage of patients aged 18 through 75 years with diabetes mellitus who had most recent LDL-C level in control (less than 100 mg/dl).

Source: http://www.cms.gov/PQRS/15_MeasuresCodes.asp#TopOfPage

Patient experience has become a recognized component of outcomes assessment. The Agency for Healthcare Research and Quality (AHRQ) has been the leader in developing surveys to capture patient experience. Initially developed to measure patients' perceptions of health plans, the Consumer Assessment of Health Care Providers and Systems (CAHPS) surveys now extend to multiple care settings. The CAHPS Clinician and Group Survey (CG-CAHPS) assesses the patient's experience of ambulatory care and covers areas such as access to care, follow-up on test results, and physician communication. While hospitals are mandated by CMS to report on the CAHPS Hospital Survey (HCAHPS), completion of the ambulatory survey remains voluntary.[18]

Quality measures serve a dual purpose: 1) they help identify gaps in care and 2) they encourage evidence-based clinical practice to fill the identified gaps. Quality measures drive improvement, inform consumer decisions, and influence payment.[17] Multiple stakeholders engage in measure development to identify gaps in care. Over the past decade, the health care industry has seen a tremendous increase in the number of quality measures available to track the clinical performance of individual providers. Professional societies are becoming more involved in measure development as a means for increasing physician participation and influencing the health care quality environment.[13]

Ambulatory Quality Measures

Healthcare Effectiveness Data Information Set (HEDIS)

As noted earlier in this chapter, the most established measurement set for ambulatory care quality is HEDIS. The National Committee for Quality Assurance (NCQA), a private not-for-profit organization dedicated to quality improvement, develops and maintains the HEDIS measures to capture effectiveness and access to care as well as utilization. Data collected through HEDIS are complied by and used for accreditation and health plan ranking.[1] At the provider or group practice level, commercial payers use HEDIS indicators as they establish metrics for value-based purchasing contracts.

Agency for Healthcare Research and Quality (AHRQ) Quality Indicators (QI)

Ambulatory providers aim to avoid hospitalization by providing appropriate care in the outpatient setting. Metrics to assess Ambulatory Care Sensitive Conditions (ACSC) by utilizing hospital administrative data were developed by AHRQ. The indicators are divided into four modules covering a broad range of care settings and aspects of quality: 1) prevention quality indicators, 2) inpatient quality indicators, 3) patient safety indicators, and 4) pediatric quality indicators. The prevention quality indicators cover conditions for which hospital admission may have been avoided through improved outpatient care. The ACSCs include chronic conditions (e.g., diabetes, heart failure) and acute conditions (e.g., pneumonia, dehydration). Reporting on these indicators provides organizations with valuable information regarding the quality of care.

Physician Quality Reporting System (PQRS)

As noted above, HEDIS assesses quality at the health-plan level and ACSC relies on hospital data. The Physician Quality Reporting System (PQRS) is the first program that assesses ambulatory quality at the physician level. Although the rising cost of health care has increased provider awareness of and interest in quality of care, there remain strong opponents who question the validity, reliability, risk-adjustment, and data collection methodology of quality metrics. In an effort to increase the value of services provided, CMS is working to transform the Medicare program from passive payer to active purchaser of high-quality health care services by linking payment to the value of services delivered.[19]

In 2007, CMS introduced the Physician Quality Reporting Initiative (PQRI), later renamed the Physician Quality Reporting System (PQRS), a financial incentive program for quality reporting. The first version of the program consisted of 74 individual quality measures that relied on the use of CPT-II billing codes to capture information on process and outcomes measures of quality (e.g., HbA1c levels for diabetes monitoring, smoking cessation counseling). The program has expanded, and, today, almost 200 performance indicators are available to physician and non-physician providers through this program. Participation in PQRS is still voluntary, but physicians who do not report on measures by 2014 will be subject to a payment differential. Also, CMS plans to increase transparency by making physician performance data available on the Physician Compare website beginning in January 2013. For further detail on PQRS, see Chapter 3.

Identification of measurement topics is guided by priorities and goals set forth by the National Priorities Partnership (NPP), a collaboration of health care stakeholders convened by the NQF to promote changes in health care delivery.[20] Among the organizations involved in measurement development are medical professional societies and the American Medical Association (AMA) Physician Consortium for Performance Improvement (PCPI), quality improvement organizations (QIOs) subcontracted by CMS, and the NCQA. Individuals with clinical expertise in the measurement area are invited to provide input on measures prior to testing and public commenting. The final step, measure endorsement by the National Quality Forum (NQF), provides validation and helps to disseminate the measure. The AQA, formerly known as the Ambulatory Care Quality Alliance, also plays a role in engaging the stakeholder community by establishing guidelines for dissemination of quality data to consumers.[21] (Figure 1, page 185)

Health Information Technology: Support for Quality Measurement

Implementation and use of health information technology (HIT) is widely seen as a key strategy for measuring and improving health care quality and safety. The Health Information Technology for Economic and Clinical Health (HITECH) Act, part of the American Recovery and Reinvestment Act (ARRA) of 2009, provides financial support for providers who achieve "Meaningful Use" criteria set forth by CMS.

Figure 1. Measurement Development Process

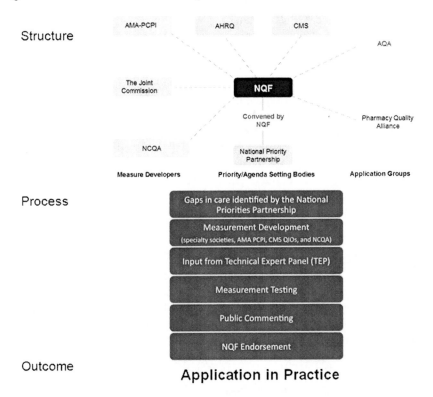

Structure

AMA-PCPI   AHRQ   CMS

AQA

The Joint Commission   **NQF**

Convened by NQF   Pharmacy Quality Alliance

NCQA   National Priority Partnership

Measure Developers   Priority/Agenda Setting Bodies   Application Groups

Process

Gaps in care identified by the National Priorities Partnership

Measurement Development
(specialty societies, AMA PCPI, CMS QIOs, and NCQA)

Input from Technical Expert Panel (TEP)

Measurement Testing

Public Commenting

NQF Endorsement

Outcome   **Application in Practice**

Adapted from: The Center for Medicare and Medicaid Services. Quality Measures Development Overview. Available at: https://www.cms.gov/qualityinitiativesgeninfo/downlaods/QualityMeasuresDevelopmentOverview.pdf

Today, most reporting on quality measures is conducted through manual review of medical records. ARRA specifies that providers who report on clinical quality measures through certified electronic health records (EHRs) and who demonstrate Meaningful Use will be eligible for incentives. To help providers meet these requirements, CMS has developed electronic measure specifications that allow quality information to be captured in discrete fields of the EHR and in electronic submissions to CMS. Electronic abstraction and calculation of the performance measures provides clinicians with real-time data to support improvements in care. Meaningful Use data allow performance to be tied to payment, thereby enhancing provider accountability through public reporting.[17] While these efforts encourage quality measurement and reporting, a number of challenges remain. One example is variable HIT adoption and use among providers, which makes it difficult to utilize the EHR as a tool for evaluation.[22]

Benefits of Accreditation

Accreditation of ambulatory care sites is voluntary, but many provider organizations elect to earn accreditation as evidence that they meet the highest standards of medical practice.[4]

Organizational commitment to providing the highest level of patient safety and quality of care when compared to national benchmarks is a recognized benefit of accreditation. Often, accreditation makes it easier for organizations to negotiate contracts with payers and to increase their competitive advantage in terms of patient referrals and recruitment and retention of staff.[23]

The accreditation process involves external peer review of the organization's compliance with established performance measures.[24] The Joint Commission (JC) and the Accreditation Association for Ambulatory Health Care (AAAHC) are non-governmental organizations that offer accreditation for ambulatory care facilities and patient-centered medical homes (PCMHs). The JC, a not-for- profit organization that has accredited hospitals across the nation since 1951, recently expanded to include ambulatory care settings. The AAAHC utilizes a procedure similar to that of the JC for accreditation of ambulatory health care organizations, including ambulatory surgery centers, multi-specialty group practices, and managed care organizations.[25]

Accreditation of health care organizations can have a positive impact on clinical outcomes of patient care.[24] Organizations that choose to obtain JC accreditation submit to an on-site survey, conducted by a team of health care professionals skilled in ambulatory care, every three years. In addition to evaluating care processes, the survey assesses the organization's adherence to JC standards and the National Patient Safety Goals. The review of care processes assists health care organizations in identifying issues and opportunities for improvement.[23]

Ambulatory Care in Times of Transition

The Impact of Health Care Reform on Ambulatory Care Quality

Health care is costly, but greater cost does not necessarily equate with better quality of care. Geographic regions that spend less per Medicare beneficiary have been shown to provide better care and achieve equal or better outcomes.[26] Current payment models based on volume of services do not support strategies aimed at reducing costs. The goal of the Patient Protection and Affordable Care Act (ACA) is to increase the value of health care by improving quality and controlling costs.[27] The ACA will impact ambulatory care delivery because it attempts to control health care spending by incentivizing primary care and prevention. The legislation includes provisions that increase payments for services to Medicare and Medicaid beneficiaries and add coverage for preventive services. The ACA also established the Center for Medicare and Medicaid Innovation to test new payment models for the ambulatory setting. Models being tested include bundled payments for episodes of care and payment for services provided by patient-centered medical homes (PCMHs). Such models would reward care coordination, a strategy known to reduce cost.

Primary care providers are being encouraged to transform their practices into PCMHs, a model that is associated with improved clinical outcomes and patient satisfaction.[28] Recognition as a PCMH requires transformation of care delivery processes and implementation of new approaches to patient care that rely on re-designed practice patterns and procedures. The traditional physician-centered approach must be replaced by a patient-centered approach wherein care is provided by a multi-disciplinary health care team. Also, providers must be prepared to expand the clinical focus to include a population-based view of patient care as supported by the PCMH model. While medical homes receive financial support from a variety of public and private stakeholders, they also require strong organizational commitment.[29]

In addition to payment reforms for PCMHs, the ACA incorporates a national, shared savings program for accountable care organizations (ACOs)—i.e., groups of providers and health care service suppliers working together to coordinate care for the Medicare patients they serve.[30] This model was developed to improve co-ordination among physicians and provide efficient care by reducing the rate of health care spending and improving quality.[31,32] The ACO model is based on lessons learned from the CMS Physician Group Practice Demonstration Project and may include physician practices and PCMHs or hospitals, nursing homes, and home health agencies.[32] ACO providers share accountability for cost reduction and quality improvement in return for a share of the savings they jointly generate for Medicare.[31,33]

Under the federal rule, physicians and health care organizations can create voluntary ACO networks to be responsible for the care of Medicare beneficiaries. In addition to receiving fee-for-service payments, the ACO network earns a share in any savings achieved if benchmarks for cost and quality indicators are met.[34] Thus, the financial reward is tied to quality of care. The final ACO rule, released by CMS in October 2011, indicates patient attribution will be prospective with retrospective reconciliation and providers will have the opportunity to select a savings track without financial risk during the initial contract period.[33]

Patient participation in ACOs is voluntary, and Medicare beneficiaries are free to seek care from any provider outside the ACO.[35] Although this arrangement limits the ACO's ability to control costs, it provides flexibility for patients who may be skeptical about how care is delivered in an ACO.[36] Concern has also been expressed about limitations on provider participation and ability to practice independently in an ACO. Providers feel such limitations would negatively impact the physician-patient relationship on which improved coordination relies.[37]

Organizational Commitment and Leadership for Quality

It is important to realize that the ability to effect change can be hindered or helped by organizations. The strategies discussed in this chapter all rely on organizational commitment to improving ambulatory quality. When the leadership sets priorities that reflect a commitment to quality, opportunities arise to drive substantial improvements. When organizational support is absent, improvement is a formidable challenge.

Conclusions

Over the past decade, great advances have been made to improve the quality of health care in the U.S. Yet, we have a long way to go before cost-effective, high-quality care is delivered in the ambulatory care setting, where patients receive more than half of their care.

Ambulatory care is a complex setting wherein multiple providers manage different aspects of an individual patient's care. A number of new strategies recognize this complexity and offer structural frameworks to improve coordination. Although ambulatory providers increasingly are being held accountable for the quality of care they provide, there are few mechanisms for measurement, and access to data remains variable. We remain hopeful that quality of care in the ambulatory setting is gaining needed attention and that a significant unrecognized value will be achieved in this setting. Allocating resources for prevention and ambulatory management will reduce the need for costly acute treatment and are likely to produce sustainable improvements in quality of care.

Study and Discussion Questions

1. Describe the major challenges facing the current U.S. health care system.
2. Describe aspects of the ACA legislation that have the potential to transform primary care.

Suggested Readings and Web Sites

Readings

Commonwealth Fund—Starting on the Path to a High-Performance Health System: Analysis of the Payment and System Reform Provisions in the Patient Protection and Affordable Care Act of 2010, http://www.commonwealthfund.org/~/media/Files/Publications/Fund%20Report/2010/Sep/1442_Davis_Payment%20and%20System%20Reform_923v2.pdf .

National Quality Forum—The ABCs of Measurement, http://www.qualityforum.org/Measuring_Performance/ABCs_of_Measurement.aspx .

Web Sites

Centers for Medicare and Medicaid Services. Physician Quality Reporting Initiative, https://www.cms.gov/PQRS/downloads/PQRI2007ReportFinal12032008CSG.pdf

National Priorities Partnership, http://www.nationalprioritiespartnership.org/

References

1. Roski J, Gregory R. Performance measurement for ambulatory care: Moving towards a new agenda. *Int J Qual Health Care*, 13(6):447-453, Dec. 2001.

2. Leas BF, Goldfarb NI, Browne RC, *et al*. Ambulatory quality improvement in academic medical centers: A changing landscape. *Am J Med Qual*, 24(4):287-94, July-Aug. 2009.

3. CDC - chronic disease - overview, http://www.cdc.gov/chronicdisease/overview/index.htm. Published July 7. Updated 2010. Accessed 11/4/2011, 2011.

4. Kovner AR, Knickman JR. *Jonas & Kovner's Health Care Delivery in the United States,* 10th ed. New York: Springer Publishing Co., LLC, 2011.

5. Van Den Bos J, Rustagi K, Gray T, *et al*. The $17.1 billion problem: The annual cost of measurable medical errors. *Health Affairs*, 30(4):596-603, Apr. 2011.

6. Institute of Medicine. *To Err Is Human: Building a Safer Health System.* Washington, DC: National Academies Press, 2000, p. 287.

7. McGlynn EA, Asch SM, Adams J, *et al*. The quality of health care delivered to adults in the United States. *N Engl J Med*, 348(26):2635-45, June 26, 2003.

8. Partnership to Fight Chronic Disease. Almanac of chronic disease 2009. Available at: http://fightchronicdisease.org/index.cfm. Accessed 10/30/2011, 2009.

9. Bodenheimer T, Lorig K, Holman H, Grumbach K. Patient self-management of chronic disease in primary care. *JAMA*, 288(19):2469-2475, Nov. 20, 2002.

10. The value of prevention. http://www.fightchronicdisease.org/sites/default/files/docs/ValueofPreventionfactsheet81009.pdf. Accessed 11/4/2011, 2011.

11. National Prevention Council. National prevention strategy: America's plan for better health and wellness. 2011(June). http://www.healthcare.gov/prevention/nphpphc/strategy/report.pdf. Accessed 11/4/2011.

12. Institute of Medicine. *Crossing the Quality Chasm: A New Health System for the 21st Century.* Washington, DC: National Academies Press; 2001.

13. Ferris TG, Vogeli C, Marder J, Sennett CS, Campbell EG. Physician specialty societies and the development of physician performance measures. *Health Aff (Millwood)*. 26(6):1712-9, Nov.-Dec. 2007.

14. Measuring and improving quality of care: A report from the American Heart Association/American College of Cardiology first scientific forum on assessment of health care quality in cardiovascular disease and stroke. *Circulation*, 101(12):1483-93, Mar. 28, 2000.

15. Donabedian A. The evaluation of medical care programs. *Bull N Y Acad Med*, 44(2): 117-24, 1968.

16. Nicolucci A, Greenfield S, Mattke S. Selecting indicators for the quality of diabetes care at the health systems level in OECD countries. *International Journal for Quality in Health Care*, 18(suppl 1):26-30, Sept. 2006.

17. ABCs of measurement. http://www.qualityforum.org/Measuring_Performance/ABCs_of_Measurement.aspx. Accessed 11/3/2011.

18. Leverage existing efforts or use a centralized approach? Two strategies for community-wide implementation of the CAHPS clinician & group survey group survey. http://www.rwjf.org/pr/product.jsp?id=71814. Published July 1. Accessed 11/4/2011.

19. Physician quality reporting initiative: 2007 reporting experience. 2011 (December 3). https://www.cms.gov/mms/Downloads/QualityMeasuresDevelopmentOverview103009.pdf. Accessed 8/17/2011.

20. National priorities partnership. http://www.nationalprioritiespartnership.org/. Accessed 11/3/2011.

21. AQA. AQA strategic plan 2010. Oct. 28, 2010.

22. Roth CP, Lim YW, Pevnick JM, *et al.* The challenge of measuring quality of care from the electronic health record. *Am J Med Qual*, 24(5):385-94, Sept.-Oct. 2009.

23. The Joint Commission. http://www.jointcommission.org/. Accessed 9/9/2011.

24. Alkhenizan A, Shaw C. Impact of accreditation on the quality of healthcare services: A systematic review of the literature. *Ann Saudi Med*, 31(4):407-16, July-Aug. 2011.

25. Accreditation Association for Ambulatory Care. http://www.aaahc.org/eweb/StartPage.aspx. Accessed 11/3/2011.

26. Fisher ES, McClellan MB, Bertko J, *et al.* Fostering accountable health care: Moving forward in medicare. *Health Aff (Millwood)*, 28(2):w219-31, Mar.-Apr. 2009.

27. Davis K, Guterman S, Collins SR, *et al.* Starting on a path to a high performance health system: Analysis of the payment and system reform provisions in the patient protection and affordable care act of 2010. http://www.commonwealthfund.org/~/media/Files/Publications/Fund%20Report/2010/Sep/1442_Davis_Payment%20and%20System%20Reform_923v2.pdf. Accessed 11/3/2011.

28. Scholle SH, Saunders RC, Tirodkar MA, *et al.* Patient-centered medical homes in the United States. *J Ambul Care Manage*, 234(1):20-32, Jan. Mar. 2011.

29. Nutting PA, Miller WL, Crabtree BF, *et al.* Initial lessons from the first national demonstration project on practice transformation to a patient-centered medical home. *Ann Fam Med*, (3):254-60, May-June 2009.

30. Accountable care organizations: Improving care coordination for people with medicare. Healthcare.gov Web site. http://www.healthcare.gov/news/factsheets/2011/03/accountablecare03312011a.html. Published March 31, 2011. Updated 2011.

31. McClellan M, McKethan AN, Lewis JL, *et al.* A national strategy to put accountable care into practice. *Health Aff (Millwood)*, 29(5):982-90, May 2010.

32. Shortell SM, Casalino LP, Fisher ES. How the Center for Medicare and Medicaid Innovation should test accountable care organizations. *Health Aff (Millwood)*, 29(7):1293-8, July 2010.

33. Berwick DM. Making good on ACOs' promise—the final rule for the Medicare shared savings program. *N Engl J Med*, 365(19):1753-6, Nov. 10, 2011.

34. Meyer H. Accountable care organization prototypes: Winners and losers? *Health Aff (Millwood)*, 30(7):1227-31, July 2011.

35. Iglehart JK. The ACO regulations—some answers, more questions. *N Engl J Med*, 364(17):e35, Apr. 28, 2011.

36. Crosson FJ. Analysis & commentary: The accountable care organization: Whatever its growing pains, the concept is too vitally important to fail. *Health Aff (Millwood)*, 0(7):1250-5, July 2011.

37. Rosenthal MB, Cutler DM, Feder J. The ACO rules—striking the balance between participation and transformative potential. *N Engl J Med*, 365(4):e6, July 28, 2011.

Chapter 12

Measuring Quality in the Pharmacy

By David Nau, RPh, PhD and Laura Cranston, RPh

Executive Summary

The focus on delivering high-quality health care has never been greater. Numerous forces have converged to accelerate the demand for evidence of quality and value in health care, and the pharmacy profession has been evolving to meet this demand. Recent milestones in U.S. health care—implementation of the Medicare Part D Prescription Drug Benefit, the Patient Protection and Affordable Care Act, and the growth of value-based purchasing initiatives—have combined to heighten the attention of the pharmacy profession to the quality of medication use in this country.

The Pharmacy Quality Alliance (PQA) brings together stakeholders from pharmacy and other health care sectors to develop, test, and endorse "quality metrics" that focus on the appropriate and safe use of medications. These quality metrics are incorporated in Medicare Part D plan ratings and accreditation programs for pharmacy-related organizations. PQA also has sponsored demonstrations to show that health plans, pharmacy benefit managers (PBMs), and community pharmacies can work collaboratively to measure and improve the quality of medication use. As health plans expand their use of these quality metrics, the front-line pharmacists in community practice have become increasingly involved with quality improvement initiatives.

This chapter highlights the rapid growth of quality measurement and quality improvement activities in ambulatory/community pharmacy and provides examples of quality metrics employed by the Centers for Medicare and Medicaid (CMS), health plans, and pharmacies to improve the quality of medication use. It also provides an overview of how quality measurement and value-based purchasing initiatives are transforming pharmacy reimbursement systems to include pay-for-performance for pharmacies.

Learning Objectives

1. Identify the drivers for increased transparency in the quality of medication utilization and the quality of pharmacy services in the ambulatory sector.

2. Describe the PQA and its impact on the measurement of quality for prescription drug plans and community pharmacies.

3. Discuss the opportunity for re-alignment of financial incentives to facilitate the participation of pharmacies in collaborative efforts to improve the quality of medication use.

Introduction

The importance of pharmaceuticals in the treatment of chronic disease has never been greater. The creation of the Medicare Part D drug benefit, combined with the growth in the number of Medicare beneficiaries, has led to significant increases in the use of medications in the United States. Employers and Medicaid programs also have seen continued increases in drug expenditures. Although great public attention has been given to the costs of these medications, less attention has been given to the quality and safety of medication use. Not surprisingly, media reports of medication errors or drug diversion occasionally grab the headlines while ongoing efforts to systematically measure and improve the quality of medication use generally go unnoticed.

Hepler and Grainger-Rousseau's conceptualization of a pharmaceutical care system offers a good framework for examining the quality of medication use.[1] This pharmaceutical care system is similar to the drug-use process described by Knapp *et al.*[2] but adds the functions of drug monitoring and management to stress the importance of ongoing attention to the patient and his or her drug regimen.

Hepler and Grainger-Rousseau suggest that there are three key elements for proper functioning of a pharmaceutical care system: 1) initiating therapy, 2) monitoring therapy, and 3) managing (i.e., correcting) therapy. Each of these elements relies on multiple professionals, as well as the patient, to ensure that the system works well. As noted by Nau and Kirking,[3] the lack of information flow between health care professionals as well as the lack of coordination across providers can inhibit quality as it relates to the use of medications. Although improvements in health information technology are helping to improve the flow of information between professionals, the coordination of care across settings and across professionals remains suboptimal. Too many patients with chronic conditions "fall through the cracks" and do not receive adequate monitoring or management of their medication therapy.

Increasingly, the quality of medication utilization is being scrutinized by accreditation bodies (e.g., The Joint Commission, National Committee on Quality Assurance) and many pay-for-performance programs now include performance measures that pertain to medications. As more hospitals, health plans and physicians are held accountable for the quality of medication utilization, there are increased opportunities for pharmacists to assist in improving medication safety and quality. While the inclusion of pharmacists on medical teams and quality initiatives within hospitals has become a "standard of care," the role of pharmacists in quality improvement within the ambulatory and community setting is less defined. The following section highlights a few of the forces that are accelerating the demand for quality measurement related to ambulatory/community pharmacy.

Driving Forces for Pharmacy Quality Measurement

Pharmacist Professionalism

Over the past 40 years, the pharmacy profession has been undergoing an evolution from "compounders" and dispensers of medications to providers of medication therapy management. This evolution has been spurred by both social and technological forces.

New drug discoveries, modern manufacturing methods, and efficient distribution systems have diminished the need for pharmacists to compound medications. Today, the art of compounding survives primarily as a niche business for a small number of pharmacists. The increasing size of the drug armamentarium, and an increased recognition of the need to tailor drug regimens on the basis of various physiological, genetic, and cultural parameters, have heightened the demand for experts in medication therapy management. Colleges of pharmacy have adapted to this changing environment by providing extensive clinical training of pharmacy students to be experts in drug therapy.

In addition to the pool of clinically trained pharmacists graduating from our nation's pharmacy schools, there has been significant growth in the number of residency-trained pharmacists and board-certified pharmacists. The Board of Pharmacy Specialties (BPS) was created in 1976 with an initial focus on certifying pharmacists in the small specialty practice of nuclear pharmacy.[4] The specialties of nutrition support and pharmacotherapy were added in 1988, followed by psychiatric and oncology specialty certifications in 1998. By 2010, there were more than 10,000 board-certified pharmacists in these specialties.

Beginning in 2011, pharmacists have been able to apply for certification as an ambulatory care pharmacist. Assuming that board-certification requirements for pharmacists follow the same path as for those for physicians, pharmacists will soon see maintenance of certification (MOC) requirements that include practice-based quality improvement programs.

Accreditation Programs

In addition to the expanded education and board-certification of individual pharmacists, there has been a rapid growth in the accreditation of pharmacy organizations, as well as growth in the use of medication-related performance metrics within health care organization accreditation programs. Both The Joint Commission and NCQA have expanded their performance measure sets to include additional medication-related measures.[5,6] In turn, this has led many accredited organizations to create expanded roles for pharmacists as medication-safety officers, compliance officers, and leaders of qualityimprovement programs. These organizations have also placed greater accountability for medication-related quality on physicians and pharmacists.

The Joint Commission, the Utilization Review Activities Committee (URAC), the National Association of Boards of Pharmacy (NABP), and others have also implemented pharmacy accreditation programs to assess and ensure minimum standards of quality for various types of pharmacies. Pharmacy accreditation programs exist for mail-service, specialty, and infusion pharmacies as well as durable medical equipment (DME) programs provided by pharmacies. PBMs have also seen the introduction of an accreditation program by URAC. Community pharmacy accreditation programs are under consideration by URAC, NABP, and the American Pharmacists Association.

The growth of pharmacy accreditation programs has led to greater demand for pharmacists who understand the principles and tools of quality improvement. Coupled with the expanded medication-related measure sets of The Joint Commission and NCQA, this has also resulted in increased availability of information about the quality and safety of medication utilization. Consumer advocates and health care purchasers are beginning to take action based on this performance information.

Medicare Part D Quality Measures

With the creation of Medicare Part D, the federal government became the largest payer in the United States for prescription drugs.[7] Of great concern after implementation of this new program was the safety and quality of medication utilization. In response, CMS implemented a performance measurement system for Medicare prescriptions drug plans (PDPs) as well as Medicare Advantage plans that provide drug coverage (MAPDs). The evaluation system for Part D includes an annual rating of each PDP and MAPD (i.e., star ratings) based on 17 measures of performance across four domains.[8] Included within the plan ratings are several measures of medication safety and adherence. In addition to annual plan ratings, CMS provides each PDP and MAPD with a monthly safety report that includes an expanded set of medication safety and adherence measures. The goal of this monthly report is to bring attention to key areas of medication safety and to facilitate quality improvement by the Medicare plans. The measures of safety and adherence were endorsed by the PQA and are described in more detail later in this chapter.

In 2012, CMS will implement a Quality Bonus Payment (QBP) system for the Medicare Advantage plans.[9] In this system, a portion of the Medicare Advantage plan's payment will be contingent upon the star rating of that plan. Thus, the MAPD plans will have greater financial accountability for medication safety and for patients' adherence to drug regimens.

The combination of public reports on Medicare plan quality combined with the new QBP system are leading the Medicare plans to look for strategies that are effective in driving improvements in safety and quality. These strategies include greater engagement of community pharmacies in quality improvement and perhaps expansion of medication therapy management (MTM) programs by those pharmacies. Many of the Medicare plans are "drilling down" to the pharmacy level in their performance measurement activities to create pharmacy report cards, and some plans have implemented pay-for-performance systems for community pharmacies.

Pharmacy Quality Alliance (PQA)

While serving as CMS Administrator, Mark McClellan stimulated the creation of the PQA with the expectation that this alliance would identify the most appropriate ways to measure the quality of pharmacy services for Medicare Part D beneficiaries as well as other patients.[10] PQA was not the first quality alliance to be established and, in fact, was preceded by both the Ambulatory Quality Alliance (AQA), which represents various physician organizations, and the Hospital Quality Alliance (HQA).

The performance measurement and reporting enterprise has grown significantly since 2004, and PQA is now a member of the Quality Alliance Steering Committee. Today, close to 70 organizations constitute the membership of the PQA, including federal agencies (CMS and FDA); America's Health Insurance Plans (AHIP); and numerous health plans, PBMs, pharmacist professional societies, and pharmaceutical research and manufacturing companies. More information on PQA is available at www.PQAalliance.org.

Given the dearth of quality measures for ambulatory pharmacy services, the PQA spent much of 2006 and 2007 identifying potential measures of pharmacy quality and pilot-testing these measures with organizations experienced in quality measurement. PQA partnered with NCQA to develop specifications for more than 30 measures that could potentially be derived from drug claims data.[11] At the conclusion of pilot-testing, 15 of these measures demonstrated favorable attributes for performance measurement and were submitted to the National Quality Forum (NQF) for consideration in 2008. Several of the measures received NQF endorsement in 2009.[12]

PQA also partnered with the American Institute for Research to develop and test a questionnaire to gather consumer perspectives on the quality of pharmacy services.[13] Although it is not a CAHPS survey instrument, the questionnaire was modeled after the CAHPS family of measures that are maintained by the Agency for Healthcare Research & Quality (AHRQ).

Several of the PQA-supported performance measures have been adopted by CMS for the Medicare Part D performance evaluation system. These include three measures that are used in the star ratings:

- High-risk medications in the elderly.

- Use of angiotensin-converting enzyme inhibitors or angiotensin-receptor blockers (ACEI/ARBs) in patients with diabetes.

- Medication adherence with cholesterol, diabetes, or ACEI/ARB medications.

Two more measures—excessive doses of oral diabetes medications and drug-drug interactions—are in the Display Measure Set.

Since PQA has determined that these same performance measures are appropriate for evaluation of individual pharmacies, CMS also provides the Part D plans with outlier reports that identify pharmacies in the plan's network that have especially poor scores on these measures. Unfortunately, these reports are not routinely provided to the network pharmacies to facilitate performance improvement by pharmacies. PQA has begun to work with numerous prescription drug plans and pharmacy providers on a standard performance report system for pharmacies that could be used to facilitate performance improvement efforts.

PQA Demonstration Projects

In the summer of 2008, PQA initiated a series of demonstration projects in five states to test the feasibility and potential impact of creating performance reports for community pharmacies.[14] The first phase of the demonstration project involved implementation of a standard report card and gathered feedback about the performance report system from hundreds of community pharmacies as well as their health plan partners. In most cases, the projects were collaborative efforts of community pharmacies, technology partners, and health plans. Two of the projects also involved state Medicaid data. The health plans and Medicaid programs provided prescription claims data to a technology partner or academic research group that aggregated the data, calculated the performance measures, and created the electronic reports for the pharmacies.

Formative evaluations and improvements were made throughout the project, and each project team shared its experiences with the other teams as part of regularly scheduled conference calls. AHRQ funded an independent evaluation of the Phase I demonstration through a contract with CNA and Thomas Jefferson University.[15]

The Phase I demonstration revealed that community pharmacists were very interested in the performance reports. The majority of pharmacists had never before seen reports on the clinically related quality of their services, so there was great curiosity about how their services compared to those of other pharmacies. The key measures included in the performance reports were the PQA-supported measures on medication adherence for diabetes and cardiovascular medication classes as well as measures of medication safety including drug-drug interactions, excessive doses of oral diabetes medications, and the dispensing of high-risk medications to elderly patients. Measures related to asthma management were included in several of the projects. Individual pharmacy staff members were able to access the electronic reports through a secure web-portal and view the "scores" for their pharmacy along with the average score for all pharmacies on each measure. Examples of the web-based pharmacy report are available from PQA.[10]

Although the pharmacists and technicians in the Phase I demonstration were willing to take ownership of their performance reports, they were often unsure how to go about modifying their services to improve performance. Most pharmacists lack training on quality improvement methods, and only a few states require community pharmacies to have quality assurance or quality improvement programs. Thus, there is a great need for additional education and training of pharmacy personnel in performance improvement and also a need for identification of best practices in improving medication safety and adherence. As a result, PQA worked with several experts to develop and disseminate a turn-key education program for pharmacy students and pharmacists regarding quality measurement and performance improvement methods. This program is available, free of charge, from PQA.

Phase II of the demonstration is under way with three teams examining different methods for pharmacists to support patients in maintaining high levels of adherence with their chronic medication regimen and/or promoting safe use of medications. Each team has implemented an innovative model for pharmacist services and is testing the impact of the services on medication adherence and subsequent outcomes. For example, the project team in Pennsylvania has implemented a point-of-dispensing intervention that involves brief screening and consultation by Rite Aid pharmacists for patients taking oral diabetes medications or one of several cardiovascular medications (beta-blockers, calcium-channel blockers, ACEI/ARBs, or cholesterol medications). Highmark (the Blue Cross/Blue Shield plan in western Pennsylvania) is providing data on prescription utilization and medical utilization for its patients in the study. Highmark patients who visit one of 125 Rite Aid stores in western Pennsylvania will receive this intervention while Highmark patients at a control group of 125 Rite Aid stores receive traditional pharmacy services. Researchers from the University of Pittsburgh and Research Triangle Institute are conducting the evaluation of this project.

Another Phase II team involves the University of Illinois-Chicago, Humana, and Jewel-Osco. This team is comparing the relative impact of MTM consultations delivered in a face-to-face manner by Jewel-Osco pharmacists, an MTM consultation delivered telephonically by Humana pharmacists, and a control group of patients who receive traditional pharmacy services. As with the Pennsylvania demonstration, the targeted patients are taking diabetes and cardiovascular medications, and the impact is being measured on medication adherence and subsequent health care utilization.

The third team in the Phase II demonstration involves the University of Tennessee, HealthSpring (a health plan based in Nashville, TN), and PharmMD. HealthSpring has contracted with PharmMD to screen HealthSpring data using PQA measures and other performance measures to identify patients with potential medication-related problems. Once identified, patients are contacted by PharmMD pharmacists via telephone to conduct an MTM consultation. Academic researchers are utilizing data from PharmMD and HealthSpring to assess the impact of the screening and consultation services on medication safety.

The demonstration projects were designed to study collaborative efforts of health plans and community pharmacies to measure and improve the quality of medication use. Given that health plans are under pressure to increase transparency, and face financial consequences regarding the quality of medication use by their members, it makes sense for health plans to re-examine their relationships with PBMs and community pharmacies with the goal of aligning incentives to improve medication-use quality.

Enabling Pharmacy Quality Improvement

To promote consistent and meaningful use of quality measures within the pharmacy sector, PQA launched the E-QuIPP Initiative in 2011. E-QuIPP is an acronym for Electronic Quality Improvement Platform for Plans and Pharmacies. The initiative employs a Web-based platform that allows multiple health plans and pharmacies to use a common set of quality measures for benchmarking performance and tracking improvement as interventions are deployed. This model for shared performance measurement and improvement is based on the successful PQA-coordinated demonstration project in Pennsylvania.

Using a common set of PQA measures, each participating health plan in the E-QuIPP initiative (or its PBM) calculates and shares the results with the E-QuIPP platform. Results from all health plans are aggregated to provide local and regional quality benchmarks. Each health plan also calculates performance measures for each of its network pharmacies so that pharmacy performance reports can be created. Because the pharmacy-level performance data are aggregated within the E-QuIPP platform, each pharmacy's report card is based on analysis of data from multiple health plans. Thus, the sample size per pharmacy is more robust than if it were derived from a single health plan, and the pharmacy is able to see the variation in performance across plans. The platform also provides pharmacies and plans with access to tools and interventions for performance improvement.

While the long-term goal of the E-QuIPP initiative is to engage all major health plans and pharmacies throughout the United States, it is being rolled out on a regional basis by securing the participation of key health plans in each state followed by the community pharmacies in the same state. Since the initiative launched shortly before the publication of this book, the long-term impact of the initiative cannot yet be assessed.

Aligning Incentives for Pharmacy Quality Improvement

The E-QuIPP initiative will provide pharmacies, PBMs, and health plans with performance feedback and tools for improvement related to medications; however, there remains a need to align the incentives of these organizations toward quality improvement. The alignment of financial incentives with improvement goals for physicians and hospitals has often been implemented through pay-for-performance (P4P) programs.[16] There are two levels at which P4P can be implemented to drive improvements in the pharmacy sector. One level is that of the PBM and/or prescription drug program, and the second level is that of the community pharmacy.

Within the Medicare Part D benefit, CMS created incentives for prescription drug plans to improve quality. These include public reporting on the quality of every drug plan (stand-alone prescription drug plans as well as Medicare Advantage [MA] plans that offer drug benefits) and encouraging Medicare beneficiaries to select a Part D plan based on the quality ratings of the plans. Thus, an indirect financial incentive is created for the plans to improve quality, since enrollment may be affected by the ratings.

For 2012, the federal government has raised the financial stakes of quality ratings for MA plans by tying a portion of the plan's revenues to its quality ratings.[9] MA plans may be able to garner up to 5 percent additional revenue for achieving a five-star quality rating from CMS.

The increasing scrutiny of drug plans concerning the quality of medication use by their enrollees should prompt multifaceted efforts to enhance quality. Health plans might pursue "carrot" or "stick" approaches to improving quality within their pharmacy networks. An example of a "stick" approach is to eliminate a poorly performing pharmacy from the health plan's network. This approach could create access issues and increase complaints from members and employers. Nonetheless, the threat of being removed from a pharmacy network based on poor quality may result in heightened attention by pharmacies to the quality of their services.

A more positive strategy for drug plans is to implement a P4P program that reward pharmacies for achieving high levels of quality or for significantly improving their quality over time. This "carrot" approach may help to facilitate quality improvement while maintaining broad access to pharmacy services for members. Appropriate rewards might include higher payments for MTM services at high-performance pharmacies or bonuses for top performers. A major impediment to this approach is the drug plans' lack of funds to create a reward pool. Although MA drug plans could reap the benefits of improved medication utilization through fewer hospitalizations of members with chronic diseases and increased payments from CMS, the stand-alone drug plans do not directly benefit from efforts to boost medication adherence or to identify patients with under-treatment of their diseases. Thus, they are less likely to create P4P programs that are focused on improving the quality of drug therapy. This issue could be addressed directly by employers and public payers by creating an incentive pool for rewarding those pharmacies that boost quality.

In light of the foregoing, there are few examples of P4P programs for pharmacies. A program implemented by Humana seeks to reward its network pharmacies for helping to increase the utilization of generic drugs.[17] The program tracks the generic dispensing rate (GDR) at each network pharmacy and issues semi-annual reports. Six-month targets for increase in GDR are based on the pharmacy's GDR for the previous six-month period. Targets for improvement are set on a sliding scale such that pharmacies with low GDR have higher targets for the percentage increase in GDR. Pharmacies that are above the network average for GDR have smaller targets for GDR increases. Pharmacies that achieve target levels for increase in GDR receive an increase in reimbursement for drugs during the following six months.

Future pharmacy P4P programs would likely include the same measures that are used to evaluate health plans and prescription drug plans. These include measures of medication safety and medication adherence that are used by CMS to evaluate Medicare Part D plans, as well as Healthcare Effectiveness Data and Information Set (HEDIS) measures used by the National Committee on Quality Assurance (NCQA) to evaluate health plans. An important consideration in the selection of performance measures is the ability of the pharmacy to affect the measure. Clearly, pharmacies can affect medication safety measures such as the drug-drug interactions measure developed by PQA. One concern with using adherence measures for P4P is that patients are ultimately in control of whether they refill a prescription or take the medication as prescribed. However, this criticism could be levied at almost any performance measure. Patients choose whether to get a flu shot, have their A1c checked, or fill their beta-blocker prescription after a heart attack. While pharmacists and physicians cannot control their patients' behaviors, they can influence them.

The difference between "control" and "influence" should influence the design of a P4P financial model. For instance, a pharmacy P4P model with adherence measures should be structured to reward measured improvement in adherence rather than current levels of adherence. Also, it may not be wise to use withhold payment as a penalty for pharmacies whose patient populations have low levels of adherence. Because the pharmacy does not control the patients' adherence, it may be unreasonable to punish a pharmacy that serves a population with poor adherence rates. However, if we assume that pharmacists can influence adherence, we may want to reward pharmacies that contribute to dramatic improvements in their patients' adherence to key medications.

Other important considerations are the amount of payment tied to performance and the distribution of the incentive payments to the pharmacy staff. The economic premise underlying P4P is the notion that providers will seek to maximize their revenue and will take actions that are in their best financial interest. Therefore, the incentive should outweigh the costs of improving performance. For example, if a pharmacy has to hire an additional technician in order for the pharmacist to spend more time on patient counseling, the incentive should be sufficient to offset the cost. The pharmacy should also consider the indirect cost associated with poor performance. When pharmacy report cards are made public, a pharmacy with low-quality performance may be perceived as inferior by the community and lose business as a result. In this case, the addition of the technician may be warranted to offset the loss of business regardless of the P4P payments.

An important consideration for pharmacy organizations is rewarding individual pharmacists who help to generate the improved performance. Staff may become more motivated to improve their performance if success is rewarded financially. Because no studies have examined this type of P4P model, it is difficult to estimate the size of reward necessary to stimulate greater attentiveness to a patient's adherence. As pressure is brought to bear on health plans to improve quality while controlling long-term costs, it is likely that drug plans will begin to experiment with these types of incentives.

Conclusion

As employers and CMS continue to move toward value-based purchasing, there will be heightened demands for transparency in the quality of care being provided. Although community pharmacies have been immune to many of these demands, reports on the quality of care provided by community pharmacists will soon be part of the public record.

Several demonstration projects sponsored by the Pharmacy Quality Alliance (PQA) have shown that the creation of pharmacy report cards is feasible. To date, these report cards have been used solely by pharmacies for quality improvement. Inevitably, there will be a call for public reporting of the report card results. Drug plans may use the reports to inform their members about the relative quality of pharmacies within their plan's network. Consumer advocacy groups may also call for the release of the report cards to better inform the public about safety issues in pharmacies.

Since quality of medication utilization is an important factor in the overall value of health care, it makes sense to offer incentives to all providers who impact the use of medications. Physicians participate in P4P programs wherein medication measures are used to determine the physician's payment. If pharmacists can affect the quality of medication use, it stands to reason that they and their pharmacy organizations should be included in P4P systems and in emerging models for accountable care organizations.

Discussion Questions

1. What are some examples of medication-quality measures that may be most useful to a pediatric population? An elderly population?

2. How might community pharmacists collaborate with primary care physicians to improve the quality of medication use in a patient population?

3. How can health plans create "shared rewards" for teams of pharmacists and physicians who collaborate to improve quality?

References

1. Hepler CD, Grainger-Rousseau TJ. Pharmaceutical care versus traditional drug treatment.Is there a difference? *Drugs*, 49(1):1-10, Jan. 1995.

2. Knapp DA, Knapp DE, Brandon BM, West S. Development and application of criteria in drug use review programs. *Am J Hosp Pharm*, 31(7):648-58, July 1974.

3. Nau DP, Kirking DM. Understanding problems in the use of medications. In Warholak TL, Nau DP, Eds. *Safety & Quality in Pharmacy Practice*. New York: McGraw-Hill, 2010.

4. Board of Pharmaceutical Specialties. http://www.bpsweb.org/about/history.cfm. Accessed July 2011.

5. The Joint Commission. Performance Measurement. http://www.jointcommission.org/performance_measurement.aspx. Accessed July 2011.

6. National Committee for Quality Assurance. HEDIS & Quality Measurement. http://www.ncqa.org/tabid/59/Default.aspx. July 2011.

7. Medicare Payment Advisory Commission. Status Report on Part D. http://www.medpac.gov/chapters/Mar10_Ch05.pdf. Accessed July 2011.

8. Center for Medicare & Medicaid Services. Part D Performance Data. http://www.cms.gov/PrescriptionDrugCovGenIn/06_PerformanceData.asp#TopOfPage. Accessed July 2011.

9. Center for Medicare & Medicaid Services. CY2012 Call Letter. http://www.cms.gov/PrescriptionDrugCovContra/Downloads/Announcement2012final.pdf. Accessed July 2011.

10. Pharmacy Quality Alliance. www.PQAalliance.org. Accessed July 2011.

11. Pillittere-Dugan, Nau DP, McDonough K, Pierre Z. Development and testing of performance measures for pharmacy services. *J Am Pharm Assoc*, 49(2):212-9, Mar.-Apr. 2009.

12. National Quality Forum. National Voluntary Consensus Standards for Medication Management. Apr. 2009. http://www.qualityforum.org/Projects/s-z/Therapeutic_Drug_Management_(2008)/National_Voluntary_Consensus_Standards_for_Medication_Management.aspx. Accessed July 2011.

13. Blalock SJ, Keller S. Consumer Assessment of Pharmacy Quality. In: Warholak TL, Nau DP, Eds. *Safety & Quality in Pharmacy Practice*. New York: McGraw-Hill, 2010.

14. Doucette WR, Conklin M, Dott DA, *et al*. Pharmacy Quality Alliance phase I demonstrations: Descriptions and lessons learned. *J Am Pharm Assoc*, 51(4):544-50, July-Aug 2011.

15. McMahon J, Pizzi L. Laying the groundwork for pharmacy quality measurement. Sept. 2010 http://www.ahrq.gov/about/annualconf10/mcmahon_pizzi/mcmahon_pizzi.HTM. Accessed July 2011.

16. Institute of Medicine. Rewarding Provider Performance: Aligning Incentives in Medicare. Washington, DC: National Academy Press, 2007.

17. Nau DP. Aligning Financial Incentives for Quality. In: Warholak TL, Nau DP, Eds. *Safety & Quality in Pharmacy Practice*. New York: McGraw-Hill, 2010.

Section IV.

Balancing Competing Perspectives: Purchasers, Physicians, Patients

Chapter 13

Value-based Purchasing

By Neil I. Goldfarb

Executive Summary

"Value-Based Purchasing" (VBP) refers to a range of activities initiated by government and private purchasers (employers) of health care to increase the quality and/or decrease the costs of care in order to improve overall value. Specific VBP strategies that purchasers may implement include collecting data on quality and utilization, publicly reporting performance data, paying providers based on performance; selectively contracting with higher quality providers and systems; designing benefit plans to promote higher value services; promoting health and disease management programs; and offering education and incentives to consumers in order to promote healthy decision making and selection of higher quality providers and higher value services. These activities place increased pressure on clinical care providers to meet or exceed quality and safety expectations but also present new incentives for providers to invest in quality measurement and improvement activities.

Learning Objectives

1. Understand the role of public and private purchasers of health benefits in the quality movement.
2. Identify specific value-based strategies being pursued by purchasers.
3. Understand how these activities impact care providers.

Key Words: Value-based purchasing, pay-for-performance, value-based insurance design, consumerism

Introduction

Purchasers of health care are the stakeholders whose money funds health care delivery. Historically, purchasers just paid the bill when patients saw clinicians.

When purchasers saw that the costs of care continued to rise, they turned to health plans to intervene more directly in the clinician-patient relationship, with an emphasis on utilization management. Most recently, purchasers have become directly involved in health policy and care delivery through "value-based purchasing" (VBP), a range of activities intended to increase the quality and/or decrease the costs of care.[1] Private purchasers (employers) led the VBP movement, but, more recently, the Centers for Medicare and Medicaid Services (CMS), as the largest government purchaser, has espoused VBP as the foundation for Medicare and Medicaid payment reform.[2] In this chapter, we will review the key VBP strategies and discuss implications for clinicians.

The Value Problem

In the U.S. health care system, purchasers typically are defined as public (government, i.e., Medicare and Medicaid) or private (employers and consumers). Roughly half of the nation's health care spending is through private sources, with the largest segment of private spending derived through employer-sponsored health insurance. Most large employers offer insurance to their employees and their family members. The likelihood of insurance being offered increases with the size of the employer organization (number of employees). Workers in small companies and/or with minimum-wage jobs are those who are most likely to not have employer-sponsored health insurance.[3] The Accountable Care Act (health reform) calls for employers with at least 50 employees to offer health insurance to their employees or to pay a financial penalty and have their employees seek insurance through Health Insurance Exchanges (HIE's). Although there are many uncertainties about this aspect of the law (which was being challenged through the courts as of fall of 2011), most policy pundits expect that the majority of mid-size and larger employers will continue to offer health benefits to their employees.

Employers who offer health benefits may be either "fully insured" or "self-insured." Full insurance refers to the employer paying premiums to the health insurer (health plan) with the insurer bearing the risk—i.e., the employer pays an actuarially based premium to the health plan, and the health plan is responsible for paying claims. If employees use more services, or more costly services, than were estimated, the plan may experience a loss (i.e., total costs of claims plus administration is less than total revenues derived from premiums); conversely, in a "good year," claims experience is lower than premium revenue and the plan makes a profit.

Because health plans build a cushion into their premiums in order to reduce their exposure to risk, most larger employers choose to be self-insured (self-funded). Under this arrangement, the employer typically contracts with a health plan to serve as a third-party administrator (TPA). The TPA's provider network, claims processing services, and other services are used, but the employer pays the insurer for actual claims experience rather than premiums. In order to reduce their exposure to risk, self-funded employers usually purchase "stop-loss" insurance, which protects them against very expensive cases or a generally high-cost year.

To consumers, whether their employer is fully insured or self-insured is usually invisible; i.e., the consumer still gets a health plan identification card and deals directly with the health plan when he or she needs access to services.

Because employers have been faced with continuing escalation in health care costs—and self-insured employers are especially at risk—they increasingly have been questioning the value of their spending. As was discussed in Chapter 1, increasing evidence demonstrates that health care quality and safety are much lower than optimal in the U.S., while spending is nearly double that of many western countries that appear to achieve equivalent or higher quality. We therefore have a value problem, where value is defined as the relationship of quality to cost (Value=Quality/Cost).

As purchasers, employers and large public programs have started to ask what can be done to improve the value of their spending. From the formula, it should be obvious that value will increase if quality increases, costs decrease, or both occur simultaneously. Value-based purchasing refers to a set of activities that purchasers have been pursuing, largely over the past 10 years and with increasing frequency today, to improve the value of health benefits spending.

VBP Strategies

Almost anything that a purchaser does to increase the quality of care or decrease the costs of care can be viewed as value-based purchasing. However, we need to remember that just cutting costs, especially short-term spending, may limit access to care or decrease quality of care and ultimately result in poorer health outcomes as well as higher costs. Therefore, VBP activities are intended to decrease costs while holding quality constant, improving quality, or holding costs constant while increasing quality. This section discusses key value-based purchasing strategies.

Data Review and Public Reporting

Many purchasers would be challenged to answer the question, "What are you spending your money on?" For this reason, developing a value-driven strategy often starts with trying to obtain data. Whether fully insured or self-funded, private purchasers often have difficulty in gaining detailed utilization data. Their insurers and TPAs may provide summary reports but deny a purchaser access to the raw data, arguing that the Health Insurance Portability and Accountability Act (HIPAA) or contractual terms restrict data access. The HIPAA barrier is usually overcome by creating a firewall between the employer's staff who use the data for population health management and those in positions to make hiring and firing decisions. Increasingly, purchasers also are negotiating contracts with insurers that will allow them access to their data.

Once data are obtained, key questions a purchaser could ask include:

- What are the most common diagnoses, procedures, reasons for hospitalization, and medications in the population?

- Which diagnoses account for the most spending?

- How many members of the population have received guideline-recommended preventive care, such as immunizations, mammograms, and colonoscopies?

- Which hospitals and physicians are providing care most often for the population?

With access to data, purchasers also can begin to look at quality and costs of care at the provider level. Just looking at provider-level data has been shown to influence provider behavior; i.e., when hospitals and clinicians know that someone is looking at their performance, they are more likely to perform at a higher value level. For this reason, as well as to increase transparency for consumers, purchasers, including CMS, have begun to publicly report performance data. For example, CMS maintains the "Hospital Compare" (www.hospitalcompare.hhs.gov) and "Nursing Home Compare" websites (www.medicare.gov/nhcompare), and the Joint Commission also reports hospital performance data through its Quality Check website (www.qualitycheck.org). Although physician-level data remain less accessible than facility-level data, the future promises to have these data available through websites and other public "report cards"—e.g., CMS' imminent launch of "Physician Compare" using data through the Physician Quality Reporting System. (See Chapter 3)

Selective Contracting and Tiered Networks

As data on facility, system, office, and individual clinician quality and safety become available, the data can be used to drive performance, as well as to steer consumers to higher quality providers. Through their health plans, purchasers may decide to drop certain poor performers from their networks and may selectively contract only with those providers who are deemed, based on measurement, to offer higher quality or value. Value-based purchasers also may develop tiered networks, paying differential rates based on quality and value (i.e., rewarding the better performers with higher rates) and/or giving consumers incentives, such as waived deductibles or reduced copayments, to seek care from the better performers.

In a related movement, some purchasers are beginning to pursue a "reference pricing" strategy. This involves determining the range of prices for a particular procedure or episode of care in a geographic region, determining the fair or market average price for the procedure, and agreeing to reimburse up to that amount regardless of the specific care providers price. For example, suppose that in a given market, the price for colonoscopy is found to range from $500 to $2500, but the median price is $1000. The purchaser could set the reference price at $1000 and make consumers aware that this is how much the health plan would cover for a colonoscopy. Consumers could be presented with the provider-specific pricing information and make their decisions accordingly, knowing that if they sought colonoscopy through a provider whose price was $1500, their out of pocket cost would be $500. In this example, the reference pricing is based solely on cost, without regard to quality. However, as the science of VBP advances, we will see quality-adjusted reference pricing, coupled with public reporting and value transparency.

Paying for Performance

The past five years have seen rapid proliferation in pay-for-performance (P4P) programs. Purchasers not only measure and publicly report on performance, but also have begun to develop clinician and facility compensation systems that pay differentially based on provider quality and efficiency. See Chapter 14 for a more complete discussion of P4P.

Value-based Insurance Design (VBID)

Value-based insurance design, also known as value-based benefit design, is concerned with redesigning benefit plans to promote the use of higher value services and to eliminate barriers to use of those services. For example, many purchasers and health plans in the past have charged copayments or even raised copayments for all drugs, regardless of perceived value of those drugs. As a result, people with asthma, diabetes, or another chronic condition may delay having a prescription filled, may not fill the prescription at all, or may not take the drug as frequently or at the dosage prescribed. This "non-adherence" ultimately may result in exacerbation of illness, leading to emergency department visits or hospitalizations. A VBID strategy would recognize the value of these controller medications, and reduce or eliminate the copayments in order to improve outpatient management and disease control and prevent the more costly and impactful episodes of illness.

Beyond lowering or eliminating pharmaceutical copayments, the next generation of VBID also is considering the value of all traditionally reimbursed services. With the growth of the science of comparative effectiveness and evidence-based medicine, look for purchasers to begin to eliminate coverage for services deemed to be of little or marginal effectiveness and/or to develop differential cost-sharing arrangements (the split of the total price between the purchaser and the consumer's out-of-pocket expense) based on the value of each clinical service.

Consumer Education and Engagement

Many of the value-based purchasing strategies discussed above are targeted toward the supply side of health care (i.e., changing provider behavior). However, influencing the demand side (i.e., changing consumer behavior) is another important strategy. In addition to redesigning co-payments under VBID, purchasers increasingly are exploring strategies for educating and empowering consumers, improving health literacy, and engaging consumers, through financial incentives, to seek care from higher value providers. Chapter 16 presents a more detailed discussion of consumerism.

Health and Disease Management

From a purchaser's perspective, the best strategy for reducing health care costs is to prevent illness and maintain the health and productivity of the workforce. The majority of employers therefore offer worksite wellness programs. A wide range of interventions fit within the broad category of "worksite wellness." Many employers have their employees complete a health risk appraisal (HRA)—a questionnaire that assesses the individual's health risks on the basis of behaviors, demographics, family history, and other factors. HRAs typically result in an individualized report that is fed back to the employee, showing how behaviors contribute to overall health risk (e.g., life expectancy) and how risk can be mitigated through behavior change. Increasingly, HRAs also include physiologic measures performed by a qualified clinician—e.g., blood pressure measurement, cholesterol test, and BMI calculation based on actual height and weight measurement. In order to promote HRA completion, employers may offer their employees a financial incentive such as a cash payment or a health insurance premium reduction for participation.

Other common worksite wellness strategies include offering on-site peer support programs (e.g., Weight Watchers®) and education programs, making an employee assistance program (EAP) available to provide counseling and support for behavioral health concerns and stress reduction, providing incentives for gym memberships or offering on-site facilities for exercise, promoting use of stairs and walking trails, redesigning cafeteria offerings and restructuring pricing of entrees in order to promote healthy eating (e.g., charging more for hamburgers and less for salads), and changing the placement and pricing of snacks in the vending machines.

Increasingly, employers are going so far as to create their own worksite-based health care facilities. On-site nurses and medical directors no longer deal solely with occupational health and safety issues. In many worksites, they now are providing primary preventive and acute care services. The proliferation of on-site clinics, for both employees and family members, is helping employers improve their access to primary care, reduce productivity loss due to care seeking from community-based providers, and improve employee satisfaction and retention. Moving forward, a key question will be how to best integrate these programs with the broader health care system so as to ensure continuity of care.

Recognizing that, no matter how effective wellness programs are, employers will continue to be faced with some segment of the employee population with chronic disease, a disease management VBP strategy also is needed. Disease management programs seek to identify the population with the disease, stratify that population based on risk of acute exacerbation, and target interventions to prevent or minimize the disease's impact. Employers may contract with disease management programs through their health plans or independently through vendors, or, in some cases, build their own in-house programs. Strategies that promote direct, personalized, and frequent contact currently appear to be more effective than general telephonic and group-based programs.

Coalitions and Multi-Stakeholder Approaches

In most regions, purchasers—even the largest employers—have limited market power and therefore limited ability to collect and analyze data on provider performance, publicly report that data, pay for performance, and influence the quality and value offered by the overall care delivery system. Because of this, local purchasers in many markets have joined together in business coalitions on health to pursue VBP strategies. The National Business Group on Health (NBGH), based in Washington, DC, consists of large national employers working together, and the National Business Coalition on Health (NBCH), also in Washington, is a national organization composed of more than 50 regional business coalitions on health. Both of these organizations seek to represent the employer community on a national level in policy discussions and in discussions with representatives of other stakeholder groups (provider, health plan, governmental, and consumer organizations) and to promote best practices for value-based purchasing. A list of NBCH member coalitions is available on the NBCH website (www.nbch.org).

Examples of VBP in Practice

There are numerous examples of how the VBP strategies delineated above are being put into practice through employers and business coalitions. In this section, we will highlight a few of these specific activities:

Pitney-Bowes: One of the earliest and most widely publicized examples of a VBID strategy comes from Pitney-Bowes (PB), the large international mail services company.[4] Several years ago, PB's benefits team was challenged by the organization's chief financial officer to develop a plan to reduce the trend of annual double-digit inflation in health care spending. After reviewing data on diagnoses and costs of care, the team decided to focus on reducing the impact of select high-prevalence, high-cost chronic diseases. Copayments for chronic management drugs for these diseases were eliminated. Simultaneously, the company offered on-site education programs, modified cafeteria and vending machine offerings, implemented an EAP, and promoted wellness. The company found that costs for the population were significantly lower over the next year and projected savings of several million dollars. Of interest, despite lowering the drug copayments for chronic management drugs, overall pharmaceutical spending went *down*; this was attributed to improved disease control, resulting in fewer hospitalizations and acute episodes, and reduced reliance on rescue medications.

Leapfrog Group on Patient Safety: After the Institute of Medicine published *To Err Is Human*, spotlighting the frequency of inpatient medical errors, a group of employers joined together as the Leapfrog Group to create "leaps forward" in inpatient safety. A literature review identified three practices that could significantly reduce hospital-based errors: using computerized order entry systems, having intensivists in the ICU, and doing evidence-based hospital referral (i.e., referring patients to hospitals that had more volume and experience with procedures rather than keeping them in house). Over the past 10 years, the Leapfrog Group's "regional rollouts" have encouraged hospitals to voluntarily report on how they meet these and other safety standards. The data on who is participating and the extent to which they meet the standards is publicly available (www.leapfroggroup.org). A growing body of evidence is demonstrating not only that the Leapfrog effort is increasing transparency about hospital-level safe practices, but also that these practices are linked to better outcomes and lower costs of care.

eValue8 Request for Information (RFI): NBCH has developed a standardized RFI to elicit information on quality and value from health plans.[5] The eValue8 tool works in tandem with the accreditation and HEDIS programs of the National Committee for Quality Assurance (NCQA), but it provides greater detail on how health plans do the work purchasers are contracting with them to do. Health plans are asked to complete the RFI before having the opportunity to meet with purchasers to review the results and identify areas for improving operations. The tool covers many areas of health plan performance, including provider network development and provider-level quality measurement and improvement activities.

Conclusion

Public and private purchasers increasingly are moving from being passive bill payers to being active participants in the health care delivery system and working with health plans, providers, and consumers to promote—or demand—quality and value. Although many of the strategies being implemented today are promising, they cannot yet be called evidence-based themselves. The proliferation of these VBP strategies in the presence of limited evidence of their effectiveness (as well as potential adverse consequences) speaks to the pressure on purchasers to maintain the current level of benefits in the face of continually escalating prices. Clinicians in practice are being impacted by these programs and undoubtedly will be impacted to a higher degree in the future. Therefore, it is essential that clinicians maintain their knowledge of national and local VBP initiatives and, where possible, become involved in multi-stakeholder collaboratives seeking to improve value.

Study and Discussion Questions

1. Do you think that employers have a right to "meddle" in the health care system?

2. Look at the Leapfrog Group's website. What do you think about its approach to measuring and improving safety? What are the challenges faced by hospitals in this movement?

References

1. Goldfarb NI, Maio V, Carter CT, *et al*. How does quality enter into health care purchasing decisions? Commonwealth Fund Issue Brief, May 2003. http://www.commonwealthfund.org/usr_doc/goldfarb_valuebased.pdf.

2. Centers for Medicare and Medicaid Services. Roadmap for Implementing Value-driven health care in the traditional Medicare fee-for-service program. https://www.cms.gov/qualityinitiativesgeninfo/downloads/VBPRoadmap_OEA_1-16_508.pdf.

3. Henry J. Kaiser Family Foundation and Health Research and Educational Trust. Employer Health Benefits 2011 Annual Survey. Report available at http://ehbs.kff.org/pdf/2011/8225.pdf.

4. Mahoney JJ. Value-based Benefit Design: Using a Predictive Modeling Approach to Improve Compliance. *J Manage Care Pharm*, 14(6 Suppl B):S3-S8, July 2008.

5. National Business Coalition on Health. http://www.nbch.org/eValue8.

Chapter 14

Public Reporting and Pay For Performance

By Flossie E. Wolf

Executive Summary

Concerns about health care quality and patient safety,[1-3] coupled with calls for transparency and accountability, have given rise to a growing interest in performance measurement.[4-6] In recent years, performance measurement initiatives such as public reporting (reporting) and pay for performance (P4P) have proliferated[7-10] and become a routine part of doing business for health plans, hospitals, and physicians.[4] As a result, today's patients, purchasers, and other health care consumers turn to numerous websites for information on health care options and performance results.

Research on performance measurement has led to enhanced risk-adjustment methodologies[11-15] and improved report designs.[16,17] Moreover, it has revealed that results can be used to increase health care quality.[16-20] Yet, there are ongoing challenges that must be addressed to make reporting and P4P more effective, and new data points and technologies must be efficiently incorporated into the process.

Due in part to conflicting interests among the various stakeholders, performance measurement remains a controversial topic. Ultimately, however, there is a common goal—to improve the quality of care provided to patients—and it appears that reporting and P4P have a strong foothold in efforts to achieve this.[5]

Learning Objectives

1. Understand the role of reporting and P4P in improving health care.

2. Become familiar with current literature on the effectiveness of reporting and P4P.

3. Assess the ongoing challenges associated with these efforts.

4. Formulate approaches to enhance reporting and P4P.

5. Identify ways in which health care providers, including clinicians, can contribute to performance measurement initiatives.

Key Words: Performance Measurement, Public Reporting, Pay-for-Performance, Quality Improvement, Health Care Quality, Performance Reporting.

Introduction

Quality of care is central to the nation's health care agenda. In recent decades, various quality improvement (QI) efforts have surfaced, including initiatives aimed at measuring and reporting health care provider performance. In theory, measuring performance and reporting the results to patients, employers, health plans, and other stakeholders improves quality by enabling each entity to make better decisions regarding health care and, in the process, encouraging providers to assess and enhance quality initiatives.[4,19,21-24] The two most visible performance measurement initiatives—public reporting and P4P—share a common goal to measure and improve quality, but their mechanisms and incentives for doing so differ.

With public reporting, performance results are prominently displayed and broadly disseminated via reports, websites, and other public media (e.g., *Newsweek, U.S. News & World Report*, and *Consumer Reports*.)[10,25] Pressure to improve performance, driven by professional and organizational pride or the desire to increase market share, is at the heart of reporting. Lower performing providers strive to improve quality in an effort to outperform their competitors. While this type of pressure may come into play, P4P programs utilize financial incentives as motivating factors to reward QI and increased efficiency.[26,27]

A pivotal event in the history of performance measurement and reporting came about in the mid-1980s with the release of hospital-specific mortality rates by the Health Care Financing Administration, now the Centers for Medicare and Medicaid Services (CMS). Although this program was eventually discontinued, it set the stage for other reporting initiatives, including:

- CMS' Hospital Compare,[28] which includes hospital results for process of care measures, select outcomes, and information on patient experience..

- National Committee for Quality Assurance's Healthcare Effectiveness Data and Information Set (HEDIS),[29] which includes widely used quality indicators on health plan performance.

- Individual state reporting initiatives.

- Other public and private efforts.

Although they are considered powerful tools for facilitating QI, public reporting and P4P have not reached their full potential.[10,30] After more than two decades of performance measurement, controversies linger regarding their importance, methodologies, effectiveness, and future use. This section addresses the questions surrounding these issues.

Why is public release of performance measurement data important?

Today's consumers demand information at every turn, from purchasing refrigerators to selecting a new car. They are unwilling to settle for goods and services that do not meet their expectations. In the current vernacular, they want transparency and accountability—and they have begun to expect the same level of transparency and accountability from the health care industry.[31,32] A consumer can go on-line to inform a decision about buying tires while an auto technician waits for an answer. It is only a matter of time before consumers demand the same transparency and accountability when making decisions about their health and well-being.

The twin concepts of transparency and accountability are central to the importance of reporting and P4P as QI tools. With increasing frequency, health care consumers—whether they are patients, health care insurers, purchasers, or other stakeholders—want to know about the available health care options, outcomes, and costs. Such concepts are changing the way we look at health care. Somewhat belatedly, we are taking a lesson from industry; i.e., transparency motivates quality and efficiency and it promotes accountability.[20,26,33] More simply put—

"The people and communities who depend on health care have a right to know how good that care is. The organizations that arrange and provide that care have a duty to tell them."[34]

What is the purpose of performance measurement data?

Public reporting and P4P initiatives are intended to stimulate improvements in health care quality by promoting behavior change, either through public forces or through financial incentives.[16,17,22,25-27,35] The expectation is that comparisons based on quality measures will inform and promote choice; stimulate demand for QI; promote efficiencies; and encourage QI by health plans, health care facilities, and individual providers.[19,23,24] High performers benefit through higher market shares or financial incentives. Low performers are likely to implement QI practices in order to regain market share or avoid a negative public image.[16,17,19,21,22,26,27]

What information is included in performance reports?

Although some states report individual physician performance for certain procedures (e.g., cardiac surgery), most public reporting focuses on publishing performance data for hospitals, health plans, and skilled nursing facilities.[36-40] Public reports on health plan performance tend to focus on member experience data and process of care measures that describe rates of adherence to care guidelines (e.g., rates for screening tests or appropriate medication use). Public reports on hospital performance might include process of care measures, but they are more likely to include patient outcome[41] measures designed to reflect results of care (e.g., patient mortality rates, readmission rates, complication rates, and length of stay) as well. Experts have stressed the importance of measuring outcomes; in particular, in achieving better results for patients.[8,42,43] This has led to the relatively new reporting and P4P efforts focused on patient safety measures such as health care-associated infections.

Often geared toward hospital and physician performance,[9] P4P initiatives generally include a mix of process of care indicators, outcomes, and cost-efficiency measures.[44] In addition, these programs often highlight indicators of patient satisfaction and information technology use.[35]

Risk Adjustment

An important aspect of reporting and P4P, risk adjustment ensures that providers receive appropriate credit for treating patients who are more seriously ill. Real or perceived inadequacies in risk adjustment have been the source of much contention. Early on, risk-adjustment discussions focused on whether administrative or billing data were sufficient. While administrative data are more readily available, they lack the necessary clinical information relevant to a patient's pathophysiological state for making a risk adjustment.[11] Furthermore, until the recent adoption of present-on-admission (POA) indicators, administrative data could not be used to distinguish between on-admission conditions and complications that occurred during a hospital stay.

Recent literature on the topic focuses on clinical elements that can be added to administrative data to enhance risk-adjustment methodologies. Findings suggest that inpatient mortality can be well predicted using risk-adjustment models that maximize objective pathophysiological data such as laboratory results.[12,13] Laboratory results, along with administrative data, and POA indicators, appear to provide appropriate risk adjustment without placing extreme burden on the data-collecting entity.[11,14,15]

Who are performance data "customers"? Who wants this information?

Performance data "customers" include: 1) individual patients, who might use the information to choose a provider; 2) employers or other purchasing groups responsible for determining insurance options; 3) insurers when establishing a network of providers; 4) primary care physicians, who might use the data to refer patients to particular hospitals or specialists; 5) physician practice groups, who might use the data to reward members for reaching certain wellness or self-management goals; and 6) hospital administrators seeking to improve care.[26]

These are valid reasons for wanting performance data, but do these groups actually use the data? Studies show that patients express interest in having comparative performance information,[19,20] but that their actual use of the information is more limited.[26,45] Often patients are unaware that the information exists or find the format in which it is presented to be too complex.[5,17,19,24,31,45,46] Producers of public reports have responded by developing user-friendly presentation formats.[46]

Although patients continue to rely on friends, family, and their primary care physicians for hospital or specialist referrals,[32,33,45] more patients report being aware of quality-related performance information,[33,47] and more appear to be seeking hospitals with high volume and low mortality.[32] Other experts express confidence that, increasingly, consumers will use the data.[48]

A major push in favor of performance measurement and reporting comes from large self-insured employers, with 78 percent indicating that they want health plans to publicly release providers' performance scores.[26] Purchasers use this information to identify high-performing, low-cost providers in hopes that their employees will gravitate toward these providers when seeking care.[26] Herein lies an example of competing perspectives among the customers of performance measurement. Conflicts arise between purchasers and providers—physicians in particular—when performance data are used to develop narrowed networks or tiered insurance products.[31] Such practices exacerbate physicians' concern that the goal of these programs might lean more toward the cost of care rather than the quality of care.[44,49]

Hospitals have been critical of performance reporting due, in large part, to concerns about measurement methods.[16,26,31] Despite this, the impact of public reporting appears strongest for this group.[24] There is evidence that hospitals use performance data to stimulate QI initiatives,[16-20] and the resulting efforts to improve ratings can lead to substantial improvements in health outcomes for patients.[31,42,46]

Physicians have been somewhat resistant to performance measurement and reporting.[24,26] Although physicians tend to be *interested* in performance measurement, they are more likely to be skeptical about the data.[8,19,32] Common objections include concerns that risk adjustment is inadequate and unease about the potential for performance measurement to result in reduced access among high-risk patients.[19,20,31,33,50-52] With regard to P4P, additional concerns noted by physicians include whether implementation is feasible, whether rewards are sufficient, and whether adherence to rigid guidelines interferes with the delicate balance required to meet the complex needs of specific patients (e.g., those with multiple chronic conditions).[49]

How effective is the reporting of performance measurement data?

Public Reporting

Evidence suggests that publicly releasing performance data stimulates QI activity at the hospital level.[18,19] A recent comprehensive review of the published evidence supports this conclusion.[20] In their work on the topic, Hibbard and colleagues[16,17] found that the hospitals included in public reports were significantly more likely to initiate QI activities than those who received confidential quality reports or no report at all.

Although reporting stimulates QI activity, the reported effects on *outcomes* are mixed. Some studies find that hospital mortality is reduced following the release of performance data; other studies report no effect.[20] This topic was the focus of extensive study after New York State released its first physician-specific outcomes report on coronary artery bypass graft (CABG) surgery in the early 1990s. Some studies reported reductions in risk-adjusted mortality rates following the release of the New York data[20,52] while others found no differences in mortality rates when comparing New York with two states that did not issue such reports at the time.[20]

In further studies of CABG mortality rates, researchers compared rates in regions with public reporting and regions without. Results from this study suggested that the public release of outcome data appears to be associated with lower risk-adjustment mortality rates for CABG surgery.[53] When Jha and Epstein[48] studied the effects of the New York CABG surgery reports 15 years after their release, they concluded that performance reports can reliably predict better-than-average performance and can help patients choose hospitals and surgeons with lower mortality.

In Pennsylvania, a state with a long history of public reporting, Hollenbeak and colleagues[54] studied the impact of reporting on six medical conditions for patients hospitalized in the state. They found that patients treated in hospitals operating within an intensive public reporting environment had significantly lower odds of in-hospital mortality when compared to similar patients treated at hospitals subjected to limited or no public reporting.

Regarding the possible effect of public reporting on market share or referral patterns, most studies report little or no evidence.[17,20,48] The evidence is mixed on the possible influence of health plan performance data on plan selection. Some studies found that the release of health plan performance information influenced plan choice, while others reported little or no effect.[20]

Pay-for-Performance (P4P)

The previous discussion focused primarily on the effectiveness of public reporting, but what about P4P? Some evidence suggests modest association between P4P and improved quality.[55] Other researchers conclude that no substantial breakthroughs in quality improvement have occurred as a result of P4P initiatives.[35,56-57] The Premier Hospital Quality Incentive Demonstration Project (PHQID), a national P4P program carried out in partnership by Premier and CMS, has generated and published research on hospital P4P programs. According to Premier, hospitals participating in this project increased their overall quality and outperformed non-participating hospitals.[58] While there is some evidence of improvement in process-based quality scores,[22,59] others reported no evidence of improved outcomes.[60,61]

More recently, Werner and colleagues[62] found that, while the performance of hospitals participating in PHQID initially improved more than non-participating hospitals, there were no significant differences between the two groups after five years. Experts who have studied P4P suggest that better design will increase the success of these efforts.[8,62-68]

Concern about Unintended Effects

A recurring question arises with respect to the possible unintended consequences of releasing performance data.[31,33,49,50,52,67] Much of the research is designed to determine whether performance reporting results in decreased access—i.e., are high-risk patients being denied care?

In their review of the published literature, Fung and colleagues[20] report that some studies identified access concerns following the release of the New York State reports on CABG surgery while others found no evidence of decreased access for high-risk-patients. In studying racial and ethnic disparities, Werner and colleagues[69] report that fewer CABG surgeries were performed among black and Hispanic patients in New York following release of these reports. They observe that, after a decade, disparities have returned to pre-report levels.

Regarding P4P, a recent study found that patients with hypertension and complex medical conditions were more likely to receive higher overall quality of care, suggesting that providers are identifying and focusing their efforts on high-risk patients.[70] Another study evaluating whether P4P decreased access for minority patients found minimal evidence that minority patients were being avoided; however, the authors advised continued monitoring.[71]

One way to address the potential for unintended consequences is to include measures on appropriateness of care.[69] Confidence in risk-adjustment methodologies might also temper these concerns.[33,49] Other avenues such as paying particular attention to disparities in designing P4P programs[67] and recognizing disparity reduction as a quality measure in these initiatives[72] have been offered as potential solutions.

Health care delivery does not occur in environments where performance reporting is the only variable in measuring change. Because so many factors are at play, it is difficult to accurately evaluate the effectiveness of performance reporting. New and improved techniques affect patient care and results, and hospitals' efforts to improve patient safety can drive QI independently of performance reporting. Additional evaluation of causal pathways may help determine whether this type of reporting actually influences quality of care.[20]

How can performance measurement and reporting be more effective?

Approaches to improve the effectiveness of performance measurement and reporting continue to be debated. A few common themes are presented here.

First, additional measures must be developed that look beyond immediate results and capture a patient's full treatment and recovery period.[5,42,43,73] Obviously, mortality rates are important measures, but so too are outcomes such as potential complications, recovery time, functional status, need for rehabilitation, whether the patient will be able to resume normal activities and how soon, and disease recurrence.[5,42,43]

Of course, this is easier said than done. Currently, outcomes are based on data that are readily available and relatively easy to collect and measure.[4,74] Developing new outcome measures would likely require new data sources and new methods for verifying and analyzing the data. This poses a dilemma for developers of performance measurement reports who want to be sensitive to the data collection demands already faced by providers. Although overcoming these data collection difficulties might be challenging, there will be an opportunity to foster interdisciplinary teamwork as attempts are made to capture data from various parts of the delivery system.[73]

Second, identifying appropriate measures is especially important in physician-based P4P initiatives. Both the measures and the incentives must be relevant to a physician's patients if the program is to be effective. It is unlikely that P4P programs will be helpful if measures apply only to a small number of the physician's patients or if the incentive is so small that making changes is not cost effective.[8,35,49,63,64] Also, the goal is to improve care on a broad level, and P4P programs should include an appropriate mix of quality measures.[27,35,49,63,64] Other key elements have been suggested for designing P4P initiatives, including:

- Rewarding both high performance and performance improvement;
- Providing incentives for reducing disparities;
- Recognizing provider circumstances such as the ability to continually invest in the program.[8,27,35,49,56,62-68]

Third, reports must be easily interpretable;[10] e.g., the identity of high and low performers should be immediately clear.[16] Inconsistencies must be minimized.[32] Although consumers have numerous websites at their disposal, they might very well find varying performance results for the same hospital. Each program is likely to use different study populations, measures, risk-adjustment techniques, and reporting periods.[5] Reducing these mixed messages will not be easy, but, in the absence of clear results, patients will likely shy away from performance data.

Fourth, reporting entities must take a few important steps:
- Engage the relevant stakeholders.
- Strive to enhance risk adjustment and be watchful of potential unintended effects.
- Acknowledge limitations in the data and in the reporting methodologies.[31]
- Make every effort to increase the timeliness of the data.[23]
- Strive to reduce the costs associated with collecting the data without compromising its accuracy and value.[31,34,64]
- Work with the media to ensure appropriate information is conveyed.[52]

Fifth, more generally, there is a need to continually re-examine expectations and modify reporting priorities to accommodate change. Those who have watched performance measurement unfold in the past 20 years would likely admit that the journey was quite different than they originally anticipated.

Finally, recognizing that health care providers—particularly physicians—are wary of performance measurement, we must find ways to increase their confidence in the reporting methods. The good news is that there appears to be broader acceptance of performance measurement among physicians.[8,51,63] Yet, in order for all health care providers to accept performance measurement as a QI tool, their concerns must be addressed. Involving them in the process as follows is a good start.

- Health care providers must be integrated into the performance measurement process. They must know the measures that are being reported as well as the goals and expected achievements for each one. They must understand the methodology and work with reporting entities to improve methods and design. They must participate on advisory committees that help shape the process and the final output. As noted by Lee and colleages,[31] "give up the role of critic for that of coauthor."

- Hospital executives, medical practice administrators, and clinicians must ensure that the data they submit to the reporting entity are good data. Work with data-reporting departments and office staff to ensure that the data are accurate and complete, including data necessary for risk adjustment.

- With regard to P4P, providers should insist on having input to ensure that measures and incentives are relevant to their patients and that they will motivate improvement.[35,61] They should take part in deciding how rewards are best distributed—i.e., to the high performers or to those who actually improve?[27]

Quality assessment and improvement will continue to be essential components of the work performed by clinicians and other health care providers. They are valued partners in ensuring that performance measurement steers QI efforts in the right direction.

Conclusion

Concerns about quality of care, together with demands for transparency and accountability, have led to increased efforts to measure and report performance results. Public reporting and P4P have been touted as effective tools for achieving improved quality.

The successful features of performance measurement include how hospitals, insurers, and health care purchasers are using the data to improve health care quality. More tepid use by individual patients and physicians might lead some to criticize the less satisfying aspects of performance measurement programs. The truth is that performance measurement has been expected to be "all things to all people". These reports are expected to incorporate competing interests of patients, insurers, purchasers, providers and policymakers, simultaneously satisfying multiple, sometimes conflicting, purposes. Purchasers and providers often disagree on how the data should be used. Patients and purchasers want user-friendly data, but providers are concerned that important data are masked by making these reports too simple. All want more timely data, but careful data collection and risk adjustment take time and resources. Measures that are most relevant might not be readily obtainable from the available data, and requiring additional data places an extra burden on the providers who are responsible for collecting it.

The challenges facing performance measurement must be addressed to make it more effective. Vigilance is needed to ensure appropriate risk adjustment and to avoid unintended consequences. We have barely touched on important quality-related issues in areas such as pediatrics and behavioral health.[75]

Although this chapter has emphasized QI, achieving health care "value"—which takes QI to the next step by adding cost to the equation [6,42]—has become an equally important component in performance measurement. Recognizing that high costs are often associated with poor quality, the concept of value makes the business case for QI, something purchasers, hospital administrators, and governing boards find appealing.[6,68,76] More recently, the term "value-based purchasing" has been used interchangeably with P4P.

Above all, there remains a common objective—improve the quality, safety, and effectiveness of care provided to the patient. While more work is needed, it appears that public reporting and P4P have a strong foothold in efforts to do just that.[5]

Case Studies

Case Study 1: Hospital Compare

Hospital Compare[28] is a national public-reporting program with a website that presents information on how well hospitals provide recommended care to their patients. It focuses mainly on adult patients undergoing treatment for heart attack, heart failure, or pneumonia or for those having surgery, although it also reports data for pediatric asthma.

The several main reporting components of Hospital Compare are:

- Process of care measures: approximately 30 measures of the frequency with which hospitals adhere to care guidelines.

- Outcome measures such as 30-day risk-adjusted mortality and 30-day risk-adjusted readmission measures for heart attack, heart failure, and pneumonia.

- Data from the CAHPS (Consumer Assessment of Healthcare Providers and Systems) hospital survey,[77] which measures patient experiences during recent inpatient hospital stays.

Studies show that hospital performance on process indicators has improved since Hospital Compare began publicly reporting these results[78] and that improved or high performance on these measures is associated with better quality outcomes.[78,79]

Case Study 2: Pennsylvania Health Care Cost Containment Council

The Pennsylvania Health Care Cost Containment Council (PHC4) is an example of a state public-reporting program.[80] Established by statute in 1986, PHC4 is charged with the collection, analysis, and public reporting of information that can be used to improve the quality and restrain the cost of health care in Pennsylvania. This state agency has a long history of reporting risk-adjusted outcome measures at both the hospital and physician levels and has also reported quality indicator and member satisfaction information for health plans. Since its inception, PHC4 has incorporated clinical findings, such as laboratory test results, into its risk-adjustment methodologies.

PHC4's *Hospital Performance Report* is a comprehensive guide featuring risk-adjusted outcomes (e.g., in-hospital mortality, readmissions, and length of stay) for approximately 50 common medical procedures and treatments. This report was the subject of a recent study that concluded that patients treated in hospitals operating under intensive public-reporting conditions have significantly lower odds of in-hospital mortality when compared to similar patients treated at hospitals with no or limited public reporting.[54]

Case Study 3: Premier Hospital Quality Incentive Demonstration Project

The Premier Hospital Quality Incentive Demonstration Project (PHQID)[58] is an example of a national P4P or value-based purchasing initiative. It represents a joint collaboration between the Centers for Medicare and Medicaid Services (CMS) and Premier Healthcare Alliance. The project, involving more than 200 hospitals, was designed to determine whether providing financial incentives to hospitals is effective in improving care. The areas of study include heart attack, coronary artery bypass graft (CABG) surgery, heart failure, pneumonia, and hip and knee replacement. The measures include a mix of approximately 30 care indicators and outcomes. Premier has reported positive results from this study.[58] Other studies have shown varying results.[22,59,60-62]

Study and Discussion Questions

1. This chapter highlighted ways for health care providers to become more involved in reporting and P4P initiatives. What opportunities do clinicians believe are most important?

2. There is much discussion in the scientific literature about expanding the current slate of commonly reported measures in an effort to make them more relevant to patients. What performance measures do clinicians want to see included in reporting and P4P initiatives, recognizing additional data collection needs likely to accompany these measures?

3. Studies suggest that patients are interested in knowing the experiences of other patients.[5,79] What effects can be expected from the onslaught of social networking websites that facilitate this type of information sharing—often

including the names of individual clinicians? How might clinicians respond to material posted on these websites?

4. What opportunities will health information technology, including electronic health records, provide in ensuring that appropriate measures and risk-adjustment data are available for performance measurement?

Suggested Readings and Websites

Agency for Healthcare Research and Quality: www.ahrq.gov

Bridges to Excellence: www.bridgestoexcellence.org

Consumer Assessment of Healthcare Providers and Systems (CAHPS): www.cahps.ahrq.gov

HealthGrades: www.healthgrades.com

Hospital Compare (Case Study 1): www.hospitalcompare.hhs.gov

Hospital Quality Alliance: www.hospitalqualityalliance.org

Leapfrog Group: www.leapfroggroup.org

National Association of Health Data Organizations (NAHDO): www.nahdo.org

National Committee for Quality Assurance: www.ncqa.org

National Quality Forum: www.qualityforum.org

Pennsylvania Health Care Cost Containment Council (Case Study 2): www.phc4.org

Pacific Business Group on Health: www.pbgh.org

Premier Hospital Quality Incentive Demonstration Project (PHQID) (Case Study 3): www.premierinc.com/quality-safety/tools-services/p4p/hqi/index.jsp

The Joint Commission: www.jointcommission.org

U.S. News and World Report (Best Hospitals): http://health.usnews.com/best-hospitals

References

1. McGlynn EA, Asch SM, Adams J, *et al*. The quality of health care delivered to adults in the United States. *N Engl J Med,* 348(26):2635-45, Jan. 26, 2003.

2. Institute of Medicine. *Crossing the Quality Chasm: A New Health System for the 21st Century.* Washington, DC: National Academies Press, 2001.

3. Chassin MR, Galvin RW, National Roundtable on Health Care Quality. The urgent need to improve health care quality: Institute of Medicine National Roundtable on Health Care Quality. *JAMA,* 280(11):1000-5, Sept. 16, 1998.

4. Clancy C. The performance of performance measurement [editorial]. *Health Services Research,* 42(5):1797-1801,Oct. 2007.

5. Rothberg MB, Morsi E, Benjamin EM, *et al*. Choosing the best hospital: the limitations of public quality reporting. *Health Affairs,* 27(6):1680-7, Nov.-Dec 2008.

6. Brook RH. The end of the quality improvement movement: long live improving value [commentary]. *JAMA,* 304(16):1831-2, Oct. 27, 2010.

7. Epstein AM. Pay for performance at the tipping point [editorial]. *N Engl J Med,* 356(5):515-7, Feb. 1, 2007.

8. Rowe JW. Pay for performance and accountability: related themes in improving health care. *Ann Intern Med,* 145(9):695-9, Nov. 7, 2006.

9. Rosenthal MB, Landon BE, Normand ST, *et al.* Pay for performance in commercial HMOs. *N Engl J Med,* 355(18):1895-902, Nov. 2, 2006.

10. Epstein AM. Rolling down the runway: the challenges ahead for quality report cards [perspective]. *JAMA,* 279(21):1691-6, June 3, 1998.

11. Pine M, Jordan HS, Elixhauser A, *et al.* Enhancement of claims data to improve risk adjustment of hospital mortality. *JAMA,* 297(1):71-76, Jan. 3, 2007.

12. Tabak YP, Sun X, Derby KG, *et al.* Development and validation of a disease-specific risk adjustment system using automated clinical data. *Health Services Research,* 45(6, part 1):1815-35, Dec. 2010.

13. Tabak YP, Johannes RS, Silber JH. Using automated clinical data for risk adjustment: development and validation of six disease-specific mortality predictive models for pay-for-performance. *Med Care,* 45(8):789-805, Aug. 2007.

14. Escobar GJ, Greene JD, Scheirer P, *et al.* Risk-adjusting hospital inpatient mortality using automated inpatient, outpatient, and laboratory databases. *Med Care,* 46(3):232-9, Mar. 2008.

15. Jordan HS, Pine M, Elixhauser A, *et al.* Cost-effective enhancement of claims data to improve comparisons of patient safety. *J Patient Safety,* 3(2):82-90, June 2007.

16. Hibbard JH, Stockard J, Tusler M. Does publicizing hospital performance stimulate quality improvement efforts? *Health Affairs,* 22(2):84-94, Mar.-Apr. 2003.

17. Hibbard JH, Stockard J, Tusler M. Hospital performance reports: impact on quality, market share, and reputation. *Health Affairs,* 24(4):1150-60, July-Aug. 2005.

18. Bentley JM, Nash DB. How Pennsylvania hospitals have responded to publicly released reports on coronary artery bypass graft surgery. *Jt Comm J Qual Improv,* 24(1):40-9, Jan. 1998.

19. Marshall MN, Shekelle PG, Leatherman S, Brook RH. The public release of performance data: what do we expect to gain? A review of the evidence. *JAMA,* 283(14):1866-74, Apr. 12, 2000.

20. Fung CH, Lim Y, Mattke S, *et al.* Systematic review: the evidence that publishing patient care performance data improves quality of care. *Ann Intern Med,* 148(2):111-23,W17-W23, Jan. 15, 2008.

21. Hibbard JH, Stockard J, Tusler M. It isn't just about choice: the potential of a public performance report to affect the public image of hospitals. *Med Care Res Rev,* 62(3):358-71, June 2005.

22. Lindenauer PK, Remus D, Roman S, *et al.* Public reporting and pay for performance in hospital quality improvement. *N Engl J Med,* 356(5):486-96, Feb. 1, 2007.

23. Romano PS, Rainwater JA, Antonius D. Grading the graders: how hospitals in California and New York perceive and interpret their report cards. *Med Care,* 37(3):295-305, Mar. 1999.

24. Epstein AM. Public release of performance data: a progress report from the front [editorial]. *JAMA,* 283(14):1884-6, Apr. 12, 2000.

25. Ferris TG, Torchiana DF. Public release of clinical outcomes data–online CABG report cards [perspective]. *N Engl J Med,* 363(17):1593-5, Oct. 12, 2010.

26. Miller TP, Brennan TA, Milstein A. How can we make more progress in measuring physicians' performance to improve the value of care? *Health Affairs*, 28(5):1429-37, Sept.-Oct. 2009.

27. Rosenthal MB, Fernandopulle R, Song HR, Landon B. Paying for quality: providers' incentives for quality improvement. *Health Affairs*, 23(2):127-41, Mar.-Apr. 2004.

28. U.S. Department of Health and Human Services. Hospital Compare Web site. w w w. hospitalcompare.hhs.gov. Accessed March 31, 2011.

29. National Committee for Quality Assurance. HEDIS Web site. www.ncqa.org/tabid/59/ default.aspx. Accessed March 31, 2011.

30. Pronovost PJ, Miller M, Wachter, RM. The GAAP in quality measurement and reporting [commentary]. *JAMA*, 298(15):1800-2,Oct. 17, 2007.

31. Lee TH, Meyer GS, Brennan TA. A middle ground on public accountability. *N Engl J Med,* 350(23):2409-12, June 3, 2004.

32. Mitka M. Ratings game: lists of "top" physicians, hospitals has unclear impact on public [perspective]. *JAMA,* 302(15):1636,1639, Oct. 21, 2009.

33. Werner RM, Asch DA. The unintended consequences of publicly reporting quality information [special communication]. *JAMA,* 293(10):1239-44, Mar. 9, 2005.

34. Berwick DM. Public performance reports and the will for change [editorial]. *JAMA,* 288(12):1523-4, Sept. 25, 2002.

35. Damberg CL, Raube K, Teleki SS, dela Cruz E. Taking stock of pay-for-performance: a candid assessment from the front lines. *Health Affairs*, 28(2):517-25, Mar.-Apr. 2009.

36. Cardiac surgery in Pennsylvania: 2007-2008. Harrisburg: Pennsylvania Health Care Cost Containment Council, 2010.

37. Adult cardiac surgery in New York State: 2006-2008. Albany: New York State Department of Health, 2010.

38. Cardiac surgery in New Jersey: 2007. Trenton: New Jersey Department of Health and Senior Services, 2010.

39. Adult coronary artery bypass graft surgery in the Commonwealth of Massachusetts: Fiscal Year 2009. Boston: Massachusetts Data Analysis Center, Department of Health Care Policy, Harvard Medical School, 2011.

40. The California report on coronary artery bypass graft: 2007 hospital data. Sacramento: California State Office of Statewide Health Planning and Development (OSHPD), 2010.

41. Ross JS, Sheth S, Krumholz HM. State-sponsored public reporting of hospital quality: results are hard to find and lack uniformity. *Health Affairs,* 29(12):2317-22, Dec. 2010.

42. Porter ME. What is value in health care? [perspective]. *N Engl J Med,* 363(26):2477-81, Dec. 23, 2010.

43. Krumholz HM, Normand ST, Spertus JA, *et al.* Measuring performance for treating heart attacks and heart failure: the case for outcomes measurement. *Health Affairs,* 26(1):75-85, Jan.-Feb 2007.

44. Rosenthal MB, Landon BE, Howitt K, *et al.* Climbing up the pay-for-performance learning curve: where are the early adopters now? *Health Affairs,* 26(6):1674-82, Nov.-Dec. 2007.

45. Schneider EC, Epstein AM. Use of public performance reports: a survey of patients undergoing cardiac surgery. *JAMA,* 279(20):1638-42, May 27, 1998.

46. Schneider EC, Lieberman T. Publicly disclosed information about the quality of health care: response of the U.S. public. *Qual Health Care,* 10:96-103, June 2001.

47. The Kaiser Family Foundation. National survey on consumers' experiences with patient safety and quality information. Web site. www.kff.org/kaiserpolls/pomr111704p-kg.cfm. Accessed March 31, 2011.

48. Jha AK, Epstein AM. The predictive accuracy of the New York state coronary artery bypass surgery report-card system. *Health Affairs,* 25(3):844-55, May-June 2006.

49. Fisher ES. Paying for performance–risks and recommendations [perspective]. *N Engl J Med,* 355(18):1845-7, Nov. 2, 2006.

50. Schneider EC, Epstein AM. Influence of cardiac-surgery performance reports on referral practices and access to care: a survey of cardiovascular specialists. *N Engl J Med,* 335(4):251-6, July 25, 1996.

51. Casalino LP, Alexander GC, Jin L, Konetzka RT. General internists' views on pay-for-performance and public reporting of quality scores: a national survey. *Health Affairs,* 26(2):492-9, Mar.-Apr. 2007.

52. Chassin MR, Hannan EL, DeBuono BA. Benefits and hazards of reporting medical outcomes publicly. *N Engl J Med,* 334(6):394-8, Feb. 8, 1996.

53. Hannan EL, Sarrazin MSV, Doran DR, Rosenthal GE. Provider profiling and quality improvement efforts in coronary artery bypass graft surgery: the effect on short-term mortality among Medicare beneficiaries. *Med Care,* 41(10):1164-72, Oct. 2003.

54. Hollenbeak CS, Gorton CP, Tabak YP, *et al.* Reductions in mortality associated with intensive public reporting of hospital outcomes. *Am J Med Qual,* 23(4):279-86,July-Aug. 2008.

55. Petersen LA, Woodard LD, Urech T, *et al.* Does pay-for-performance improve the quality of health care? *Ann Intern Med,* 145(4):265-72, , Aug. 15, 2006.

56. Rosenthal MB, Frank RG, Li Z, Epstein AM. Early experience with pay-for-performance: from concept to practice. *JAMA,* 294(14):1788-93, Oct. 12, 2005.

57. Pearson SD, Schneider EC, Kleinman KP, *et al.* The impact of pay-for-performance on health care quality in Massachusetts, 2001-2003. *Health Affairs,* 27(4):1167-76, July-Aug. 2008.

58. CMS-Premier Hospital Quality Incentive Demonstration Project Website. www.premierinc.com/quality-safety/tools-services/p4p/hqi/index.jsp. Accessed March 31, 2011.

59. Grossbart SR. What's the return? Assessing the effect of "pay-for-performance" initiatives on the quality of care delivery. *Med Care Res Rev,* 63:1(suppl):29S-48S, Feb. 2006.

60. Glickman SW, Ou F, DeLong ER, *et al.* Pay for performance, quality of care, and outcomes in acute myocardial infarction. *JAMA,* 297(21):2373-80, June 6, 2007.

61. Ryan AM. Effects of the Premier Hospital Quality Incentive Demonstration on Medicare patient mortality and cost. *Health Services Research,* 44(3):821-42, June 2009.

62. Werner RM, Kolstad JT, Stuart EA, Polsky D. The effect of pay-for-performance in hospitals: lessons for quality improvement. *Health Affairs,* 30(4):690-8, Apr. 2011.

63. Rosenthal MB, Dudley RA. Pay-for-performance: will the latest payment trend improve care? [commentary]. *JAMA,* 297(7):740-4, Feb. 21, 2007.

64. Epstein AM, Lee TH, Hamel MB. Paying physicians for high-quality care. *N Engl J Med,* 350(4):406-10, Jan. 22, 2004.

65. Dudley RA. Pay-for-performance research: how to learn what clinicians and policy makers need to know [editorial]. *JAMA,* 294(14):1821-3, Oct. 12, 2005.

66. Werner RM, Dudley RA. Making the "pay" matter in pay-for-performance: implications for payment strategies. *Health Affairs,* 28(5):1498-508, Sept.-Oct. 2009.

67. Casalino LP, Elster A, Eisenberg A, *et al.* Will pay-for-performance and quality reporting affect health care disparities? *Health Affairs,* 26(3):w405-w414, May-June 007.

68. Young GJ, White B, Burgess JF Jr, *et al.* Conceptual issues in the design and implementation of pay-for-quality programs. *Am J Med Qual,* 20(3):144-50, May-June 2005.

69. Werner RM, Asch DA, Polsky D. Racial profiling: the unintended consequences of coronary artery bypass graft report cards. *Circulation,* 111(10):1257-63, Mar. 15, 2005.

70. Petersen LA, Woodard LD, Henderson LM, *et al.* Will hypertension performance measures used for pay-for-performance programs penalize those who care for medically complex patients? *Circulation,* 119(23):2978-85, June 16, 2009.

71. Ryan, AM. Has pay-for-performance decreased access for minority patients? *Health Services Research,* 45(1):6-23, Feb. 2010.

72. Ho K, Moy E, Clancy CM. Can incentives to improve quality reduce disparities? [editorial]. *Health Services Research,* 45(1):1-5, Feb. 2010.

73. Lee TH. Putting the value framework to work [perspective]. *N Engl J Med,* 363(26):2481-3, Dec. 23, 2010.

74. Porter ME. Measuring health outcomes: the outcome hierarchy. *N Engl J Med,* 363(26, suppl 2),S1-S19, Dec. 23, 2010.

75. Romano PS. Improving the quality of hospital care in America [editorial]. *N Engl J Med,* 353(3):302-4, July 21, 2005.

76. Clough J, Nash DB. Health care governance for quality and safety: the new agenda. *Am J Med Qual,* 22(3):203-13, May-June 2007.

77. US Department of Health and Human Services. Hospital Consumer Assessment of Healthcare Providers and Systems (HCAHPS) Website. www.cms.gov/HospitalQualityInits/30_HospitalHCAHPS.asp. Accessed March 31, 2011.

78. Werner RM, Bradlow ET. Public reporting on hospital process improvements is linked to better patient outcomes. *Health Affairs,* 29(7):1319-24, July 2010.

79. Jha AK, Orav EJ, Li Z, Epstein AM. The inverse relationship between mortality rates and performance in the Hospital Quality Alliance measures. *Health Affairs,* 26(4):1104-10, July-Aug. 2007.

80. Pennsylvania Health Care Cost Containment Council Web site. www.phc4.org. Accessed March 31, 2011.

81. Fanjiang G, von Glahn T, Chang H, *et al.* Providing patients web-based data to inform physician choice: if you build it, will they come? *J Gen Intern Med,* 22(10):1463-6, Oct. 22, 2007.

Chapter 15

The Importance of Patient Safety Organizations

By Michael C. Doering, MBA

Executive Summary

The primary objective of patient safety organizations is to improve health care facility processes based on guidance developed from the analysis of reported data. Additionally, information developed from this analysis should enable patients to make informed decisions and better steward their health care.

All patient safety organizations collect data on patient safety events. Depending on the jurisdiction and type of organization, data collection may be voluntary or mandatory. Upon receipt of the reported information, patient safety organizations analyze the reports to: identify issues and trends; identify potentially actionable information; communicate with facilities, providers, and consumers; communicate to governments; make recommendations for changes; and educate and train providers and patients. As patient safety organizations evolve, their missions should expand to include things such as dissemination of preventive recommendations, adoption of recommendations by industry change-agents, and achieving buy-in and support from clinical staff.

The states, rather than the federal government, set the trend in developing patient safety reporting programs and, by 2008, 26 states required some form of patient safety event reporting. State reporting requirements vary significantly regarding the number and definitions of reportable events, the threshold level of harm necessary for reporting, the primary use of the information, the issues of accountability versus confidentiality and mandatory versus voluntary reporting, and what type of facilities should report.

In 2009, the federal government completed regulations for formally recognized Patient Safety Organizations (PSOs). The PSOs conduct non-mandatory data collection from their member facilities using AHRQ common formats.

The Pennsylvania Patient Safety Authority (PaPSA) collects more than a quarter-million patient safety events a year from more than 1,200 Pennsylvania health care facilities. Utilizing the analysis of this information, the PaPSA publishes the Patient Safety Advisory, a peer-reviewed quarterly journal promoting evidence-based guidance to more than 5,000 subscribers in Pennsylvania and an additional 2,500 national and worldwide readers. It also developed educational programs that reach approximately 4,000 health care workers annually in person and many others through electronic media.

Learning Objectives

1. Understand a high-level history of patient safety organizations and the role event reporting played in shaping these organizations.

2. Understand some of the basic characteristics of patient safety event reporting.

3. Understand the potential activities of a mature patient safety organization.

Key Words: Patient Safety Organization, Patient Safety, Patient Safety Act, AHRQ, Patient Safety Event Reporting, Pennsylvania Patient Safety Authority, Patient Safety Rule

Introduction

Since the publication of the Institute of Medicine's *To Err Is Human*, there has been a proliferation of organizations that, collectively, can be called patient safety organizations (PSOs). This chapter looks at the history of PSOs, the role of event reporting in shaping their activities, their defining characteristics, and recent federal expansion of the concept through a formal Patient Safety Organization designation and certification.

PSOs work to protect the safety of patients receiving medical care. These organizations collect information about adverse events—and, in some cases, near miss or non-harmful events—from reporting facilities. The ultimate objective is to get facilities and providers to modify processes based on guidance developed from analysis of the collected information. In addition, many PSOs provide information to consumers/patients so they can make informed decisions and be better stewards of their health care.

All PSOs collect data regarding patient safety events. Most of this information is provided by reporting facilities voluntarily or, in many cases, to comply with state law. Upon receipt of the information, the PSO performs some or all of the following:

- Analyze the reports to identify issues, trends, and potentially actionable information.

- Communicate with facilities, providers, and/or consumers through published material, regular reports, and direct contact.

- Communicate to governments to ensure appropriate applications of law and to inform future legislation regarding health care facilities.

- Make recommendations for changes in facilities' and providers' infrastructure, policies and procedures, or work processes.

- Educate and train providers and patients on how to make safer the care they provide or receive.

While monitoring for safety concerns, analyzing data on patient safety events, and producing recommendations for prevention are necessary steps in achieving a safer healthcare system, these are only the first few steps. Although many PSOs have reached this level in their evolution, there is a larger chain of events that must occur in order for the system to become safer. Subsequent steps in the chain include dissemination of the preventive recommendations, adoption of these recommendations by change agents within health care organizations, achieving the buy-in and support of clinical staff as well as administration, allocation of adequate resources where necessary, and flawless execution. To be successful in actually improving care at the bedside, PSOs require the consent, cooperation, and collaboration of the organizations and individuals who provide the care.

Characteristics of Patient Safety Organizations and Reporting Programs

The 1999 Institute of Medicine (IOM) seminal report, *"To Err Is Human: Building a Safer Health Care System,"* significantly increased the focus on patient safety.[1] The report promoted patient safety event reporting and identified specific characteristics that should be included in a reporting system. The IOM believed that state governments should collect adverse event information that could be used to develop a national adverse events system.

States, rather than the federal government, took the lead in developing patient safety reporting programs. At the time the IOM report was published, 12 states required some form of patient safety event reporting using the National Academy of State Health Policy's (NASHP) tightened 2007 criteria for comparison purposes.[2] By January, 2008, the number of states with requirements had increased to 26.[1]

State reporting requirements vary significantly in the following ways:

Volume: Due to the differences in reporting requirements, reports collected annually differed substantially. Many state government-run programs implemented a list of 29 Serious Reportable Events (SREs) promulgated by the National Quality Forum (NQF), a national standards-setting body. Other states (e.g., New York) established their own lists of defined event types that must be reported. Still others (e.g., Pennsylvania) have established broad definitions of reportable events based on the level of injury and the patient outcome.

Level of harm: Some systems accommodate near miss and low level of harm reporting while many only accept the reporting of events that resulted in serious injury or patient death.

Primary end use of the information: Many systems are implemented to hold reporting facilities accountable for actively identifying patient safety events with the potential for making all information transparent to the public. There is a tension between efforts to change provider performance through transparency and accountability versus efforts to change it through quality improvement and education while keeping reported events confidential.

Confidentiality: A long-held belief is that facilities are more likely to report patient safety events if the information contained in a particular report is kept confidential. Particularly in systems that aim to collect reports of near miss and non-harm events, confidentiality is necessary to induce providers to report events that may otherwise be unknown, unobservable, and not available for analysis.

Mandatory versus Voluntary: Some states require reporting of certain events while others have merely established a system for data collection with reporting volume being completely dependent on voluntary submission by facilities. However, even in mandatory reporting programs, there is a sense in which all reporting is voluntary. Agencies collecting these data have put the majority of their effort into analyzing the reports they do receive rather than auditing to find the ones they don't receive.

Who Reports? Most patient safety data reporting systems focus on hospitals, though many go beyond this to include other settings of care. [2]

Expansion of state-required reporting led to an increase in PSOs. The type and number of events reported in a particular state differ significantly. Some states require the reporting of certain outcomes or very specific events. Ohio requires the reporting of any postoperative respiratory failure. Pennsylvania requires the reporting of 217 separate classifications of event types. In many cases, the level of harm is a contributing factor in determining whether an event is reported. Different types of events can be placed on a continuum as in Figure 1.

Figure 1. Continuum of Patient Safety Events by Severity

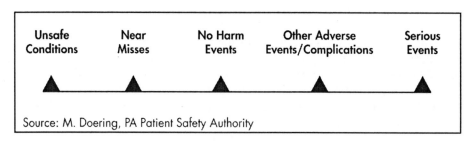

| Unsafe Conditions | Near Misses | No Harm Events | Other Adverse Events/Complications | Serious Events |

Source: M. Doering, PA Patient Safety Authority

Serious Reportable Events (SREs) are well-defined events that are considered egregious because they are of high severity and are believed to be preventable. Examples are performing the wrong surgical procedure on a patient, discharge of an infant to the wrong family, and stage 3 or 4 decubitus ulcers. Developed by the NQF, they were once known as *never events* because they "should never happen to a patient."

Other adverse events and complications cause harm to a patient but are not included in the list of SREs or do not cause enough harm to be considered an SRE.

No harm events are patient safety events that reach the patient but do not cause harm. An example would be giving the patient the wrong medication but without causing an adverse impact on the patient. This type of event is important as it can be a precursor to a similar event that could cause serious harm.

Near misses are patient safety events that do not reach the patient due to the intervention of a checking process or an alert health care worker. If an incorrect medication is dispensed but intercepted by the bedside nurse, this event is considered a near miss. This type of event is important because, without intervention, a near miss might cause serious harm to a patient.

An unsafe condition is a condition that could easily lead to a more serious patient safety event if the situation is not addressed. Storing side by side, look-alike medications that are known to be mistaken for one other is an example of an unsafe condition.

The Office of Inspector General reported that, of 26 states with reporting systems, three base reporting solely on SREs, while eight use a modified version of the SREs.[1] The remaining states utilize a host of other diverse event reporting requirements. This variation in reporting requirements has led to large differences in the number of reports submitted in a given state—from 305 in Minnesota in 2010[3] to more than 250,000 in Pennsylvania for the same year.[4]

The Importance of Reporting Near Misses and Other Non-Harmful Events

In November 2003, the IOM released a report calling for a standardized reporting format to facilitate data aggregation between states.[5] This report also recommended that near misses and events that reach the patient but do not cause harm be included in reporting. Some consider non-harm reporting to be a waste of resources, arguing that a facility might spend all its time collecting events rather than working on improving processes. However, there are some clear benefits to collecting non-harm events.

- Non-harm events provide a relatively benign learning opportunity. A near miss event can identify a problem that needs to be addressed without waiting for a potentially catastrophic event with serious patient injury. In addition, a report of an actual wrong site surgery informs the reader as to the potential cause of the error while a report of a near miss can identify not only the cause, but the intervention used to keep the event from reaching the patient.

- Because some SREs happen quite infrequently, there may be insufficient reports to develop a substantive determination of possible causes and potential guidance for improvement. Near miss reports add to the body of information used for these purposes.

A near miss can be more informative than an SRE. When the Pennsylvania Patient Safety Authority (PaPSA) published information regarding the frequency of wrong site surgery in Pennsylvania, a reporter called to ask me if any specific events were interesting or stood out. I told him about a report on a patient who was supposed to have surgery to repair a ligament in the right knee. The surgeon who spoke with the patient pre-operatively said he wanted to confirm surgery on the left knee. The patient did not correct the surgeon. A few minutes later, the patient called a nurse over and said he believed the surgeon was going to operate on the wrong knee. The nurse asked why the patient didn't correct the surgeon. The patient replied, "Because he's a doctor."

The reporter asked what happened to the patient. I said that the nurse made sure everyone was aware of what knee was to be repaired and surgery was completed properly. The reporter responded, "So the patient was OK? That's not interesting." But it was interesting to us. If the patient had never said anything and merely hoped that the correct knee would be repaired, an SRE could have occurred. Because this near miss was reported, we learned a great deal—including the existence of a communication barrier between a surgeon and her patient.

Challenges to Patient Safety Reporting Programs

All patient safety organizations utilize some type of patient safety reporting system. According to Harper and Helmreich, "…the purposes of these reporting systems are to 1) collect patient safety information by providing care providers with the means to report events or errors, and 2) enable organizations to use this information to create changes to reduce the likelihood of the reoccurrence of the error."[6] While reporting has proliferated, there are several issues associated with reporting systems:

- Reporting facilities can view patient safety event reporting as a burden on resources. Many larger facilities already track adverse events and potential adverse events internally for risk management and other purposes. Reporting to external organizations can require multiple entries of the same event; for instance, facilities may be required to report the same event to the Centers for Medicare and Medicaid Services, state agencies, and one or more accreditation organizations. In addition, each of these organizations may require different information, and thus unique handling, of the same event.

- The same event can be classified differently depending on the reporting system. For example, an anesthesia block performed on the wrong side of the patient is considered a wrong site surgery in some reporting systems, but not in others.

- Reporting systems may not yield an accurate representation of event rates; for example:

  o A patient safety event contributes to the numerator of a rate equation (e.g., wrong site surgery per 10,000 surgeries performed). However, most reporting systems do not collect the corresponding denominator to enable completion of the equation.

  o State requirements can lead to variable interpretations by reporters (e.g., to be reportable in Pennsylvania, a patient safety event needs to be "unanticipated,"[7] but, unfortunately, the word "unanticipated" is not defined or clarified in the corresponding Pennsylvania statute, resulting in differing interpretations by reporting facilities).

  o Because of under-reporting, one cannot be certain that all reports of all events have been received by any reporting system. Different facilities report at differing rates due to the maturity of the culture of safety within the facility, which affects the dedication and willingness to report these events. Individual health care workers may not report events. When surveyed regarding potential under-reporting, health care workers agreed with the following statements between 10 and 28 percent of the time.

    — "I did not think my report would result in any changes being made."

    — "I did not have the time."

    — "I did not want anything negative to happen to the people I work with."

    — "I did not want my name to be attached to a report."

Many patient safety event reports are filed by nursing personnel. However, it is important for physicians to report as well. If physicians believe in the importance of reporting, other facility staff will be more comfortable with reporting. Why don't more physicians report? The five self-reported barriers to event reporting for physicians are:[8]

1. No feedback on event follow-up—57.7 percent

2. Form too long; lack of time—54.2 percent

3. Event seemed trivial—51.2 percent

4. Was busy or forgot—47.3 percent

5. Not sure who is responsible to make report—37.9 percent

Given the issues associated with reporting, a commonly asked question is whether there is value in reporting systems and PSOs. Another typical question raised is why hospitals are required to report to PSOs if they are monitoring events reported internally. Several important reasons are listed below.

Aggregation of rare events: A wrong site surgery event may happen only once in three years in a medium sized hospital, but it happens across the Commonwealth of Pennsylvania more than once a week.[9] Aggregation of numerous, yet relatively rare, events allows a patient safety organization to analyze the causes of events and release more generalized improvement guidance.

Prompting facilities to focus on patient safety: Not all facilities have cultures that are conducive to patient safety improvement. Many might not focus on identifying patient safety events without a requirement that they do so.

Transparency: Reporting patient safety events promotes transparency within the facility, which benefits both staff and patients.

The Joint Commission states that aggregation and analysis of data collected through reporting systems could result in the reduction of medical errors.[6] As with any type of reporting system, the mere reporting of events does not guarantee success. Success comes from using the reported and aggregated information to drive changes in process, procedure, policy, and practice to improve patient safety.

The Federal Government Introduces Formal Patient Safety Organizations

Due in part to the IOM's recommendation to capture information to assist in reducing harm to patients, the U.S. Congress passed the Patient Safety and Quality Improvement Act of 2005 (Patient Safety Act)[1] which mandated several items to assist in improving safety for patients, including the development of a national patient safety database and the establishment of a network of formal PSOs.

To implement the Patient Safety Act, the Department of Health and Human Services promulgated the Patient Safety and Quality Improvement Final Rule (Patient Safety Rule) in January 2009.[10] The Agency for Healthcare Research and Quality (AHRQ) is one of the agencies charged with implementation of The Patient Safety Act through administration of the Patient Safety Rule. AHRQ is responsible for PSO operations.

According to AHRQ, "A PSO is an entity or a component of another organization that is listed by AHRQ based upon a self-attestation by the entity that it meets certain criteria established in the Patient Safety Rule. The primary activity of an entity seeking to be listed as a PSO must be to conduct activities to improve patient safety and health care quality. A PSO's workforce must have expertise in analyzing patient safety events, such as the identification, analysis, prevention, and reduction or elimination of the risks and hazards associated with the delivery of patient care."[11]

To qualify as a PSO, an entity must satisfy numerous requirements related to preservation of confidentiality, security of data, utilization of qualified staff, data collection using common formats, and development and dissemination of guidance to member facilities. As of November 2011, there were 78 listed qualifying PSOs.[12] PSOs can differ in their scope and organization. They may serve hospitals in a particular state (e.g., the Maryland Patient Safety Center PSO), a specific specialty or event type (e.g., the Institute for Safe Medication Practices, which is limited to medication-related events), a certain facility type (e.g., academic medical centers or rehabilitation hospitals), or a group of affiliated hospitals or a hospital system.

PSOs are reassessed periodically to determine if they continue to meet the qualifications for certification. One requirement is that a PSO must be "active"; i.e., have evidence of contracts with member facilities. Lack of business is one reason why, as of November 2011, 29 entities were de-listed because they no longer qualified as PSOs.[13]

In theory, PSOs could be a winning proposition for all parties. The federal government wants standardized information for the national patient safety database, and it assumes that the PSOs (which must use the AHRQ common formats for data reporting) will voluntarily submit reports. Facilities that participate in PSOs benefit from generous confidentiality provisions that apply to anything classified as patient safety work product, and stand to benefit from any patient safety improvements brought about by the efforts of the particular PSO. These benefits are likely to appear over time as the system matures. Facilities will have to determine the value of membership in a particular PSO with an eye to cost of participation. Time will tell how successful the PSO network will be.

The Pennsylvania Experience

The Pennsylvania Patient Safety Authority (PaPSA) received a report about the following near miss event in 2005:

> [C]linicians nearly failed to rescue a patient who had a cardiopulmonary arrest because the patient had been incorrectly designated as "DNR" (do not resuscitate). The source of the confusion was that a nurse had incorrectly placed a yellow wristband on the patient. In this hospital, the color yellow signified that the patient should not be resuscitated. At a nearby hospital, in which this nurse also worked, yellow signified "restricted extremity," meaning that this arm is not to be used for drawing blood or obtaining IV access.

> Fortunately, in this case, another clinician identified the mistake, and the patient was resuscitated. However, this "near miss" highlights a potential source of error and an opportunity to improve patient safety by re-evaluating the use of color-coded wristbands.[14]

The facility reported this patient safety event to the PaPSA in accordance with Pennsylvania law. While there was no harm to the patient, the result could easily have been catastrophic. The patient safety analyst reviewing the event was curious as to what extent wristbands cause error in Pennsylvania. PaPSA conducted a survey of Pennsylvania hospitals to determine which colors were used to denote different meanings. The results are presented in Figure 2, page 238. In the sample of facilities that returned the survey, blue wristbands were used to identify 13 different meanings including DNR and allergy to latex. DNR or limited DNR could have been represented by five different colors.

Figure 2. Variety of Medical Messages and Colors Used on Patient Wristbands in PA Facilities[14]

Message \ Colors	Purple	Blue	Teal	Green	Red	Pink	Orange	Yellow	White
DNR									
Limited DNR									
Fall Risk									
Restricted Extremity									
Allergy (other than latex)									
Allergy to Latex									
Tape Allergy									
Procedure Site									
Blood Type/Blood Bank ID									
No Blood Products									
Outpatient or ER Patient									
Pediatrics/Mother-Child Match									
Parent/guardian									
Similar Name									
Observation									
Isolation									
Elopement									
Pacemaker									
Anticoagulants									
Nothing by Mouth (NPO)									
Dietary Restrictions									
Diabetics									

Reprinted with permission of PA Patient Safety Authority

The PaPSA published this information in a supplemental Pennsylvania Patient Safety Advisory and distributed it to all patient safety officers in the Commonwealth. A group of facilities in the northeast region of the Commonwealth formed a working group, *The Color of Safety Task Force*, to develop standardized colors for use by many types of facilities. The Authority and the Hospital and Healthsystem Association of Pennsylvania supported the effort.

While not necessarily recommending the use of colored wristbands, the PaPSA did advocate limiting the number of wristbands in use, standardizing the meanings associated with the colors, pre-printing or embossing the meaning on the wristband, and other practices. Numerous facilities in Pennsylvania adopted the Authority's suggested practices, including standardizing the meanings of the colors. The cause was taken up by many other PSOs around the country and, with one small change (also accepted by Pennsylvania), the recommendations of *The Color of Safety Task Force* have been adopted in more than 38 states[15] and has been endorsed by the American Hospital Association.[16] The reporting of one non-harm event led to changes that are taking place nationwide.

The foregoing is an example of how PSOs are supposed to work. Information is submitted to a PSO through a reporting system. The PSO conducts analysis and conveys feedback to participating facilities. Recommendations and/or guidance can also be given to facilities. These activities can be conducted solely by the PSO or in conjunction with collaborative partners. It also illustrates the point that reporting, by itself, will not improve patient safety. Improvement is dependent on what is done with the information that is reported.

Established by Pennsylvania's MCARE Act of 2002, the PaPSA is an independent state agency charged with taking steps to reduce and eliminate medical errors by identifying problems and recommending solutions that promote patient safety. It is governed by an 11-member Board appointed by the Governor and the legislature. In June 2004, hospitals, ambulatory surgery facilities, and birthing centers began reporting patient safety events to PaPSA through the Pennsylvania Patient Safety Reporting System (PA-PSRS). In 2006, abortion facilities began reporting and, in 2008, nursing homes began reporting all health care-associated infections (HAI) to the PaPSA. The PaPSA focuses on data collection, analysis, guidance, education, and training related to patient safety in Pennsylvania. PaPSA is non-regulatory and is independent of the PA Department of Health, which is charged with providing regulatory oversight.

Pennsylvania law mandates the reporting of patient safety events through PA-PSRS regardless of whether the event caused harm to the patient. As of November 2011, the PPSA has received more than 1.5 million reports from Pennsylvania facilities and more than 250,000 reports in 2010 alone.[4] Excluding HAI, 7,508 (approximately 3.3 percent) of all reports cause harm to the patient. Figure 3 summarizes the reports received in PA-PSRS during 2010.

Figure 3. Summary of Reports Submitted in PA-PSRS (2010)

Facility Type	Harm	No Harm	NH HAI	Total
Acute Hospital	5,500	188,165		193,665
Other Hospital	747	27,443		28,190
Ambulatory Surgery Centers	1,244	2,405		3,649
Other	17	103		120
Nursing Homes			27,869	27,869
Total	7,508	218,116	27,869	253,493

Source: M. Doering, PA Patient Safety Authority

When a report is submitted to PA-PSRS, it is subjected to an electronic triage process that prioritizes the report and places it in an appropriate queue for patient safety analysts to review. PPSA patient safety analysts include nurses, attorneys, biomedical engineers, pharmacists, statisticians, and physicians. Utilizing the data, the analysts develop articles for the *Pennsylvania Patient Safety Advisory*.

Articles in the *Advisory* draw on PA-PSRS data to frame a specific patient safety issue using statistics and narrative. The articles promote evidence-based guidance as found in the current clinical literature. The Authority's web site (separate from the reporting system) receives about 22,000 unique visits and 75,000 separate page hits per month.

The Patient Safety Rule states that no entity using a mandatory reporting system can qualify as a PSO.[17] While the PaPSA cannot have the formal federal PSO designation, it is widely considered to be one of the most mature, broadly functioning patient safety organizations in the country. In 2008, the PaPSA's Board chose to significantly expand the agency's efforts in education and collaboration and, by 2011, many supporting programs had been implemented.

The following are examples of the programs and activities conducted by the PaPSA. These are the types of activities that PSOs could be implementing.

- Regional and hospital-specific educational programs that train approximately 4,000 Pennsylvania health care workers annually.

- Regional patient safety liaisons employed by PaPSA visit facility patient safety officers, conduct training, facilitate communication and sharing between facilities, disseminate guidance, and encourage adoption of safety practices.

- Management of and participation in numerous collaborative projects with 98 hospitals and partners, including the members of the PA chapter of the National Surgical Quality Improvement Program (PA-NSQIP), regional quality alliances such as southeastern PA's Health Care Improvement Foundation, and the Hospital and Healthsystem Association of PA.

- Educating hospital trustees on their role in encouraging a culture of safety and in challenging management to adopt safe practices.

- Educating patients on the importance of taking a more active role in their health care and on the safety practices they should expect when interacting with health care providers. These efforts include the development and distribution of consumer tips based on selected articles from the Advisory on topics where consumers can potentially influence providers' adherence to best practice (e.g., hand washing).

Conclusion

The federal government, states, patient safety organizations (federally certified or not), and individual facilities are focusing numerous resources on improving the safety of patients in the health care environment. However, the fluidity of health care treatment and the absence of absolute and comparable data make it difficult to measure and make conclusions regarding the success these organizations have in improving patient safety. Marking the 10th anniversary of the IOM report, Dr. Robert Wachter graded overall improvement in patient safety a B minus utilizing 10 factors of measurement.[18] While this grade increased from a C five years earlier, it still highlights that significant work is still required.

While an overall patient safety measurement statistic may be elusive, improvement has been demonstrated in specific areas. The following are examples from Pennsylvania.

- Pennsylvania has comprehensive health care-associated infection (HAI) reporting requirements for hospitals and nursing homes. The Patient Safety Authority, the Department of Health, and the Pennsylvania Healthcare Cost Containment Counsel all utilize the data to facilitate improvement activities. Since Pennsylvania's focus on HAI reduction began, significant progress has been made. Hospital central line-associated bloodstream infection (CLABSI) rates have been reduced in hospitals by 24.4 percent from 2009 to 2010[19] and are reportedly approximately one-third lower than the national average.[20]

- The Philadelphia-based Health Care Improvement Foundation sponsored a collaborative in which participating hospitals achieved a 72 percent reduction in wrong site surgery.[20]

- Wrong site surgery persists in Pennsylvania hospitals, but the severity of the cases has been reduced as a greater proportion of events now consist of wrong-side regional anesthesia blocks.[20]

These are just a few examples of what can be accomplished. With continued efforts and focus, harm to patients can be further reduced and, for some events, hopefully eliminated.

Study and Discussion Questions

1. Should patient safety reporting be voluntary or mandatory?

2. What do you believe are the benefits to a national database of patient safety reports? Can this system be used to monitor the rate of incidence of patient safety events?

3. Are PSOs beneficial in improving patient safety or should facilities be left to individual patient safety improvement programs?

4. Do higher rates of reporting events with patient harm indicate a facility that is less safe or a facility that has a good culture of safety and reporting? Is your answer the same for near misses?

5. Are you comfortable reporting patient safety events?

Suggested Readings and Web Sites

Readings:

HHS PSO Final Rule—http://edocket.access.gpo.gov/2008/pdf/E8-27475.pdf

Pennsylvania Patient Safety Authority 2010 Annual Report—
http://www.patientsafetyauthority.org/PatientSafetyAuthority/Documents/2010_Annual_Report.pdf

National Academy for State Health Policy, patient safety publications—
http://www.nashp.org/pst-nashp

GAO report to Congress on implementation of Patient Safety Act—
http://www.gao.gov/new.items/d10281.pdf

Web Sites:

AHRQ Patient Safety Page—http://www.ahrq.gov/qual/

AHRQ PSO website—http://www.pso.ahrq.gov

Pennsylvania Patient Safety Authority—http://www.patientsafetyauthority.org/Pages/Default.aspx

NASHP—http://www.nashp.org/

National Quality Forum patient safety page—
http://www.qualityforum.org/Topics/Safety_pages/Patient_Safety.aspx

ECRI Institute PSO website—
https://www.ecri.org/products/patientsafetyqualityriskmanagement/PSO/Pages/default.aspx

Institute for Safe Medication Practices PSO—http://www.ismp.org/about/pso.asp

References

1. Office of Inspector General. *Adverse Events in Hospitals: State Reporting Systems.* Washington, DC: Department of Health and Human Services, Dec. 2008.

2. Rosenthal, J and Takach, M. *2007 Guide to State Adverse Event Reporting Systems. State Health Policy Survey Report.* Washington, DC: National Academy for State Health Policy, Dec. 2007.

3. Division of Health Policy. *Adverse Health Events in Minnesota, Seventh Annual Public Report.* St. Paul, MN: Department of Health, Jan. 2011.

4. Pennsylvania Patient Safety Authority. *2010 Annual Report.* Harrisburg, PA: PA Patient Safety Authority, 2011.

5. Institute of Medicine Committee on Data Standards for Patient Safety. *Patient Safety: Achieving A New Standard for Care.* Washington, DC: National Academies Press, Nov. 2003.

6. Harper ML, Helmreich RL. Identifying Barriers to the Success of a Reporting System. In Henriksen K, Battles JB, Marks ES, Lewin DI, ed. *Advances in Patient Safety: From Research to Implementation,* Vol. 3: Implementation Issues. Rockville, MD: Agency for Healthcare Research and Quality, Feb. 2005.

7. Medical Care Availability and Reduction of Error (MCARE) Act. Act of Mar. 20, 2002. Pennsylvania, P.L. 154, No. 13, Sec. 302. 2002.

8. Evans SM, Berry JG, Smith BJ, *et al.* Attitudes and barriers to incident reporting: a collaborative hospital study. *Qual Saf Health Care* 15(1):39-43, Feb. 2006.

9. Pennsylvania Patient Safety Authority. Doing the "Right" Things to Correct Wrong Site Surgery. *PA PSRS Patient Saf Advis* 4(2):29,32-45, 2007.

10. Agency for Healthcare Research and Quality. *Patient Safety Organization Information,* May 27, 2011. http://www.pso.ahrq.gov/psos/overview.htm.

11. Agency for Healthcare Research and Quality. *Legislation, Regulations, and Guidance.* May 27, 2011. http://www.pso.ahrq.gov/regulations/regulations.htm.

12. Agency for Healthcare Research and Quality. *Geographic Directory of Listed Patient Safety Organizations.* May 27, 2011. http://www.psa.ahrq.gov/listing/geolist.htm.

13. Agency for Healthcare Research and Quality. *Delisted Patient Safety Organizations.* May 27, 2011. http://www.pso.ahrq.gov/dellisted.delistedpsos.htm.

14. Pennsylvania Patient Safety Authority. Use of color-coded wristbands creates unnecessary risk. *PA PSRS Patient Saf Advis,* 4(2):29,32-45, 2005. http://www.patientsafetyauthority.org/Advisories/AdvisoryLibrary/2005/dec14_2(suppl2)/Pages/dec14;2(suppl2).aspx.

15. The St. John Companies. *State color-coded wristband standardization,* March 2011. http://www.patientidexpert.com/material/us_colorcode_implementation.pdf.

16. American Hospital Association. *Implementing Standardized Colors for Patient Alert Wristbands.* Sept. 2008. http://www.aha.org/advocacy-issues/tools-resources/advisory/2008/080904-quality-adv.pdf.

17. Agency for Healthcare Research and Quality. Patient Safety and Quality Improvement Act of 2005. *http://www.pso.ahrq.gov/statute/pl109-41.htm.*

18. Wachter RM. Patient safety at ten: unmistakable progress, troubling gaps. *Health Affairs,* 29(1):165-73, Jan.-Feb. 2010. (published online Dec. 1, 2009; 10.1377/hlthaff.2009.0785).

19. Pennsylvania Department of Health. *Healthcare-associated Infections in Pennsylvania, 2010 Report.* Harrisburg, September 2011: 4, 52.

20. Marella WM. Commentary: Signs of Safety Improvement in Pennsylvania's Healthcare Community. *PA PSRS Patient Saf Advis* 8(1):41-3, 2011. http://patientsafetyauthority.org/ADVISORIES/AdvisoryLibrary/2011/mar8(1)/Pages/41.aspx.

Chapter 16

An Evidence-based Approach to Engaging Patients

By Judith Hibbard, DrPH and Mary Minniti, CPHQ

Executive Summary

Current health care policy directions, including innovations such as the PCMH, that seek to engage patients in their own care recognize the critical role that patients play in determining health outcomes and health care costs. Activated or engaged patients can be an important resource for improving health care quality and outcomes. Activation refers to the degree to which an individual understands his or her own role in maintaining and promoting personal health and the extent to which he or she possesses a sense of self-efficacy for taking on this role. In this chapter we examine what is meant by patient activation or engagement, why it is important, how it is measured, and strategies that clinicians can use to support patient engagement or patient activation. Two case studies are presented that illustrate how clinicians and teams of clinicians can use measurement to better engage with their patients and improve outcomes.

Learning Objectives

1. Define patient activation, identify how to measure it, and delineate how it is different from patient compliance.

2. Describe the levels of activation and what they mean.

3. Describe the methods by which clinicians can use measurement to better engage their patients.

Key Words: Patient Activation, Patient Engagement, Behavior Change

Introduction

The triple aims of health care reform are to improve the quality of care, to improve population health, and to constrain costs. These aims are beginning to be reflected in how providers are paid; i.e., rewarding providers who deliver high-quality care, demonstrate better outcomes, and do it a lower cost.[1] With so much at stake, attention has also focused on patients and the role they play in achieving these goals. After all, what patients do in their everyday lives has a tremendous impact on their health and the outcomes of care, not to mention their need for care. In effect, patients can be an important resource in achieving the triple aims. This is particularly true for activated patients, those patients who have the knowledge and skills to manage their health.

Recognition of the patient's role in health outcomes and health costs is manifested in current health care policy directions, including such innovations as the PCMH, which seeks to engage patients in their own care, and the linking of provider payments to patient experience scores.

In this chapter we examine what is meant by patient activation or engagement, why it is important, and strategies that clinicians can use to support patient engagement or patient activation.

What Is Meant by Patient Engagement or Patient Activation?

In this chapter we use the terms patient activation and patient engagement interchangeably, referring to the same idea. Activation or engagement is the degree to which an individual understands his or her own role in maintaining and promoting personal health and the extent to which he or she possesses a sense of self-efficacy for taking on this role. It is a global construct reflecting an individual's overall knowledge, skill, and confidence for self-management. Thus, the concept involves beliefs about one's role as well as knowledge and self-efficacy for being a steward of one's own health.

Being an activated patient implies more than simply following medical advice; it means taking a proactive role in one's own health. This construct is measured using the Patient Activation Measure (PAM),[2-3] a 13-item questionnaire that measures the latent concept of activation[4] on a scale of 0-100. Activation or engagement appear to be developmental; i.e., individuals go through different phases or levels as they become more competent self-managers over time.[5]

How does this concept differ from what clinicians have been doing all along? Clinicians already give patients information so that they can make better choices and change behaviors that put them at risk. Providers have always played a role in encouraging positive behavior changes in patients, but activating patients is a different approach.

Supporting behavior change focuses on getting patients to "comply" with medical advice or to change a specific risk behavior. In contrast, patient activation or engagement focuses on facilitating the skills, knowledge, and confidence necessary for an individual to take an active role. To be proactive, patients must feel a certain level of ownership and a sense of control over events related to their health and health care. Building confidence through experiential learning and small steps is the key strategy for increasing activation.

Why Is Patient Activation Important?

Studies of different populations in a variety of settings indicate that patient activation, as measured by the Patient Activation Measure (PAM), is correlated with a full range of health behaviors and many health outcomes. For example, the PAM score is significantly correlated with most preventive behaviors (e.g., screenings, immunizations), healthy behaviors such as healthy diet and regular exercise, health information-seeking behaviors, and disease-specific self-management behaviors (e.g., medication adherence, condition monitoring).[4-9]Higher activation scores also have been linked with patients' having fewer unmet medical needs, a regular source of care, and higher participation rates in physical therapy after spine surgery.[8-10] The findings remain statistically significant even after controlling for socio-demographic factors and insurance status. Furthermore, studies conducted in several countries have replicated the findings.[11-14]

Activation scores are predictive of outcomes within condition-specific patient groups, including multiple chronic conditions, serious mental health diagnoses, heart disease, multiple sclerosis, chronic obstructive pulmonary disease, cancer, inflammatory bowel syndrome, hypertension, asthma, and diabetes.[7,15-17]

Lower activation scores have been correlated with higher use of costly health care services—e.g., emergency department use, hospitalization, and re-hospitalization within 30 days of discharge.[18] One longitudinal study examined whether activation scores could predict future behavioral and health outcomes for diabetes patients. This Kaiser Permanente study following diabetic patients from 10 states over a two-year period found that baseline PAM scores were significant predictors of glycemic control, adherence to diabetic testing, and hospitalizations in a subsequent two-year period.[19]

In addition to linking activation level with behaviors, research findings also indicate that certain behaviors are unlikely to occur until people become more activated. Behaviors that are more complex, that require sustained action, or that require a more proactive approach are unlikely to occur until people are at the highest levels of activation. For example, knowing about treatment guidelines for a chronic condition, or being persistent in asking questions when providers are unclear, occurs almost exclusively among the most activated patients.[20]

What Does a PAM Score Indicate?

PAM scores indicate where an individual falls on a continuum of activation or engagement. As indicated above, the PAM score gives the clinician insight into a range of behaviors and behavioral tendencies. Without an intervention or special effort to change, PAM scores are relatively stable. A number of studies have documented interventions that increase activation scores. Research also shows that when PAM scores increase, multiple behaviors improve.[5] As patients begin to feel more "in charge" of their health, they apparently do many things differently, an indication that increased activation is an important intermediate outcome of care in itself.

Empirical evidence also reveals four activation levels (based on PAM scores) that individuals go through in the process of becoming fully competent managers of their own health.

Level 1: Patients may still be passive recipients of care and not understand the importance of playing active roles in their own health.

- They may lack good problem-solving skills.
- They are less likely to believe that they can positively influence their own health.
- They are more likely to report difficulty in handling stress in a healthy way than people at higher levels of activation.

Level 2: Patients may lack confidence or a basic understanding of their health status and recommended health regimens.

- They may have difficulty handling stress.
- They are less optimistic about their ability to positively influencing their own health.

Level 3: Although patients have the basic information and are beginning to take action, they may still lack some skills for making changes.

Level 4: Patients have adopted many necessary behaviors but may not be able to maintain them over time or in the face of life stressors.[3]

The value of identifying the activation level is to gain insight into possible strategies for supporting self-management among patients at different points along the activation continuum. The score is important in that a change of only a few points is linked with behavioral changes.[6] The level is useful for designing effective interventions and communications that will meet patients' needs, and the score is most useful for tracking progress.

Measuring patients' activation levels gives clinicians three key advantages in supporting patients. First, it provides an assessment to help clinicians tailor the type and amount of support necessary for an individual patient. It lets clinicians know where a patient is on this continuum and enables them to meet the patient there. Second, the score provides guidance on the type and amount of support that is likely to be helpful to the patient. Third, it provides a metric to track progress for an individual patient or a population of patients.

Four Levels of Patient Activation:

- Level 1 — Patients tend to be passive and feel overwhelmed with managing their own health.

- Level 2 — Patients may lack knowledge and confidence for managing their health.

- Level 3 — Patients appear to be beginning to take action but may still lack confidence and skill to support their behaviors.

- Level 4 — People have adopted many of the behaviors to support their health but may not be able to maintain them in the face of life stressors

Tailoring Support to Activation Levels:

- At **level 1**, focus on building self-awareness and understanding behavior patterns, and begin to build confidence through small steps.

- At **level 2**, work with patients, continuing in small steps that are "pre-behaviors," such as adding a new fruit or vegetable each week to their diet; reducing portion sizes at two meals daily; and beginning to build basic knowledge.

- At **level 3**, work with patients to adopt new behaviors and to ensure some level of condition-specific knowledge and skills. Supporting the initiation of new "full" behaviors (e.g., 30 minutes of exercise three times a week) and working on the development of problem solving skills.

- At **level 4**, the focus is on relapse prevention and handling new or challenging situations as they arise. Problem solving and planning for difficult situations help patients maintain their behaviors.

What Can Clinicians Do to Support Activation Gains in Patients?

Most clinicians prefer that everyone on their team has the necessary skills to function as a team member. If patients are "on the team" too, it is important to gauge their ability to function in that role. Assessing a patient's activation level provides valuable information on the patient's ability to self-manage. It also suggests how the clinician can best support the patient in gaining knowledge, skill, and confidence for doing so. Clinicians currently using the PAM to assess patients consider it an additional *vital sign* that provides essential information for working effectively with the patient.

Tailoring support to a patient's activation level simply means focusing on the challenges typically faced by people at their level of activation. Based on empirical findings, it is possible to identify and encourage specific behaviors that are realistic for people at a particular level.[20] For example, at Level 1, the typical challenges are lack of self-confidence in affecting own health, no or limited problem-solving skills, difficulty managing stress, overwhelmed by the task of managing their health, and inadequate grasp of their crucial role in the care process. An appropriate action plan will focus on self-awareness and mindfulness of behaviors, role delineation, and stress management, along with small behavioral action steps.

A small step is one that is likely achievable and will provide the patient an opportunity to experience success. The step may not be meaningful in a clinical sense, but success will build the patient's confidence. Taking the stairs at work three times during the coming week is an example of a small step.

A clinician can support actions that reduce the patient's feelings of being overwhelmed by giving the patient "permission" not to make all the necessary changes at once and by encouraging the patient to focus on a single change before tackling anything else. To avoid the common practice of providing people with too much information, a clinician might ask the patient what he or she would like to know more about.

At Level 2, patients are more likely to understand that they must play an active role, but they may lack the knowledge or the confidence to do so. It is essential to ensure that these patients understand the basics of their condition, their treatments, and the specifics of their role in care. Equally important is building a sense of competence by continuing to encourage small steps and reducing feelings of being overwhelmed.

Patients at Level 3 are beginning to be more active managers. An appropriate action plan is one that focuses on supporting the initiation of a new "full behavior," such as exercising for a half hour three times a week. Focusing on a single behavior at a time is beneficial.

Although they differ from those at earlier levels, patients at Level 4 face challenges of coping with new or unfamiliar situations as they arise, and maintaining behaviors already adopted even when routines change or during times of stress. Acquiring coping and problem-solving skills along with gaining awareness of environmental and situational factors that undermine the maintenance of behaviors are important at this level.

For patients in each level, experiencing a series of successes with the particular challenges they face builds a sense of self-efficacy and increases activation.[21-22] Encouraging realistic behaviors is part of enabling these successes. Acquiring the basic knowledge, beliefs, and skills in the earlier levels of activation is necessary in order to build a sense of efficacy for the self-management tasks in the later levels.

When a patient is permitted to choose the focus of behavior change, it helps the individual take ownership of his or her health. Also, because the individual is more motivated to make the change, it is more likely that she or he will succeed. With each success, the individual is likely to feel more competent to take on the next challenge. Experiencing success builds motivation to move forward. Thus, starting with behaviors the individual chooses (not necessarily the behaviors viewed as the most important clinically) will "kick start" the process of taking ownership and building a sense of competence.

The clinician might begin a conversation with a patient by asking, "If you were going to do something to improve your health starting today, what would you want to do?" Whatever the patient says, whether it be losing 50 pounds or not eating fast food every day, the clinician can help the patient focus on a step that will move him or her in the desired direction—a step that is realistic for the patient's level of activation.

For example, a patient at Level 1 says that cutting back on fast food is a good idea. Scaling the immediate action step to a small goal—one that can be achieved realistically in the near term—is a proven strategy. Engaging the patient in a conversation to select the target goal is essential; for instance, "I understand you are interested in eating less fast food. Instead of trying to do it all at once, why don't you think about doing it over time?" If the patient agrees, ask, "During the next week, would you be able to cut out fast food on two days?" Once the patient selects a goal, explore her or his confidence by asking, "How confident are you that this is doable?" The patient has chosen the goal, but the clinician has helped to scale it back to something that is likely achievable by the patient.

This tailored approach to support patient engagement was tested in a quasi-experimental study carried out in a disease management program. Using the patient's PAM score to tailor support, health coaches were trained and given guidelines to customize telephone coaching based on the patient's activation level. The goal was to ask patients to do things at which they could succeed to build confidence in their ability to manage their health. Another group of patients was coached in the usual way (without benefit of patient PAM scores).

The findings showed significant improvements in activation scores, adherence to treatment, clinical indicators (e.g., blood pressure and LDL), and reductions in utilization in the form of lower emergency department use and fewer hospitalizations during the six-month intervention. These improved outcomes were in comparison to those receiving "usual coaching."[23]

What Can Clinical Teams Do to Support Activation Gains in Patients?

The PCMH emphasizes team-based care and a population-based approach to care, both of which are designed to increase the quality of care and improve the health of patients.

Team-based care is an ideal platform for supporting patient activation. When a team-based approach is employed, all members of the health care team can use a patient's PAM score for consistency and better coordination of their interactions with and support of patients. Team members all know that a patient at level 2 should not be given reams of paper to read or a long list of behavior changes to make. Understanding the challenges faced by patients at different levels of activation, all team members reinforce the same messages and approaches. Hearing the same message from the dietician, the nurse, and the physician is more powerful than hearing it from a single clinician.

Team-based care is also more efficient, with resources being deployed according to specific needs of different populations rather than in a one-size-fits-all approach. For example, because low-activated patients are more passive, it may be necessary to reach out to them with a "high-touch" approach. Allocating additional staff time and/or determining the right mix of support services for low-activated patients are other ways in which teams use existing resources more efficiently. The more activated the patients, the more motivated and ready they are to use relevant information and pursue appropriate referrals.

The bottom line—by segmenting patient populations, it is possible to achieve better outcomes with the same amount of resources.

Two Case Studies Using Measurement to Guide Support for Patients in the Clinical Setting

1. Pursuing Perfection in Whatcom County, WA

In 2001, the Robert Wood Johnson Foundation responded to the Institute of Medicine's report *Crossing the Quality Chasm* by initiating a $20 million program called *Pursuing Perfection.*[24] Its intent was to stimulate innovation across the health care industry by focusing on six aims outlined in the report: patient-centered, efficient, timely, safe, evidence-based, and equitable. Whatcom County, north of Seattle, was one of seven elite organizations selected to "pursue perfection." Unlike other grantees, this was a consortium of community health care providers, independent of one another, yet collaborative in their approach to health care quality. The organizations included two not-for-profits (PeaceHealth St. Joseph Hospital and SeaMar), a federally qualified health center, three for-profit independents (key primary care providers, Family Care Network, and Madrona Clinic), as well as a specialty practice (Cascade Cardiology). Two insurers (Group Health and Regence) participated in all aspects of the effort, providing data to track the potential costs and benefits of the effort.[25] In some ways, this collaboration was an early version of what is now called an "accountable care organization."[26]

Whatcom County's aim was to create a patient-centered chronic care management system across the community. As patients on the grant planning team explained, "We don't live within health care organizations; we live in the community and need support regardless of which organization(s) from whom we might be receiving care." During the planning grant, in partnership with patient advisors, a clinical care specialist role was created. These positions were a shared resource in the community, i.e., unaffiliated with a specific practice site and hiring was done by patient advisors as well as representatives of the health care organizations. The nurses filling the positions had extensive experience in both hospital and outpatient settings. The medical director of the federally qualified health center provided clinical oversight, and the grant project director provided program supervision.

In the ongoing work with patients as advisors to the chronic care program, a philosophy emerged that the patient was the most important member of the care team. From this perspective, each patient had a "virtual care" team with members working in various organizations. This was especially true for patients who had multiple conditions and providers.

As implementation and referral to services for complex patients began in 2002, the priority became patients with diabetes and congestive heart failure. In the spirit of patient-centered care, the health issues, concerns, and needs of the patient determined how the clinical care specialists spent their time—a key strategy for engaging patients to align their goals and long-term health outcomes. Once a referral was made, the clinical care specialist completed an in-person assessment with the patient. Patient activation was a critical component and vital to the long-term success of the program. The PAM was used as part of a comprehensive assessment that included standard screenings for depression, quality of life, and functional outcomes.

Once the PAM was completed, patient responses were reviewed during the initial interview to explore topics identified as gaps in knowledge, skills, and/or confidence. For instance, if a patient disagreed with the statement, "I know what each of my prescribed medications do?" the RN elicited more detail with respect to the patient's understanding and identified opportunities to fill in the gaps. Since the survey questions were organized from easiest to most difficult to achieve, the patient's responses guided the RN in identifying needs for additional support. This approach built rapport quickly, allowing the RN to build on strengths identified by the patient and to help ensure the patient's success in taking the next steps.

The patient's patient activation level was re-surveyed every six months. To the surprise of the clinical care specialists, there was a dynamic change in the activation levels based on a variety of factors. There were some patients whose activation levels appeared to be high initially, despite referrals from community doctors who found their medical management challenging. When this population was re-measured after the first three to six months, their PAM scores decreased. The reason became clear in conversations with the patients. In some cases patients admitted that, because they had gained a better understanding of what it took to be actively managing their conditions, they rated themselves more critically in the second PAM. In other cases, patients reported either that they didn't understand the question or that they rated themselves higher because they didn't know the RN. In the absence of a trusting relationship with her, they were less honest in answering the questions. In a follow up conversation with the RN, one patient responded, "I thought I should know what my medications should do, so I didn't want you to think I didn't."

When a new health crisis and/or change in life circumstance emerged, a decrease among the "most activated" patients occurred—especially when physical function decreased significantly. This was an important learning because, once activation had been measured, services and the intensity of interventions were organized around the activation level. For a patient whose activation level was Level 4, support and outreach from the RN was less frequent than for a patient whose activation score was Level 2. As part of the program, the RNs were notified when patients accessed the emergency department (ED). In one such case, a Level 4 patient's recent ED visit prompted the RN to re-measure the individual's activation and found it to be Level 2. The patient had not been on a rigorous monitoring schedule because of the previously measured high activation level. As a result of this experience, it became standard practice to have monthly monitoring calls for patients with high activation levels but complex lives and/or conditions regardless of their most recent PAM.

Because the concept of patient activation was not widely understood or accepted, the RNs often received referrals of patients labeled "non-compliant" by the doctors. In most cases, closer assessment revealed that the individuals were very much interested in better health and quality of life but lacked the knowledge, resources, skills, and/or confidence to follow doctor's orders. As the RNs became more attuned to the concept of activation, they understood that "non-compliance" was an incorrect, disrespectful way to characterize patients—the antithesis of a truly patient-centered culture.

One nurse in the *Pursuing Perfection Program* in Whatcom County stated, "When people are trying to help an individual improve their health and self- manage it, knowing a patient's activation level and integrating this knowledge into the care provided is fundamental. Without it, the impact of any intervention is severely compromised. Unknowingly the caregiver and the patient are unprepared to achieve the improved health outcomes they both seek."

2. Team Fillingame, PeaceHealth Medical Group, Eugene, Oregon

From 2006 to 2007, Regence partnered with Peach Health Medical Group (PHMG) to fund small tests of change focused on improving diabetes care, increasing patient activation, and exploring opportunities to provide support to patients outside the primary care setting. In 2008, Regence invited PeaceHealth to develop a model of primary care that could be tested with a panel of patients to determine if transformation of primary care could meet the triple aims.[27] To that end, PHMG identified a physician champion, Ralph Fillingame, to work in collaboration with the PeaceHealth system and region to research and understand some of the best practices across the country.

A grant was submitted with the dual purpose of improving primary care delivery using a team-based approach and actively engaging the patient in managing her or his own care. The overarching goal was to reinvent *all* of primary care—not just how primary care manages chronic disease. The key was putting patients at the center of health care and enabling them to be the drivers of care rather than passive recipients.

To bring about this radical transformation, PHMG proposed a model wherein caregivers working together would improve access to primary care; reduce costs; execute evidence-based practices; and, together with the patient, achieve transformative results in health status. Two basic principles guided the Innovation Pilot ("Team Fillingame") design: "Make it easy to do the right thing for the patient" and "All should be working at the top of their license."

In the fully loaded team model, there are 2.5 health coaches, a 0.6 full-time equivalent (FTE) nurse practitioner, a 0.8 FTE RN care manager, a 0.75 FTE physician, one FTE care facilitator, and a 0.25 FTE wellness coordinator. This team has established protocols, clarified roles, and attended to training needs of team members to ensure effectiveness in their expanded roles.

The relationship of the physician to other team members has been changed substantially. By using protocols, explicit teams roles, and appropriate training, the physician has moved out of the "bottleneck" position emphasized by the traditional model. This reduces the burden on the physician, freeing him or her to focus on more complex situations that require diagnostic and clinical skills sets.

Team members serve patients on the basis of agreed-upon evidence-based standards and licensure. Any member of the team can refer to another team member without asking the physician. Because roles are well understood by all team members, questions are encouraged and freely asked to clarify roles and approaches in new situations. Such proactive support among all team members, including the physician, allows the team to continually improve care of patients.

The pilot program invited patients and their families to begin and/or expand their roles with Team Fillingame. A variety of outreach activities, coupled with ongoing verbal and written communications, supported patients' shift from passive recipients of services to active team members.

All team members, including the doctor, were trained in the concepts of activation and health coaching. Team Fillingame used the PAM to assess activation and organize services to better support patients. This "vital sign" along with other staff tools (e.g., a Coaching for Activation [CFA] website) were foundational elements that remain important today. The CFA website became a key component in expanding the capacity of the health coaches (i.e., "up-skilled" medical assistants) to access appropriate tools for supporting patient goal setting that is aligned with patient activation levels.

A goal of this patient engagement innovation was to increase the health coaching skills of all team members and to enhance their understanding of what activation is and how it impacts lifestyle and behavior choices. Beginning with assessments of activation levels for at-risk patients, the process has moved toward assessing activation levels for all patients on a yearly basis.

Re-measurement occurs more frequently if scores and significant team coaching time indicate a need. This provides valuable feedback to staff regarding their effectiveness in helping patients improve the confidence, skills, and knowledge needed to manage their health. Individuals with high levels of activation are more likely to adhere to medication regimens, actively pursue healthy lifestyle choices, and maintain focus on their health goals even under stress.

The team has found activation to be a critical piece of information for organizing appropriate follow-up and outreach activities with patients. Currently, activation level information is used in daily practice huddles. Any patient who has not completed a PAM in the previous year is re-measured. PAM scores are used to make on-the-spot changes to the office visit and subsequent follow-up. All team member assignments are informed by the patient's activation level. The domains of acuity and activation determine which team members are involved in follow up and what the plan of action entails.

Health coaches follow up on select patients with low acuity and activation Levels of 3 and 4. The RN care manager and/or the wellness coordinator (with behavioral health expertise) follow up on patients with higher levels of acuity and/or lower activation levels. This segmentation allows team members to work at the top of their licenses and meet patient needs. The goal is to improve patient's activation over time through targeted support, outreach, and assistance in goal setting.

The RN care manager provides direct care to complex patients in the practice as well as providing support and mentoring the health coaches on the team. According to the present RN care manager, assessing activation affects the care manager's ability to be an effective member of the care team: "Interestingly, learning about and using the PAM materials and tools has broadened my sense of who patients are and how they may perceive their place on the care team. Low knowledge and confidence about a disease process is often also reflected in how patients interact within the team environment. Building rapport and trust is so important in a team environment, with patients and with other team members."

Since nursing in primary care settings is very fast-paced and task-oriented, utilizing the PAM has changed relationships with patients as well as the interactions between team members and patients. The current RN care manger notes: "I may *know* what they need to do, but using the PAM activation level coupled with the PAM materials has allowed me to individualize the approach I take with patients. Understanding a patient's knowledge about and confidence in caring for a condition takes the traditional *jump-in-and-fix-it* approach out of an interaction with the patient."

During the pilot phase (2009-2010), at least two surveys were completed on 232 patients. Since patient activation changes on the basis of multiple factors, the team anticipated some movement. It was hoped that subsequent patient scores would show an increase over the baseline and that the improvements would be significant. To a great extent, this is what preliminary data revealed. (Figure 2 and Figure 3) Although some patients had small declines in their PAM scores, a larger group increased in activation over time. A smaller group had no change between surveys.

Figure 1. Coaching for Activation — How We Used Patient Activation Scores to Segment Population and Ensure Right Resource for Patient Needs

Activation Level ↓			
4	Care Facilitator / Peer Support	Health Coach RN, WC	NP + Team
3	Health Coach	NP + Team	NP, RN, WC
2	Wellness Coordinator	RN, WC, NP	MD, RN, WC
1	RN Care Mgr	NP	MD, RN
Acuity ⟶	Low	Medium	High

Table created by M. Minniti

Figure 2. Number of Patients with Changes on PAM Scores

Ranges in points	# Patients with Improved PAM	# Patients with Decline PAM
<10	62	59
10-20	30	27
20-45	25	7

Average Positive Variance	11
Median Positive Variance	7
Average Negative Variance	-10
Median Negative Variance	-7

Percentage of Patients with Improvement	47%
Percentage of Patients with Decline	39%
Percentage of Patients who stayed the same	14%

Figure 3. Distribution of Score Changes on PAM

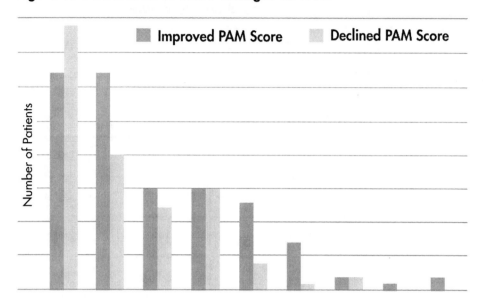

Unlike the previous case study, this one increased the competency of an entire primary care team in patient engagement and activation. This is a fundamentally different approach to primary care, especially for a physician in a traditional primary care practice. In reflecting on his experience with patient activation, Ralph Fillingame, MD, responded: "Assessing patient activation and applying it to motivational interviewing with the patient may be the secret sauce needed to make the patient-centered medical home work. I realized I have been delivering the same message in the same way to all my patients over the past 25 years as if all patients are the same. Obviously they are not. I am now less likely to 'lecture' to patients and more likely to explore with them the barriers to achieving the good health we both want for them. Giving up the concept that I am in control of what my patients do is frightening and freeing at the same time."

The typical metrics of outcomes, finances, and patient/team satisfaction have also been tracked. Preliminary data show improvement in commonly measured clinical outcomes such as hemoglobin A1C and hypertension control. A review of metrics revealed improvement in 8 of 10 clinical measures for the population; 50 percent of the improvements were statistically significant. For example, the percentage of patients with hypertension under control (i.e., <140/85) improved by 20 percent between 2009 (56 percent) and 2010 (76 percent).

Team Fillingame patients' monthly use of emergency department and/or urgent care for conditions appropriately treated by primary care decreased by 46 percent between December 2009 and December 2010. For overall ED usage, Team Fillingame observed a 54 percent decrease from the baseline year (2008) to 2010.

In addition to clinical outcomes, patient experience of care and organizational health were tracked. In both areas, there were significant improvements from baseline to the measurements in 2011. To understand staff satisfaction in this team model, the team was measured separately from other departments within PHMG. Staff scores improved in each of the yearly measurement periods. In the most recent survey (late winter of 2011), Team Fillingame improved its overall score and demonstrated stronger organizational health than 85 percent of the organization. In addition, Team Fillingame results have consistently improved each quarter on surveys of patient experience of care.

The Team Fillingame experience has been featured at national conferences on medical home and practice redesign, and the innovations are being implemented across PeaceHealth Medical Group, including the use of patient activation in daily practice as part of patient-centered primary care home efforts. It received the 2010 Society of Teachers of Family Management Practice Award and been highlighted as a case study at the Center for Health Professions website.

Study and Discussion Questions

1. What are some strategies that clinicians currently use to engage patients? Do you think they would work with patients of all levels of activation? Why or why not?

2. Are there ways that the current delivery system tends to "de-activate" patients? What are they?

3. If you were going to design motivational messages for patients at each level of activation, what would those messages be?

4. If a patient is not ready to take on all the tasks that they need to do to manage their health, how do you negotiate a realistic care plan that balances their behavioral and clinical needs?

5. What are some ways using a team can more efficiently do their work if they know a patient's activation level?

Additional Resources and Readings

Deen D, Lu WH, Rothstein D, et al. Asking questions: The effect of a brief intervention in community health centers on patient activation. *Patient Education and Counseling.* 84(2):257-60. Aug. 2011.

Dixon A, Hibbard JH, Tusler M. How do people with different levels of activation self-manage their chronic conditions? *The Patient.* 2(4):257-68, Dec. 1, 2009.

Donald M, Ware R, Ozolins I, et al. The role of patient activation in frequent attendance at primary care: A population-based study of people with chronic disease. *Patient Education and Counseling.* 83(2):217-21, May 11, 2011.

Frosch DL, Rincon D, Ochoa S. Mangione CM. Activating Seniors to Improve Chronic Disease Care: Results from a Pilot Intervention Study. *Journal of the American Geriatric Society.* 58(8):1476-503, Aug. 2010.

Greene J, Hibbard JH, Tusler M. How Much Do Health Literacy and Patient Activation Contribute to Older Adults' Ability to Manage their Health? *AARP Public Policy Institute*, June 2005.

Hibbard JH. Community-Based Participation Approaches and Individual Health Activation. *Journal of Ambulatory Care Management.* 32(2):275-7, Oct.-Dec 2009.

Hibbard JH and Mahoney ER. Toward a Theory of Patient and Consumer Activation. *Patient Education and Counseling.* 28(3):377-81, Mar. 2010.

Hibbard JH, Collins P, Mahoney E, Baker L. The Development and Testing of a Measure Assessing Physician Beliefs about Patient Self-Management. *Health Expectations.* 13(1):65-72, Mar. 2010.

Hibbard JH. Using Systematic Measurement to Target Consumer Activation Strategies. *Medical Care Research and Review.* 66(1, Suppl):9S-27S, Feb. 2009.

Hibbard JH, Greene J, Tusler M. Plan design and active involvement of consumers in their own health and health care. *American Journal of Managed Care.* 14(11):729-36, Nov. 2008..

Hibbard JH, Greene J, Painter M, *et al.* Racial/Ethnic Disparities and Consumer Activation in Health. *Health Affairs.* 27(5):1442-53, Sept.-Oct. 2008.

References

1. Fisher ES, McClellan MB, Bertko J, *et al.* Fostering Accountable Health Care: Moving Forward in Medicare. *Health Aff* (Millwood). 28(2):w219-w231, Mar.-Apr. 2009.

2. Hibbard JH, Stockard J, Mahoney ER, Tusler M. Development of the Patient Activation Measure (PAM): conceptualizing and measuring activation in patients and consumers. *Health Services Research.* 39(4, part 1): 1005-26, Aug. 2004.

3. Hibbard JH, Stockard J, Mahoney ER, Tusler M. Development and testing of a short form of the Patient Activation Measure. *Health Services Research.* 40(4, part 1):1918-30, Dec. 2005.

4. Hibbard JH, Mahoney ER. Toward a theory of patient and consumer activation. *Patient Education and Counseling.* 78(3):377-81, Mar. 2010.

5. Hibbard JH, Mahoney E, Stock R, Tusler M. Do increases in patient activation result in improved self-management behaviors? *Health Services Research.* 42(4):1443-63, Aug. 2007.

6. Fowles J, Terry P, Xi M, *et al.* Measuring self-management of patients' and employees' health: Further validation of the Patient Activation Measure (PAM) based on its relation to employee characteristics. *Patient Education and Counseling.*77(1): 116-22, Oct. 2009.

7. Mosen D, Schmittdiel J, Hibbard JH, *et al.* Is patient activation associated with outcomes of care for adults with chronic conditions? *Journal of Ambulatory Care Management.* 30(1):21-9, Jan.-Mar. 2007.

8. Becker E, Roblin D. Translating primary care practice climate into patient activation: The role of patient trust in physician. *Medical Care.* 46(8):795-805, Aug. 2008.

9. Hibbard JH, Cunningham P. How engaged are consumers in their health and health care, and why does it matter? *Research Briefs.* (8), Oct. 2008.

10. Skolasky RL, Mackenzie EJ, Wegener ST, Lee HR. Patient activation and adherence to physical therapy in persons undergoing spine surgery. *Spine.* 33(21):E784-91, Oct. 1, 2008.

11. Maindal T, Sokolowski I, Vedsted P. Translation, adaptation and validation of the American short form Patient Activation Measure (PAM13) in a Danish version. *BMC Public Health*, 2009: 9:209, June 29, 2009.

12. Steinsbekk A. Måling av effekt av pasientopplæring [Norwegian version of Patient Activation Measure (PAM)]. *Tidsskr Nor Laegeforen.* 128(20):2316-8, Oct. 23, 2008.

13. Fujita E, Kuno E, Kato D, *et al.* Development and validation of the Japanese version of the Patient Activation Measure 13 for mental health. *Seishinigaku (Clinical Psychiatry).* 5:765-72, 2010.

14. Coulter A, Ellins J. How engaged are people in their health care? Picker Institute Europe, Nov. 2005. http://www.pickereurope.org/item/document/36. [cited 2011 March 7]

15. Stepleman LM, Rutter C, Hibbard JH, *et al.* Validation of the Patient Activation Measure (PAM) in a Multiple Sclerosis clinic sample and implications for care. *Disability and Rehabilitation.* 32(19):1558-67, 2010.

16. Green CA, Perrin NA, Polen MR, *et al.* Development of the Patient Activation Measure for Mental Health (PAM-MH). *Administration & Policy in Mental Health and Mental Health Services Research.* 37(4):327-33, July 2010.

17. Munson, GW, Wallston, KA, Dittus RS, *et al.* Activation and perceived expectancies: Correlations with health outcomes among veterans with inflammatory bowel disease. *Journal of Internal Medicine.*24(7): 809-15, July 2009.

18. AARP Public Policy Institute. Beyond 50.09 Chronic Care: A Call to Action for Health Reform. 2009. http://assets.aarp.org/rgcenter/health/beyond_50_hcr.pdf. [cited 2011 March 7]

19. Remmers C, Hibbard JH, Mosen DM, *et al.* Is patient activation associated with future health outcomes and health care utilization among patients with diabetes? *J Ambul Care Manage.* 32(4):320-7, Oct.-Dec. 2009.

20. Hibbard JH. Using systematic measurement to target consumer activation strategies. *Medical Care Research and Review.* 6(1 Suppl):9S-27S, Feb. 2009.

21. Bandura, A. Health promotion by social cognitive means. *Health Education & Behavior.* 31(2):143-64, Apr. 2004.

22. Battersby MW, Ask A, Reece MM, *et al.* The Partners in Health Scale: the development and psychometric properties of a generic assessment scale for chronic condition self-management. *Australian Journal of Primary Health.* 9(3):41-52, Aug. 1, 2003.

23. Hibbard JH, Greene J, Tusler M. Improving the outcomes of disease-management by tailoring care to the patient's level of activation. *Am J Managed Care.* 15(6):353-60, June 2009.

24. Kabcenell A, Nolan T, Martin L, Gill Y. Innovation Series 2010, Pursuing Perfection Initiative: Lessons on Transforming Healthcare. Cambridge, MA: Institute for Healthcare Improvement, 2010.

25. Homer J, Hirsch G, Minniti M, Pierson M. Models for Collaboration: How Systems Dynamics helped a Community Organize Cost-effective Care for Chronic Illness. *Systems Dynamics Review.* 20(3):199-222, Fall 2004.

26. Minniti M. The healthcare crisis: are communities the solution?"*Oregon's Future*, Summer 2005.

27. Berwick DM, Nolan TW, Whittington J. The Triple Aim: Care, health, and cost. *Health Affairs*. 27(3):759-69, May-June 2008.

28. Blash L, Chapman S, Dower C. *Peacehealth's Team Fillingame Uses Patient Activation Measure to Customize the Medical Home.* San Francisco, CA: Center for Health Profession s, May 30, 2011. http://www.hwic.org/resources/details.php?id=9006

Chapter 17

Organizational Impact of Quality and Safety

By Rangaraj Ramanujam, PhD and Alon Peltz, MD, MBA

Executive Summary

Quality improvement (QI) interventions are often implemented without an accompanying effort to ensure proper alignment between the intervention and the organizational context. As a result several QI initiatives fail to deliver on their promise. This chapter provides a framework for understanding the impact of organizational context on QI and discusses the implications for implementing QI.

Learning Objectives

1. Recognize the critical impact of organizational context on the effectiveness of QI initiatives.
2. Utilize a framework of organizational performance for understanding the effects of the various contextual features of an organization.
3. Identify strategies for effectively managing the implementation of QI initiatives.

Key Words: Organizational Structure, Mission, Implementation, Structure, Nature of Work, Congruence

Introduction

The following case study clearly illustrates the impact of organizational context on QI initiatives.

In 2002, Cedars-Sinai, the world-renowned teaching hospital in Los Angeles, implemented a computerized order entry system (CPOE) that was internally developed over a three-year period at a cost of $34 million. It was designed to automatically check for drug-drug interactions, verify medication dosages, and enhance the accuracy of patient accounting bills. After being piloted in one department earlier that year, the system was subsequently launched simultaneously across all business units of this 877-bed facility with 1,800 practicing physicians. Within three months of the "implementation day," the administration was forced to pull the plug on the CPOE as a result of intense resistance from physicians who disliked the system. The well-intended and carefully planned quality improvement (QI) initiative was a spectacular failure.[1,2,3]

Unfortunately, Cedars' experience with CPOE is all too common in health care, where several carefully planned QI efforts have failed to live up to their promise.[4] (Table 1, page 265)

Such cases offer a sobering reminder of how organizational context can undermine the success of even the most carefully planned QI intervention. The CPOE was developed in response to growing evidence that proper utilization of electronic decision support software could facilitate medication management, reduce costs and errors, improve chronic disease management, and decrease unnecessary laboratory testing.[1,2,3] *The CPOE system at Cedars was tested with more than 20,000 test orders prior to launch. The subsequent organization-wide implementation, however, was flawed in many respects. The organization did not anticipate that the majority of clinicians would view the new system as representing a drastic change from the status quo or that they would remain skeptical about the promised downstream benefits of CPOE. Few clinicians had been involved in the design of the new system, and the level of training provided to clinicians was widely viewed as inadequate. Moreover, the all-at-once roll out did not provide a phase for trial and error, which is critical for learning any new complex technology. As the Chief Medical Officer of Cedars wrote in 2003, "[o]ne of the most important lessons learned to date is that the complexity of human change management may be easily underestimated."*[2]

Cases such as this raise an important question that is the focus of this chapter: If a technically sound improvement tool works in one clinical setting, shouldn't it also work in all other settings? In other words, how does organizational context shape the success or failure of a QI initiative?

To address this question, we present an influential framework of organizational performance and change[5] to identify the various features of their organizational context and their interrelationships. Using this framework, we discuss how these features can aid or enhance the effectiveness of QI interventions. We then discuss implications for developing effective implementation strategies.

Table 1. Examples of Implementation Failure in Health Care

QI Intervention	Description	Example	QI Outcome
Clinical Practice Guideline	Systematically developed, evidence-based statements designed to assist with decision making for specific clinical situations; improves care by increasing the use of appropriate interventions in a timely manner	The Ottawa Ankle Rules, a diagnostic clinical practice algorithm used in emergency medicine to help determine with high sensitivity, which patients may forgo radiography without risk of missing a clinically important fracture	A survey found that although 90% of US physicians reported awareness of the Ottawa Ankle Rules, only 35% of respondents reported using it daily in their clinical practices. (Lang, 2007)
Multidisciplinary Patient Rounds	An activity that promotes structured communication among members of a multi-disciplinary care team.	Bedside patient rounds at which professionals from multiple specialties come together to communicate, coordinate, make joint decisions, and set mutual goals for individual patients	There can be limited participation by "lower-status" health care professionals in multidisciplinary rounds (Corley, 1998)
Error Reporting System	Voluntary reporting of adverse events, errors, and near misses via formal systems such as computer programs and incident reports; allows organizations to learn from errors systematically	A national survey of clinicians investigated the hypothetical attitudes of clinicians toward using an error reporting system and their actual reporting or real errors.	Most (73%) physicians reported an inclination to report a hypothetical minor error; however, few (17.8%) had actually reported an actual minor error, and a similar number (16.9%) acknowledged not reporting an actual minor error. Slightly more than half of physicians knew how to use the error reporting system at their workplace. (Kaldjian, 2008)
Pay for Performance	Provider compensation that is contingent on adopting specified structures, performing specified processes, or achieving designated outcomes	A pay-for-performance initiative at a large west coast health plan sought to provide participating medical groups with financial benefits for meeting or exceeding 10 clinical quality goals.	The initiative showed very modest quality gains despite a significant financial investment. (Longo, 2005)

Adapted from Nembhard et al. 2009

Organizational Performance Framework

Important systematic approaches to QI were discussed in the preceding chapters: identifying problems, studying root causes, developing solutions, and examining outcomes. However, QI does not operate in a vacuum; it occurs in an organizational setting.[6] Too often, the make-up of the organization to which an improvement initiative is applied determines the success or failure of an initiative. An influential framework of organizational performance provides a systematic way to think about the various contextual features of an organization and their interrelationships (Figure 1). We will use this framework to help guide our understanding of organizations, their impact on QI, and the importance of tailoring a quality initiative to ensure consistency with the organization.

Figure 1. Congruency Model of Organizations

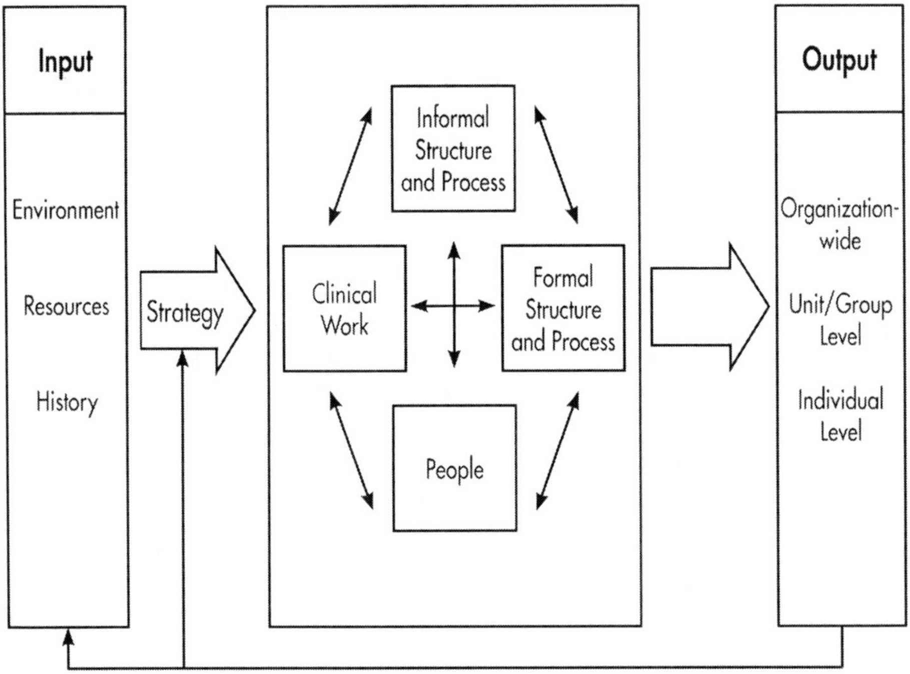

Adapted from Nadler and Tushman 1989

According to this framework, an organization is essentially a complex system that—given a set of limited resources, an external environment, and history—develops a strategy to convert inputs to a set of desired outputs or performance outcomes. The conversion process relies on four distinct yet mutually interacting components: work, people, formal structures and processes, and informal structures and processes. Before we elaborate on these components, which are especially relevant for our discussion of QI, we should note the following implications of this framework.

First, QI can be measured at different levels of analysis (e.g., a team of care providers, a micro-system, or a hospital). The configuration of the organizational components that enhances quality at one level may not necessarily improve quality at another level. For instance, an organizational context that promotes the quality of outcomes of individual employees may include a work design that emphasizes independent tasks and activities, organizational structure that demarcates roles and responsibilities of individuals, and organizationally shared values that emphasize individual contributions. This set of features may not be as effective in promoting quality at the group level. Similarly, a work design that focuses exclusively on promoting group performance may pose challenges for enforcing individual accountability. Therefore, a combination of approaches is required to promote performance across multiple levels. Identifying the system level that is targeted for QI is important for designing appropriate interventions for implementing the proposed system. This is also important for measuring learning and performance at the appropriate level.

Second, effective performance depends not only on features of work (i.e., clinical processes and outcomes) but also on their alignment or "congruence" with the organizational strategy and other organizational components. For instance, given competing strategic priorities, such as increasing revenues, reducing costs, and promoting safety, if the organizational design and processes are primarily aligned with cost reduction, the organization is more likely to respond to cost-related performance measures. Moreover, even when improvement on clinical performance is viewed as a priority, there may be competing priorities among various clinical processes and outcomes. This is especially likely as the proposed set of clinical performance measures widens. Thus, performance improvement will depend not only on the proposed QI but also on the extent to which it is congruent with the organizational strategy (e.g., how QI, as captured by specific peformance measures, fits into the organization's strategic agenda) and other organizational components (e.g., whether the roles and responsibilities of care providers are consistent with the requirements of the proposed measurement system). Absent such congruence, QI implementation may not translate into performance improvement as expected.

Third, to maintain congruence, a major change in any organizational component will require corresponding changes in the other components. In other words, effective implementation of the proposed system may require health care organizations to initiate corresponding changes in their strategies; formal and informal organizational structures and processes; design of care delivery processes; and the roles, responsibilities, skills, and attitudes of their employees. In short, it may require transformational change. Given these implications, we now turn to each of the four components that constitute the organization.

The Nature of Clinical Work

The characteristics of clinical work powerfully shape the cognitive, emotional, and social demands that clinicians routinely encounter while delivering care. Clinical work is increasingly complex, uncertain, time-pressured, risky, and interdependent.[6]

The unrelenting advances in knowledge of clinical, diagnostic, and therapeutic domains contribute to the growing complexity of practice. Yet, despite such advances, clinical work continues to be highly uncertain, with clinicians routinely encountering ambiguous situations that fall outside the scope of current knowledge.[7] Health care delivery is also risky in that mistakes can potentially have life or death consequences for patients and huge emotional and financial costs for providers.[8] This discourages the trial and error learning that is so essential for implementing any new QI intervention.[9] Primary care physician attitude to risk has been shown to negatively correlate to their willingness to utilize electronic information resources, such as MEDLINE, to guide their clinical decision-making.

In addition, health care delivery is time-sensitive, in that most treatment options cannot be deferred to accommodate other activities such implementing new QI interventions. Further, the trend toward increased workload also means that most clinicians have limited time for activities such as engaging in continuous QI. In the Cedars-Sinai case one of the reasons that clinicians rejected the initiative was it increased their already time-constrained workload.[2] Over and above all these features, clinical work is also unavoidably interdependent with some estimates suggesting that providing care to a single hospital patient involves 20 different health professionals.[7] This means that the effectiveness of QI efforts requires ongoing collaboration, communication, and coordination among the various participants in the continuum of care. Together, the various characteristics of clinical work pose a formidable set of challenges for creating the motivation, capabilities, and opportunities for care providers to regularly participate in QI.

People

The participants in the health care delivery system represent another important context. In health care, the workforce is *highly inter-professional* and, even within professions, *highly specialized.* In effect, the interdependent clinical work is jointly carried out by people with different professional backgrounds, such as physicians, nurses, pharmacists, and technicians, and different professional specialties. For example, a single patient may be evaluated and treated by respiratory therapists, an acute care nurse practitioner, a physician assistant, patient care technicians, registered nurses, and phlebotomists.[10] Physicians can choose to specialize in more than 140 different disciplines.[11]

The highly specialized inter-professional workforce poses major challenges for teamwork that is so critical for effective care delivery.[4] Differences in training, skills, and even technical language across professionals and specialties increase the risk of miscommunication, conflict, and misunderstanding during the regular course of work. The effects may be exacerbated when these team members are required to jointly embrace a QI intervention. The absence of collaboration and open communication contributes to quality errors and moral distress among health care workers.[12-15]

Another implication of relying on professionals is that their professional identity—i.e., their self-understanding of who they are, what they do, and what is (and is not) their work—is strongly shaped by their formative professional training.[6] Unlike workers who typically fulfill a defined task and responsibility, professionals are defined more globally by their qualifications, their memberships in organizations, and/or by their training.[16] Most professionals value autonomy and expect to be able to control the design and implementation of their work. A professional identity and values, which come with professional membership, promote meaningful job attachment and responsibility. However, if QI is not viewed as an inherent part of the professional role, it could lead some professionals to treat QI as an activity for which they have no professional obligation.

Formal structure

Another critical contextual feature of an organization is its structure—i.e., the arrangement of roles, responsibilities, and reporting relationships that is typically represented in the form of an organizational chart. Consider two characteristics of a formal structure—hierarchy and departmentalization. By hierarchy, we refer to the number of different levels in the chain of command. Hierarchies that are more vertical create status gradients that can inhibit upward communication flow. They present a considerable challenge to QI because the effectiveness of many QI initiatives relies on a team-based, bottom-up process that is enacted by front-line employees who are lower in the hierarchy. In many health care environments communication must typically transverse multiple "status" levels before ultimately reaching the top—which is usually assumed to be the physician. As a result, the hierarchy is vertical and individualistic. While all members of the professional team share control for the patient experience, in many health systems top-down communication challenges often continue to predominate.[12]

Organizational structure affects not only the division of labor but also the flow of information and the allocation of attention and resources in an organization.[17] For example, an organization in which activities are grouped by specialties (e.g., pediatrics, urology) can limit ongoing interactions between specialties and thus make it difficult for people to work across specialties. By contrast, an organization wherein activities are grouped around service (e.g., women's health) requires different specialists to regularly interact with one another. Implementing a QI program that requires ongoing collaboration will be more challenging than the first scenario.

Informal Relations (Culture)

The final contextual feature that exerts strong but invisible effects is the culture of an organization—i.e., the shared values, assumptions, and attitudes of the members of an organization.[18] The strength of a culture depends on the extent to which members share such a common understanding. Culture determines what people view as important and unimportant and what they view as acceptable or unacceptable. For instance, a strong organizational culture that values deference to authority (e.g., the physician) will not value inputs from front-line employees that are critical for QI.

Although culture is often considered an "intangible" characteristic, there is growing evidence that organizational culture impacts patient outcomes and worker satisfaction.[19-21] For example, an organizational culture with an exclusive focus on the bottom line and productivity may not be consistent with continuous improvement. Organizational culture has a major impact on how people in organizations choose from among competing priorities. Such situations are encountered routinely in health care, where the very notion of effective delivery is defined in terms of multiple criteria (i.e., efficacious, efficient, safe, timely, equitable, and patient-centered) that can often be in conflict. Therefore, the likelihood that people in the organization will consistently choose actions that enhance safety will depend on the extent to which the culture values safety as a priority relative to other criteria. In most hospitals, the culture values so called production pressures over safety and quality. In such a context, implementing a QI program can be problematic.

For QI to become embedded in day-to-day activities, the organizational culture must emphasize quality.[19] For example, the Virginia Mason Medical Center, in Seattle, Washington, has an institutional culture of quality. The vision of Virginia Mason is to "become a Quality Leader and transform health care". The culture of Virginia Mason is quality–and the hospital employees are united by a drive to eliminate patient harm and to improve quality. Each of the medical center's 5,000 employees is empowered by the leadership to act as a "patient safety inspector" and is encouraged to openly discuss concerns and to use the Patient Safety Alert system, the hospital's blame-free error reporting system.[18]

Implications for Implementing QI initiatives

So far, we have discussed the contextual features linked to each of the four organizational components separately. However, organizational context is really the interplay of these various contextual features. The impact of context on QI depends on the extent to which the context is congruent with the organizational requirements for QI intervention under consideration. This means that the implementation success of a QI initiative depends much less on any single strategy but rather on an integrated bundle of interrelated strategies that are aimed at enhancing the readiness of an organization to adopt an innovation such as a QI intervention. Readiness is related to whether the organization's members share in needs assessment of the current problem, understand how the innovation will fit with the current values of the organization, appreciate the implications of the innovation, and have dedicated resources and support for the intervention.[22] If the staff isn't concerned about an area, or if they do not see tangible benefits arising from the initiative, they, as the members of the system, are less likely to accept the initiative. Similarly, as has been discussed in previous chapters, the challenge of a QI initiative is to design it so that adequate time and resources are dedicated to the initiative. Regardless of how cleverly designed an improvement initiative, if the system is not ready to accept the initiative, it will not have the same benefits that are envisioned on paper.

The following are some strategies for enhancing the readiness of an organization to successfully adopt QI:

1. *Enable non-threatening experimentation and adaptation of QI.*

   Recall that we started our discussion of the nature of work by discussing the impact of four characteristics (uncertainty, risk, time-pressure, and interdependence) on the reluctance or inability of care providers to engage in the trial-and-error learning that is critical for QI. To encourage such experimentation, organizations should consider framing the QI intervention in terms of learning rather than performance. Research in psychology suggests that when new tasks are framed as a learning challenge, people are much more likely to explore new actions and relationships, change their current patterns of interpersonal interactions, and feel psychologically safer in sharing ideas with one another.[23] In contrast, when new tasks are primarily framed as a performance challenge, people tend to become risk-averse and are less likely to experiment or persist with the task long enough to gain competence.

   In addition to framing QI as learning, it is also important to create non-threatening opportunities such as pilot projects and simulations for employees to develop familiarity with a QI innovation. Such opportunities encourage experimentation because failures in this setting carry no risk of harm to patients. In addition, such opportunities help staff to directly experience the benefits of the QI intervention. This can significantly increase their subsequent commitment to this intervention.

   It is critical to provide additional time and resources for people to adapt to the QI intervention after it is implemented. One of the reasons the CPOE example at the start of the chapter failed was because the physicians were unprepared to spend a longer time using the computer to enter an order when they merely scribbled a drug abbreviation and dosage in the past.[2] Also of importance is making sure that project champions and leaders are allowed to dedicate sufficient time to the QI project—otherwise, the project will take a "back burner" to their many other responsibilities.

2. *Create formal structures to foster teamwork and collaboration.*

   As discussed earlier, highly specialized workplaces also present special challenges for implementing QI initiatives. Often, highly specialized units are not team-oriented structures and communication can suffer. In addition, the inherent vertical structure of health care makes bottom-up QI a challenge. Ease of communication between all levels of the responsibility chain requires flat communication channels. Examples of flat organization structures include structured team-oriented bedside rounds where all members of the health care team are afforded the opportunity to provide input into patient care decisions. While the physician ultimately will dictate the final course and treatment plan, this open communication allows all members to contribute.

In general, formal structures that routinely bring together various interdependent care providers and professionals during the process of delivering care increase the likely success of QI because of ongoing opportunities for information exchange that is critical for coordination and for the early detection of problems and opportunities at work. For instance, the high-performance health care system envisioned by the Institute of Medicine is less vertical and more horizontal and team-oriented. This style of collaboration, termed "expertise diversity," involves many different individuals, each with a specialized knowledge and skill level, who collectively bring together various perspectives through open communication channels.[10]

3. *Develop capabilities for transformational leadership and teamwork at all levels to elicit ongoing employee commitment.*

Transformational leadership refers to a set of processes that enables organizational leaders to elicit employee commitment to organizational goals. Transformational leaders shift the focus of organizational members from their individual or specialty-specific goals to broader collective goals such as safety and quality. They do so by being intellectually stimulating, charismatic, and considerate and by modeling collaborative behaviors. These processes can enable employees to recognize the overlap between their individual goals and the organization's collective goals. For instance, when leaders show consideration by ensuring that an employee's need for individual development is being fulfilled while working toward organizational goals, the employee tends to respond by voluntarily engaging in so-called citizenship behaviors (e.g., helping co-workers adapt to the new QI intervention) that, although not formally required by their job descriptions, are critical for successful implementation. Moreover, transformational leadership facilitates open communication, an essential pre-condition for the success of QI initiatives. Finally, transformational leaders often provide the support that is essential for employees to persist with QI in the face of competing priorities and setbacks during implementation.

Organizations can promote transformational leadership in at least a couple of different ways. First, they can hire leaders who have demonstrated transformational leadership in other organizations. Second, they can set up leadership development programs to train current leaders in the appropriate use of transformational leadership processes. Although the overall effectiveness of such programs in changing entrenched leadership styles remains an open question, there is growing evidence that such programs can change several specific leadership behaviors, such as communication style, which is critical for the success of QI efforts.

Transformational leadership is necessary at all levels in the hierarchy. At senior levels, it helps set the organizational priorities that become the basis for decisions and actions further down the hierarchy. Transformational leadership is necessary closer to the front line as well as in order to enlist care providers' ongoing commitment to the QI initiative.

4. *Create culture of quality.*

The long-term success of QI in any organization requires a culture that values quality and infuses this value in every other component. As Kotter writes, "... [u]ntil new behaviors are rooted in social norms and shared values, they are subject to degradation as soon as the pressure for change is removed."[24]

Because it is inherently intangible, culture cannot be the direct target of any implementation strategy. Rather, culture is the outcome of the integrated set of changes that are initiated in other organizational components. A culture of quality emerges over time as top management begins to routinely view quality as a major organizational priority, as leaders at all levels increasingly rely on transformational leadership styles to gain employee commitment to QI, as organizational structures shift toward arrangements that routinely warrant inter-professional collaboration, and as employees begin to participate more frequently in learning activities such as experimentation. This means that culture is not limited to any single QI intervention; rather it shapes and is shaped by all the various QI related activities of an organization.

Figure 2. The Emergence of Safety Culture

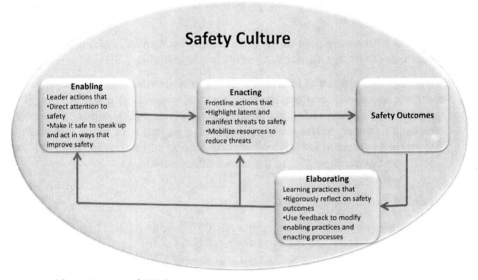

Adapted from *Vogus et al 2010*

A recent framework of safety culture (Figure 2) provides a way to think about the emergence of culture in terms of the various strategies we discussed above: "Safety culture involves actions that single out and focus safety-relevant premises and cultural practices that reduce harm.[19] This entails: a) enabling, which consolidates the premises for a safety culture; b) enacting, which translates consolidated premises into concrete practices that prioritize safety; and c) elaborating, which enlarges and refines the consolidation and translation."

Conclusion

There is growing recognition that, in order to more effectively fulfill their missions, health care organizations must implement a set of fundamental and wide-ranging changes in their care delivery processes, technology, people, structures, and the cultures. In other words, transformational change is indispensable for health care organizations to realize the promised gains from continuous QI.

QI efforts must necessarily address questions about: 1) the relationship between QI and the local organizational context (e.g., how the proposed performance measurement will affect and be affected by the formal and informal organizational structures and processes at the point of care), and 2) the implementation of the proposed system (e.g., how we can get health care organizations to adopt and utilize the proposed system).

Study and Discussion Questions

1. Consider any hospital that you are familiar with. Try to describe its organizational context in terms of various contextual features and organizational components. To what extent is the context congruent with the organizational requirements of a collaborative continuous QI process such as the Toyota Production System?

2. Based on your assessment of the congruence, what specific changes will you recommend to ensure the success of QI implementation?

3. Given that this chapter is intended to serve as an introduction to thinking about organizational context, the discussion of various contextual features is necessarily limited. Can you think of other contextual features associated with each of the organizational components (e.g., nature of work, culture) that might be relevant for QI? What is the impact of these features, and how would you devise strategies to manage it effectively?

Suggestions Readings and Web Site

National Healthcare Quality Report. 2010. AHRQ Publication No. 11-0004, Rockville, MD: Agency for Healthcare Research and Quality.

Institute of Medicine. *Crossing the Quality Chasm: A New System for the 21st Century.* Washington, DC: National Academies Press, 2001.

Kaplan GS, Patterson SH. Seeking perfection in healthcare: a case study in adopting Toyota production system methods. *Healthcare Executive.* 23 (3) 16-21, May/June, 2008.

Leape LL, Berwick DM. Five years after *To Err Is Human*: what have we learned? *JAMA.* 293(19):2384-90, May 18, 2005.

Weick, KE., Sutcliffe, KM. *Managing the Unexpected—Assuring High Performance in an Age of Complexity.* San Francisco, CA: Jossey-Bass, 2001.

Goleman D, Boyatzis RE, McKee A. *Primal Leadership: Learning to Lead with Emotional Intelligence.* Boston, MA: Harvard Business School Press, 2002.

References

1. Connolly, C. Cedars-Sinai doctors cling to pen and paper. *Washington Post*. Mar 23, 2005, p. A01.

2. Morrissey J. Harmonic divergence. Cedars-Sinai joins others in holding off on CPOE. *Modern Healthcare*. 34(8):16, Feb. 23, 2004.

3. Kass-Bartelmes BL, Ortiz E, Rutherford MK. Using informatics for better and safer health care. *Research in Action*, Issue 6. AHRQ Pub. No. 02-0031. Rockville, MD: Agency for Healthcare Research and Quality, 2002.

4. Nembhard IM, Alexander J, Hoff T, Ramanujam R. Why does the quality of health care continue to lag? Insights from management research. *Academy of Management Perspectives*. 2009, 23(1):24-42, 2009.

5. Nadler DA, Tushman ML. Organizational frame bending: principles for managing re-orientation. *Academy of Management Executive*, 3(3): 194, 1989.

6. Ramanujam R, Rousseau DM. The challenges are organizational not just clinical. *Journal of Organizational Behavior*. 27(7):811-27, 2006.

7. Bohmer, RMJ, Knopp, CI. The challenge facing the U.S. healthcare delivery system. (Case No. 9-606-096). Boston, MA: Harvard Business School Publishing, 2007.

8. Leape LL, Berwick DM. Five years after *To Err Is Human*: what have we learned? *JAMA*. 293(19):2384-90, May 18, 2005.

9. Tucker AL, Nembhard IM, Edmondson AC. Implementing new practices: an empirical study of organizational learning in hospital intensive care units. *Management Science*. 53(6):894-907, 2007.

10. van Der Vegt GS, Bunderson JS. Learning and performance in multidisciplinary teams: the importance of collective team identification. *The Academy of Management Journal*. 48(3):532-47, June 2005.

11. Accreditation Council for Graduate Medical Education (ACGME). List of ACGME-Accredited Specialties and Subspecialties, 2011.

12. Institute of Medicine. *Crossing the Quality Chasm: A New System for the 21st Century*. Washington, DC: National Academies Press, 2001.

13. Barnard, A. Doctors were unsure of roles as boy died at Children's. *Boston Globe*. September 19, 2003, p. A1.

14. Blatt R, Christianson MK, Sutcliffe KM, Rosenthal MM. A sensemaking lens on reliability. *Journal of Organizational Behavior*. 27(7):897–917, 2006.

15. Knifed E, Goyal A, Bernstein M. Moral angst for surgical residents: a qualitative study. *Am J Surg*. 199(4):571-6, Apr. 2010.

16. Drach-Zahavy. The proficiency trap: how to balance enriched job designs and the team's need for support. *Journal of Organizational Behavior*. 25(8):979-96, 2004.

17. White, KR, Griffith JR. *The Well-Managed Healthcare Organization*, Seventh Edition, Ann Arbor, MI: AUPHA/HAP.

18. Kaplan GS, Patterson SH. Seeking perfection in healthcare: a case study in adopting Toyota production system methods. *Healthcare Executive*. 23(3):16-21, May/June 2008.

19. Vogus TJ, Sutcliffe KM, Weick KE. Doing no harm: enabling, enacting, and elaborating a culture of safety in health care. *Academy of Management Perspectives*, 24(4):60-77, 2010.

20. Laschinger HK, Almost J, Tuer-Hodes D. Workplace empowerment and magnet hospital characteristics: making the link. *J Nurs Adm*. 33(7-8):410-22, May/June 2008.

21. Aiken LH, Clarke SP, Sloane DM, *et al*. Effects of hospital care environment on patient mortality and nurse outcomes. *J Nurs Adm*. 38(5):223-9, May 2008.

22. Greenhalgh T, Robert G, Macfarlane F, *et al*. Diffusion of innovations in service organizations: systematic review and recommendations. *Milbank Q*. 82(4):581-629, 2004.

23. Edmondson, AC Speaking up in the operating room: How team leaders promote learning in interdisciplinary action teams. *Journal of Management Studies*. 40(6):1419-52, 2003.

24. Kotter, JP. Why transformation efforts fail. *Harvard Business Review*. March–April 1995, pp. 59-67.

Section V.

Improving Health Care Quality: The National Agenda

Chapter 18

Tools for Quality Improvement: Six Sigma

By Yosef D. Dlugacz, PhD and Carolyn Sweetapple, RN, CPA, MBA

Executive Summary

Improving quality requires change, but, for many organizations, change is difficult to implement. It is easy to talk about changing the culture so that all employees embrace quality; i.e., open communication, transparent results of valid measures, organizational and personal accountability, and embracing a methodology to improve. However, in practice, such change is difficult to achieve.[1] Companies that succeeded in changing their organizational cultures (e.g., General Electric [GE]) used an objective statistical method to improve production, increase efficiency, and optimize positive results.[2] In this chapter we will discuss Six Sigma as a method for change and address some of the issues involved in generating and sustaining change for quality improvement.

Significant change is essential if health care organizations are to meet federal expectations (e.g., from Centers for Medicare and Medicaid Services [CMS]) that contain soaring medical costs, provide access to the uninsured, and reduce poor outcomes for patients.[3] Billions of dollars in incentive payments are being offered to health care organizations and providers to improve care by reducing variation, developing order sets to standardize processes, adopting computerized medical records, and using a methodology to create effective medical services.[4]

To meet the needs of today's health care agenda, health care organizations must have the ability to create databases, generate sophisticated analytics, and develop methodologies and tools to manage the new expectations to determine the effectiveness of processes and services. Organizations that develop and deploy methods for addressing quality outcomes, patient safety issues, efficiency and waste analyses, prevention strategies, the public demand for transparency, and the selection of services based on results will survive in the increasingly competitive health care marketplace.[5]

Learning Objectives

1. Understand the role of data in assessing and improving processes.

2. Describe how Six Sigma can be used to change organizational culture.

3. Define the issues involved in applying Six Sigma to health care.

Key Words: Organizational Change, Process Improvement, Quality Methodology, Data

Introduction

The Value of Data

Data, statistical measurements, and analytics are among the tools necessary for cultural change as well as being crucial to working within a contemporary health care environment. Increasing demands from chief financial officers (CFOs) for quality data and explanations of quality measurements drive organizations to rely on methodology. Recognizing this, graduate level curricula in health care education programs offer (and often require) courses in operational statistics, methods, control charts, developing variables, regression analysis, sampling, and more.[6] The value of understanding and being able to work with complex data and databases no longer engenders arguments or advocacy. And with the advent of the electronic medical record and computerized physician order entry, data will be increasingly available and abundant.[7]

Quality of care is measured via data. Quality improvements are monitored via data.[8] Government and regulatory agencies require data to ensure that the standard of care is delivered. Increasingly, reimbursement will involve data with a focus on *how* care is provided rather than on *how much* care is provided. Because data are so integral to health care, chief executive officers (CEOs) have begun to insist that hospital managers and clinicians learn to work with data in order to explain their quality of care in comparison with the quality of other organizations.[9]

What is Six Sigma?

A quality methodology that originated in the manufacturing industry, Six Sigma relies on data and statistical analyses to help businesses link improved quality with increased profit. In the 1980s, an engineer for Motorola (Mikel Harry) realized that the products with the fewest defects, or those products that deviated the least from the standard, performed best after delivery to the customer. He developed the basic structure of Six Sigma, reducing defects through a defined series of steps (DMAIC):

- **D**efine the problem and the customer's goals.

- **M**easure key aspects of the current process while collecting data.

- Analyze the data to understand cause-effect relationships and identify the root cause of the defect being investigated.

- Improve the process based on data.

- Control deviations from the process and monitor continuously.

Motorola and then General Electric (GE) developed and adopted Six Sigma as both their quality methodology and their business strategy.[10] The Motorola CEO, Bob Galvin, hoped to achieve a culture of continual improvement with zero product defects by adopting Six Sigma. Importantly, he required everyone at the company to be responsible for, and to, each other in achieving this goal. In 1988, the company, which had been floundering financially due to poor quality, won the prestigious Malcolm Baldrige National Quality Award. This award evaluates an organization's team approach, level of accountability, reliance on data for decision-making, and analytics to improve processes and work redesign.

Realizing that GE would save approximately $10 billion by improving quality to the level of Six Sigma, CEO Jack Welch launched Six Sigma at the company in 1996. His goal was to accomplish what Motorola had done but within a shorter time frame. Welch's contribution to Six Sigma as a business model was to involve leadership and to reward success with incentives. The financial incentives inspired employees to participate in quality performance improvements and to become involved in Six Sigma. Welch also directed that any employee in a position of manager or higher be specifically trained in Six Sigma tools and processes. Moreover, he insisted that corporate executives lead the quality charge. All employees at all levels had to buy into the quality improvement methodology.[11]

Among the reasons that Six Sigma appealed so strongly to Jack Welch was that it uses a very practical and applied (rather than theoretical) approach to quality problems and solutions. He liked the concept of identifying and eliminating defects to ensure improved quality and conformity to the standard. Without defects, customers would be satisfied and recalls, maintenance problems, and waste would be reduced, with a concomitant rise in profits—a "win-win" proposition.

Six Sigma and Culture Change

In 1998, Mark Chassin, now president of The Joint Commission, wrote an article entitled: "Is Health Care Ready for Six Sigma?" for the *Milbank Quarterly.*[12] In it, he stressed the necessity of understanding the underlying causes of problems before adopting Six Sigma in the health care environment:

> *"Serious, widespread problems exist in the quality of U.S. health care: too many patients are exposed to the risks of unnecessary services; opportunities to use effective care are missed; and preventable errors lead to injuries. Advanced practitioners of industrial quality management like Motorola and General Electric have committed themselves to reducing the frequency of defects in their business processes to fewer than 3.4 per million, a strategy*

*known as Six Sigma Quality. In health care, quality problems frequently oc-
cur at rates of 20 to 50 percent, or 200,000 to 500,000 per million. In order
to approach Six Sigma levels of quality, the health care sector must address
the underlying causes of error and make important changes: adopting new
educational models; devising strategies to increase consumer awareness;
and encouraging public and private investment in quality improvement."*
[Abstract]

Massive culture change must occur before health care organizations are able to
integrate quality into every level of care. Six Sigma is not a magic bullet or a quick
fix for a broken process. Although a powerful statistical tool and rigorous process,
the real strength of employing Six Sigma lies in promoting new ways of thinking
about old problems. Answering the following questions can lead to making necessary changes:

- What are the root causes of the defect, and what are the ramifications of the
  improvement?

- What is stopping the organization from fixing an existing problem?

- What factors are needed to bring Six Sigma (or any sophisticated quality
  methodology) into the health care organization?

- How can the organization use Six Sigma as a force to change culture?

The Role of Leadership

Fundamental organizational change comes from the top. When introducing Six
Sigma to change organizational culture, leadership commitment is the most important aspect. If the CEO directs that quality be introduced into every level of
the organization and that every employee be held accountable for defects, the organization will undergo positive change. Establishing accountability for change
and adopting a model of change based on quality is the responsibility of senior
staff. The national organizations wrestling with the challenges of health care—
e.g., the Institute for Healthcare Improvement, the Institute of Medicine, the National Quality Foundation—all agree that improving quality and safety requires
the CEO's complete commitment.

The CEO must invest in training employees to be Six Sigma experts, and such
training takes time. The goal of the training is not only to teach statistical tools to
talented people but to actually make an impact on the way issues and problems
are viewed. Individuals who receive training in Six Sigma should be encouraged
to work on varied projects throughout the organization for several years before
assuming leadership positions and guiding others.

It should be noted that, as quality theorist Joseph Juran pointed out, identifying
experts to facilitate quality improvements is not a new concept.[13] However, the
deliberate and focused training and support of leadership makes these facilitators
more potent in the organization.

Six Sigma training has various degrees of expertise. The CEO and other top organization leaders that compose the Executive Leadership set a vision for Six Sigma implementation and provide resources for improvements. The Executive Leadership identifies Champions from upper management who are responsible for integrating Six Sigma into projects across the organization. The Champions identify Master Black Belts whose sole responsibility is to act as coaches for Six Sigma projects. Under their supervision, Black Belts apply Six Sigma methods to specific projects, focusing on the execution of the project. Green Belts work under the guidance of Black Belts to implement Six Sigma projects.

Six Sigma Training

At the North Shore-Long Island Jewish (LIJ) Health System, certain individuals in management and leadership roles were identified by senior leadership as being of high potential for more responsible leadership roles. Several years of extensive training prepared these targeted individuals for advancement in this large diverse health system. Using an applied learning model, education was focused on team building and communication skills, analytic skills, Six Sigma methodology, and change management.

In the process of changing the way a person considers problems, Six Sigma training changes the individual's internal culture, which, in turn, becomes a key component in changing the organizational culture. Health care professionals know that data are necessary for intelligent decision-making and that methodology should be applied to problem-solving.[14] But Six Sigma training helps incorporate statistical information as a more subjective experience. Defects and errors become unacceptable issues that must be eliminated. Six Sigma training encourages professionals to view problems with a new mind set. For example, most clinicians accept that a certain percentage of hospitalized patients will develop decubitus ulcers (bedsores) as a consequence of underlying disease.[15] However, to a Six Sigma-trained professional, decubiti are defined as unacceptable defects in a process, and the goal is to eliminate them rather than accept their incidence and explain their causation.

When organizational challenges occur, Six Sigma training on how to listen and process information is extremely valuable. The training helps focus one's energy and skill on understanding and responding to the "voice of the customer"—i.e., identifying the goals that should be met, the issues that surround that goal, and the requirements for meeting those needs. Additionally, Six Sigma Black Belts know how to build an appropriate team of stakeholders, ask crucial questions, and garner the resources necessary to drive the improvement effort. The value of formal and frequent communication is in delivering the right message to the right people at the right time.

Six Sigma training provides the tools necessary for supervising effective improvements. The more tools in the toolbox, and the more experience one has in using those tools, the more confident and comfortable individuals become in leadership roles. By following a deliberate and systematic process, a Black Belt can use his or her skills effectively and efficiently to make a positive difference in the way others react to improvements. But the entire organization must be committed to the methodology for true success.

To ensure enculturation, the CEO must invest in generating enthusiasm among all employees for improving quality. The workforce should be expected to improve operations through a methodology that measures results rather than through the traditional route of experience. The message must be clear and the agenda for senior staff established: "Learn and support the new method or you're out!" Leaders who reward improvements with incentives tend to get increased buy-in. With combined enthusiasm from the CEO and the CFO, who recognizes that increased quality (or reduced defects) brings increased profits, and with rewards for improved performance, the organizational transformation begins.

Applying Six Sigma

In order to introduce Six Sigma into a health care organization, specific questions must be addressed:

- Who are the customers and what are they buying? Are customers expecting a cure or a service performed with a hospitalization? Are they patients or members of the professional staff?

- What are the customers' specifications for satisfaction regarding the product being delivered? Satisfaction might involve competence, civility, safety, cleanliness, timeliness, and recovery.

- What processes are used in the delivery of the product? Medication, surgery, office visit, hospitalization?

- How do the processes work? Are they planned or unplanned? What is the process flow?

- Which personnel are involved? In health care, the physician is key for defining the process. Many other health professionals are also involved.

- How much time is involved? Once the process is defined, a baseline will be developed with goals that measure timeliness.

- Is there duplication, redundancy, or waste inherent in the way the process is designed? Are the steps of the process clearly defined? Are they effective?

- What measures should be defined to evaluate improvements to the process? Have reliable measures been developed to monitor whether a process is in control? What is the distance from the benchmark?

- How can improvements be sustained? Have the physician and other participants bought into the process and reached agreement on methods and desired outcomes? Are processes in place to evaluate sustained improvements over time? What is the accountability and report-out structure?

When all parties involved have access to the same set of facts, and agree on the facts, they can begin to shape plans for improvement.

In health care, the product or unit of analysis is a moving target. For example, is the focus on the process of diagnosis, or on a specific diagnosis associated with a select group of patients? Complexity does not preclude improving quality in appropriate situations. Although not all processes or services benefit from a Six Sigma improvement project, there is a range of processes and practices to which it can be applied. With data available via the EMR and other sources, defects are more easily recognized, defined (through root cause analyses, regression analysis, and other established quality management tools), and improved based on federal and state expectations (e.g., Hospital Compare).

Six Sigma is useful in reducing variation in a defined process to ensure predictable performance and eliminate unnecessary costs. It can be applied to operational processes, such as billing or missed appointments, or clinical processes such as medication administration.[16] For example; compliance with the IHI protocols for preventing central-line infections can be measured. Deviation from the protocol can be tracked and/or a bottleneck in the process can be identified. The "defect" in the "product" in this example is infection. Such a defect will be unsatisfactory to customers—be they physicians, hospital administrators, insurers, or patients.

It is important to recognize that one organization's successful process improvement project is not always generalizable to another organization. Each organization must assess where Six Sigma project improvements are likely to be most useful and productive. Individual stakeholders determine where to place their Six Sigma efforts for maximum return.

More than a set of statistical tools and formulaic routines for process improvements and increased profitability, Six Sigma is a process that can be used to transform organizations, to change the way things are into the way they should be. In addition to the enculturation of employees to do things the right way and to become involved in improvements, Six Sigma requires effective methods of communication across the entire organization.

In health care organizations, much information is transferred subjectively and unreliably. Communication breakdowns are cited as contributing factors in most adverse events that occur in hospitals.[18,19] Informal communication is inadequate for a quality organization. Formal communication must be adopted to ensure adequate and effective transfer of information. The health care industry has begun to adopt checklists, similar to those relied upon by the airline industry, and has implemented TeamSTEPPS[20] to improve communication and eradicate the information silos that are characteristic of traditional health care organizations.

Carolyn Pexton, the former director of communications at GE health care and an authority on Six Sigma, lists hospitals and health care organizations that have deployed Six Sigma to advantage across the United States[17]:

- Projects at Thibodaux Regional Medical Center (Louisiana) have yielded more than $4 million in revenue growth, cash flow improvement, and cost savings.

- A range of projects at Commonwealth Health Corporation (Kentucky) resulted in more than $7 million in savings while improving quality and staff and patient satisfaction.

- Good Samaritan Hospital (California) reduced registry expenses by mapping multiple process drivers and achieved cost savings between $5.5 and $6 million.

- At Rapides Regional Medical Center (Louisiana), emergency department projects have led to reduced wait time, fewer patients leaving without being seen, higher satisfaction and an annualized savings potential of $957,000.

- Virtua Health (New Jersey) has had a vigorous Six Sigma program in place for several years as part of its Star Initiative to achieve operational excellence. In one project focused on congestive heart failure, length of stay was reduced from 6 to 4 days, patient education improved from 27 to 80 percent, and chart consistency improved from 67 to 93 percent.

- Valley Baptist Health System (Texas) reduced surgical cycle time, added 1,100 cases per year to its capacity, thereby raising potential revenue by more than $1.3 million annually.

- Yale-New Haven Medical Center (Connecticut) achieved a 75 percent reduction in bloodstream infection rates in the Surgical Intensive Care Unit, with $1.2 million annually in estimated savings.

- Boston Medical Center (Massachusetts) improved diagnostic imaging throughput, with a potential impact of more than $2.2 million in cost savings and revenue growth.

- A project at the University of Pittsburgh Medical Center's (Pennsylvania) catheterization laboratory increased available capacity by 2.08 patients per lab per weekday, with a potential revenue impact of $5.2 million annually.

- Providence Health System (Washington) has been implementing Six Sigma and change management on an enterprise-wide basis across four regions. Total savings achieved as a result of completed projects covering various operational and clinical issues exceeds $40 million.

- The Women and Infants Hospital of Rhode Island successfully used Six Sigma and change management to standardize operating procedures for embryo transfer, yielding a 35 percent increase in implantation rates.

Sustaining change presents its own set of challenges. When leadership changes, during economic downturns, or with staff turnover, the investment in quality must remain intact for improvements to be sustained. At the North Shore-Long Island Jewish Health System, the CEO established the Center for Learning and Innovation (CLI) to transform the culture of individuality into one of teamwork and to provide training in quality and safety issues. CLI has been educating its 30,000 employees for the past decade.

Case Study: Improving Organizational Processes

Define

How can Six Sigma be used to improve a faulty process? With leadership's commitment to employing Six Sigma and trained personnel, the Black Belt change agents identify and prioritize an improvement project. During the initial *Define* phase, the project charter is established in which the customers of and stakeholders in the process are identified, the scope of the project is described, and a business case for the improvement is made. A team is formed, including people who work closely with the process and people outside the process. The combination of "old hands" and "fresh eyes" provides balance and objectivity in assessing the process. Process deficiencies are defined and the impact of the deficiencies on the customer is described.

For example, at one system hospital, data alerted administrative leadership that patients who were being discharged to nursing homes had an increased length of stay (LOS). A delay in the discharge process has an impact on patient safety because it can compromise an already vulnerable patient by prolonging exposure to hospital-acquired conditions such as infection. Timely discharge also has an impact on bed throughput, resulting in increased organizational costs.

For this improvement project, the most invested stakeholders were the case managers who are responsible for spearheading the discharge planning process. Other members of the team included physicians, nurses, physical therapists, medical records staff, and administrative leadership.

As in any Six Sigma project, once a team is chartered and the project is delineated, the Black Belt project leader facilitates the team's movement through the phases of Six Sigma. Each of these phases (*Define, Measure, Analyze, Improve,* and *Control*) is structured with established deliverables and tools.

Measure

In this step, the team learns how the process works and, most important, how it is deviating from customer expectations. To understand the process, the team "maps" the process, using Suppliers, Input, Process, Output, and Customer (SIPOC). (Figure 1, page 288)

Figure 1. High Level Process Map — SIPOC
Discharge Planning for Rehabilitation

Supplier	Input	Process	Output	Customer
Physician, Case Manager, Nurse, Patient and family	Medical Record, Patient status	Initiates discharge plan	Order for assessment for rehabilitation services	Case manager, Physical Therapist
Case Manager, Physical Therapist	Order for assessment for rehabilitation services	Reviews patient information, eligibility and makes referral	Referral, Progress Notes	Social Worker, Physician
Social Worker	Referral, Progress Notes	Opens a case, reviews record, interviews patient and family	Discharge Plan	Registered Nurse, Patient and family
Registered Nurse	Discharge Plan, Medical Record	Completes Patient Review Instrument (PRI)and sends to nursing home	Patient Review Instrument (PRI)	Nursing Home Admissions Officer
Nursing Home Admissions Officer	Patient Review Instrument (PRI)	Reviews documents and accepts patient	Acceptance , Bed Offer	Social Worker, Physician, case Manager, Physical Therapist, Patient and family

The process is analyzed at a high level to identify key elements:

- Who are the suppliers?
- What is their input to the process?
- What are the steps to the process?
- What is the output of the process?
- Who are the customers that benefit?

The process transforms inputs from suppliers to outputs that are used by the customer. The goal of mapping is to ensure that every member of the team has common information, agrees on the categories, and shares a common mindset as to how the process works.

In this example, the physician, one of several suppliers, inputs an order identifying the patient as a candidate for rehabilitation services. The customer of this order is the case manager responsible for assessing the patient and making appropriate referrals.

Figure 2. CTQ Tree

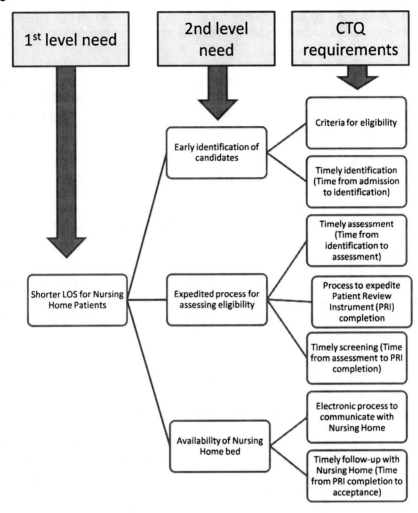

Once identified, customers are asked about their experiences with the process. This helps define the "critical to quality" (CTQ) elements for the process and customer expectations for performance. In Six Sigma terminology, this is obtaining the "voice of the customer." After the CTQ elements are identified, variables are defined (Figure 2). The CTQ tree is an algorithm that transforms the voice of the customer into specific, quantifiable variables. Through this algorithm, subjective information is converted into objectively defined variables.

When the mapping is complete and the voice of the customer is heard, the dependent variable (i.e., the metric that will set the standard for process performance) is defined. For instance, a customer taking a car for repair might expect the mechanic to be knowledgeable and competent, the pricing for the repair to be competitive with other service shops, and the repair to be made quickly. Interviewed customers might expect the repaired car to be returned within several hours of drop-off–e.g., a car brought in at 8 a.m. should be repaired and ready for pick up by 3 p.m. From this information, the Six Sigma team develops a variable for timeliness, the turnaround time of repair.

In the *Measure* phase, baseline data are collected to evaluate the current process performance—in this example, the time customers wait for repair. That number is compared to the benchmark established by the customer's expectation. If the present turnaround time is two days and the benchmark is one day, the team acknowledges a variance or "defect" of one day.

For the discharge planning improvement process, the dependent variable metric was LOS for patients discharged to nursing homes for rehabilitation. The process analysis revealed that the LOS for this patient population was 20 days. The goal of the improvement was to discharge patients at 10 days (a 50 percent reduction), reduce cost, and increase patient and caregiver satisfaction.

Analyze

In this phase, the team members become "detectives" as they dissect the process for variables that potentially contribute to the process variance. For the LOS improvement project, process mapping and time-value analyses were conducted in addition to data collection and analyses.

During this discovery phase of *Analyze*, the team is expected to "walk the process"—to experience the process in the way a patient/customer would. In the car repair example, the team would consider the way the mechanic interacted with the car and question why there was a gap in time between diagnosis and repair.

At this stage of the process, variations caused by lack of standardized operating policies and procedures, bottlenecks, hand-offs, and communication gaps are identified. If the team identifies 20 problems with the process, a prioritization filter must be used to determine which problems are most critical. Using the Pareto principle of 80/20 rule, the team considers that, for many events, 80 percent of the effects may be caused by 20 percent of the problems. To get the biggest bang for the improvement buck, the variables with the most significant impact on the overall process must be identified using statistical testing such as multiple regression analyses, T tests, or chi squares. Of course, the agents of change must be educated in statistics and methods.

In the LOS example, analysis of the discharge problem highlighted the importance of examining the entire situation before determining where to focus the improvement effort. Looking at the universe of patients who were discharged to nursing homes, the team was able to identify three distinct groups: 1) a group of patients needing long-term care (long term–new), 2) a group of patients who were admitted to the hospital from nursing homes to the hospital due to an acute health episode (long term–existing), and 3) a group of patients who required nursing home care for short-term rehabilitation (short term–subacute) (Figure 3).

Figure 3. Frequency Distribution

Segment	N	Percent	Mean LOS	SD
Long term- new	109	23%	28.10	29.86
Long term- existing	114	24%	10.85	11.33
Short term- sub acute	**248**	**53%**	**20.07**	**13.36**
All Nursing facility discharges	471	100%	19.70	19.10

When all nursing home referrals were analyzed, data revealed that the patients who were admitted from and returned to nursing homes (long-term–existing) had the lowest mean LOS. Patients who were newly referred to nursing homes for long-term care (long-term–new) had relatively long LOS with a high standard deviation (SD), indicating a great deal of variation. This could be attributed to the complex insurance issues and financial documentation involved in discharge planning for this group.

The team had assumed that the long-term–new group would be the focus of the improvement efforts. To the surprise of everyone involved, the short-term–acute group of patients, which accounted for more than 50 percent of the nursing home discharges, had the right combination of long LOS, high SD, and no obvious reason. Clearly if 50 percent of the LOS could be reduced, the problem would be reduced as well.

One of the great advantages of Six Sigma and other quality methodologies is that data analysis generates new ideas and helps focus on the most critical issues, in many cases overriding well-entrenched, preconceived notions. Case managers had been focusing on outliers (the new nursing home patients) rather than on the plentiful low-hanging fruit.

With the problem patient population identified, the next step was to question, analyze, and identify the causes of the extended LOS for the short-term patients. Analysis revealed that no criteria existed by which discharge planners could identify patients who were eligible for short-term rehab. Without standardization, there was a great deal of practitioner variance with regard to referrals. Once the patients were identified and the referral was sent to the nursing home, there was inadequate communication between the hospital and the nursing home. Also, there was no electronic process to ensure that the referral was received and no appropriate follow-up procedure.

To further understand the situation, the team invited the nursing home admissions coordinators to explain the nursing home's process for identifying and accepting candidates for rehabilitation to the hospital case managers. This exchange uncovered the fact that, because case managers were using Fax for communication with nursing homes, the hospital patient referrals were mixed in with hundreds of other daily faxes and not receiving timely attention.

Another discovery was that the patient review instrument (PRI), an important element in the documentation required for nursing home acceptance, was delayed because of hospital staffing issues and the lack of a procedure to prioritize short-term rehab patients.

In sum, issues identified in the *Analyze* phase were poor eligibility criteria, inadequate process to prioritize PRI completion, and inefficient (manual) process tracking. These three elements contributed to eight days of delay in the discharge planning process for patients who constituted 50 percent of the nursing home referral population.

Improve

With the problems identified, the team moved into the *Improve* phase wherein various solutions are explored for effectiveness. Each potential solution is tested through pilot or designed experiments, and data are collected to assess effectiveness. The information leads to redefined processes. Once solutions are identified, stakeholders are informed, the staff is appropriately educated, and a full-scale improvement implementation is planned.

To improve the LOS delay, the team and nursing home personnel established criteria to identify candidates for rehabilitation early in the patient's hospitalization. Once patients were identified, an existing automated system was used to alert the social work department of a need to expedite the PRI completion. A process for a standardized turnaround time was established with the nursing home. The nursing home staff specified the information and format needed from hospital case managers and requested a follow-up phone call after faxing a referral. Thus, by leveraging existing technology and existing staff, streamlining the process, and establishing standard operating procedures and criteria, LOS was reduced by 10 days. The goal of the initiative was met.

Control

In this final phase, statistical process control procedures are established. Ownership and accountability for process performance are established as well. The process is reviewed to assess rigorousness, including use of failure mode and effect analysis, error proofing, and risk evaluation.

One issue regarding Six Sigma that raises suspicion among health care leaders is sustainability. A quick fix is effective in the short term but is generally not long-lasting. Most Six Sigma "failures" occur when insufficient time, energy, or rigor is devoted to identifying the independent variables in the *Analyze* phase. The challenge for sustainable improvement is to redesign a flawed process for immediate implementation while allowing sufficient flexibility for continuous redesign and evolution as changes in technology and staffing occur.

In this example, the staff closest to the work redesigned the processes and therefore had a vested interest in the ongoing success of the redesign. People involved in the process redesign should be specially trained to think in a Six Sigma framework. The reduced LOS was sustained in this project because accountability was established in high-performing department managers who were trained in Six Sigma methodologies and change management. Since the launch of this project, improvement has been maintained for more than six years.

Conclusion

Today's health care organizations must focus on the relationships among quality, outcomes, and processes and respond to a national reform agenda that includes pay for performance, value-based purchasing, and patient satisfaction. These elements cannot be productively addressed without a rigorous methodology that centers on database creation, understanding and defining relevant variables, and statistical analyses to create standards of care that explain variation from best practices. Most important, health care professionals require a change in mind-set such that: errors are unacceptable; processes are subject to improvements; rigorous methodology is applied to assess, monitor, and improve care; and dialogue is ongoing and productively applied to a shared agenda of excellence.

Discussion questions

1. What are the advantages and disadvantages of employing Six Sigma to change organizational processes?

2. Once a problem has been "fixed" through a Six Sigma improvement initiative, what steps should be taken to ensure sustainability of the improvement?

3. What is the role of statistics in making decisions in health care processes?

References

1. Schein, EH. *Organizational Culture and Leadership*, 4th ed. San Francisco, CA: Jossey-Bass, 2004.

2. Ulrich D, Kerr S, Ashkenas R. *The GE Work-Out : How to Implement GE's Revolutionary Method for Busting Bureaucracy & Attacking Organizational Problem*. New York, NY: McGraw-Hill, 2002.

3. Scott T, Mannion R, Davies TO, Marshall, MN. Implementing culture change in health care: theory and practice. *Int J Qual Health Care.* 15(2):111-8, Apr. 2003.

4. U.S. Department of Health and Human Services, Centers for Medicare and Medicaid Services. *EHR Incentive Program.* http://www.cms.gov/ehrincentiveprograms/, May 2011.

5. Porter ME, Teisberg EO. *Redefining Health Care: Creating Value-Based Competition on Results.* Boston, MA: Harvard Business School Press, 2006.

6. Institute of Medicine. *Health Professions Education: a Bridge to Quality.* Washington, DC: National Academies Press, 2001.

7. Hillestad R, Bigelow J, Bower A, et al. Can electronic medical record systems transform health care? Potential health benefits, savings, and costs. *Health Affairs.* 24(5):1103-17, Sept.-Oct. 2005.

8. Iezzoni LI. Measuring quality, outcomes, and cost of care using large databases:Oroceedingsof the Sixth Regenstrief Conference Assessing Quality Using Administrative Data. *Annals of Internal Medicine.* 127(8, Part 2):666-74, Oct. 15, 1997.

9. Dlugacz, YD. *Value-Based Health Care: Linking Finance and* Quality. San Francisco, CA: Jossey-Bass, 2010.

10. Pande PS, Neuman RP, Cavanagh RR. *The Six Sigma Way: How GE, Motorola, and Other Top Companies Are Honing Their Performance.* New York, NY: McGraw-Hill, 2000.

11. Slater R. *Jack Welch and the GE Way: Management Insights and Leadership Secrets of the Legendary CEO.* New York, NY: McGraw-Hill, 1999.

12. Chassin M. Is health care ready for six sigma? *Milbank Quarterly.* 76(4):565-91, 1998.

13. Paton, S M. Juran: A lifetime of quality. *Quality Digest,* 2006. http://www.quality-digest.com/aug02/articles/01_article.shtml.

14. Dlugacz YD. *Measuring Health Care: Using Quality Data for Operational, Financial, and Clinical Improvement.* San Francisco, CA: Jossey-Bass, 2006.

15. Witkowski JA, Parish LC. The decubitus ulcer: skin failure and destructive behavior. *International Journal of Dermatology.* 39(12):894–6, Dec. 2009.

16. Revere, L., Black, K. Integrating six sigma with total quality management: A case example for measuring medication errors. *Journal of Healthcare Management.* 48(6):377-91, Nov.-Dec. 2003.

17. Pexton C. Measuring Six Sigma results in the health care industry, iSixSigma.com, http://health care.isixsigma.com/library/content/c040623a.asp. Accessed March 19, 2007.

18. Sutcliffe KM, Lewton E, Rosenthal M. Communication failures: an insidious contributor to medical mishaps. *Acad Med.* 79(2):186-94, Feb. 2004.

19. Lingard L, Espin S, Whyte S, *et al.* Communication failures in the operating room: an observational classification of recurrent types and effects. *Qual Saf Health Care.* 13(5):330-334, Oct. 2004.

20. King HB, Battles J, Baker DP, *et al.* TeamSTEPPS™: Team Strategies and Tools to Enhance Performance and Patient Safety. In: Henriksen K, Battles JB, Keyes MA, Grady ML, eds. *Advances in Patient Safety: New Directions and Alternative Approaches,* Vol. 3. Rockville, MD: Agency for Healthcare Research and Quality (US), 2008

Chapter 19

Role of Health IT in Measurement and Improvement

By Harm J. Scherpbier, MD

Executive Summary

The fundamental building blocks of the health information technology infrastructure are electronic medical records (EMRs) in hospitals and physician offices. These systems help improve the quality and efficiency of care. Driven by incentives in the American Recovery and Reinvestment Act, EMRs increasingly support clinicians in every step of patient care. These systems are becoming smarter, using clinical decision support to provide guidance to physicians at the point of care.

EMRs are becoming interconnected through health information exchanges—exchanging data between organizations and creating a more complete picture of the patient. Finally, through personal health records and patient portals, the data in EMRs are becoming easily available to patients and their families, engaging them to a greater degree in their care decisions. Health informatics are in a period of rapid development and deployment, changing the way we provide care at every stage of the process.

Learning Objectives

1. Identify current applications of informatics in health care and analyze their impact on quality improvement and patient safety initiatives.

2. Recognize organizational and governance structures for leading and guiding health informatics projects.

3. Analyze the impact of government policy, specifically the ARRA HITECH Act, on health care information projects.

4. Understand the importance of health care information technology standards on the ability to exchange health information and on usability of data for population health purposes.

5. Understand the impact of the consumer on health care delivery and how informatics enable the consumer.

Key Words: American Recovery and Reinvestment Act (ARRA), Barcode Medication Administration Systems (BCMA), Computerized Physician Order Entry (CPOE), Consumer Driven Healthcare, Electronic Health Record (EHR), Electronic Medical Record (EMR), Health Information Technology (Health IT), Health Information Exchange (HIE), Health Level 7 Standards (HL7), Meaningful Use, Outcome measures, Performance measures, Personal Health Record (PHR), Unintended Consequences

Introduction

This chapter reviews the role of health care information technology (Health IT) in health care delivery, particularly its essential role both in measuring outcomes and quality of care and in helping to improve care at the point of care. Recent years have seen a strong increase in the use of electronic medical records (EMRs) in physician offices and hospitals—and in the connections between them via the health information exchange (HIE). This increase is largely a result of government stimulus money that rewards physicians and hospitals for implementing EMRs and achieving Meaningful Use of these systems. At the same time, patients are using information systems to manage their own care. All these factors create a fast-changing world of Health IT.

Health IT Impact On Care Delivery

In their work on patient safety opportunities for clinical informatics, Kilbridge and Classen[1] outline the three fundamental ways in which Health IT impacts the quality and safety of care along three major axes. These will serve as a structure for this chapter.

First, Health IT tools aid in avoiding errors at the point of care. For example, physicians use computer systems when they prescribe medications and nurses use computer systems when they administer medications to patients in the hospital. These systems alert the clinician when they are about to make a mistake in ordering a medication: for example, one to which the patient is allergic, one that might cause an interaction with a current medication, or one written for the wrong patient or in the wrong dose.

Second, Health IT plays an important role in gathering and analyzing data for measuring patient safety and for tracking the impact of quality improvement initiatives. With more and more data available electronically, in structured format suitable for analysis, we now have an opportunity to use larger and more comprehensive databases with clinical data in addition to billing data for outcomes analysis. Using these databases, we can measure the impact of different methods of care delivery and analyze the outcomes. The analysis can occur within one organization (e.g., a physician practice or a hospital), across or between organizations, at regional or state levels, or at a population level. All of these entities use data gathered from EMRs, and all rely on Health IT principles to prepare the data for analysis.

The third way in which Health IT affects the quality and safety of care is quite different from the other two; now that more care is delivered with the help of information systems, the information systems themselves can become the source of errors. An important aspect of Health IT is to identify potential mistakes and avoid or limit the impact of these "unintended consequences."

The three ways described above apply within health care organizations. A fourth way in which Health IT impacts care delivery occurs mostly outside the walls of health care organizations—for example, by giving patients and families direct access to their health information and to a wide array of health information. Such access is rapidly changing the way patients and families manage their care and also how they relate to and communicate with care providers.

Improving Quality at the Point of Care

Each report in the Institute of Medicine's series on Quality of Care (*To Err is Human: Building a Safer Health System* [1999]; *Crossing the Quality Chasm: a New Health System for the 21st Century* [2001]; and, most recently, *Health IT and Patient Safety: Building Safer Systems for Better Care* [2011]), recommends using point of care information systems to help physicians, nurses, and other practitioners make the best decisions and avoid errors. While the transition from paper charts to EMRs in physician offices and hospitals is taking longer than expected, the American Recovery and Reinvestment Act (ARRA) initiatives provided a strong boost. The move to point-of-care computing is well under way.

The most common way in which computers help improve quality and avoid errors at the point of care is through e-prescribing and computerized physician order entry (CPOE). Long considered a major milestone in the implementation of hospital EMRs, CPOE is a key Meaningful Use requirement. By inserting information systems into the process of ordering tests and medications for patients, CPOE gives organizations some control over the physician's order-writing pen. CPOE systems check all physician orders, alerting the user if a medication is ordered for a patient who is allergic, if a dosage is incorrect, if there are potential drug-to-drug interactions, duplicate medications, and/or other potentially avoidable errors. (Figure 1, page 298)

Figure 1. Drug/drug interaction alert in CPOE Session

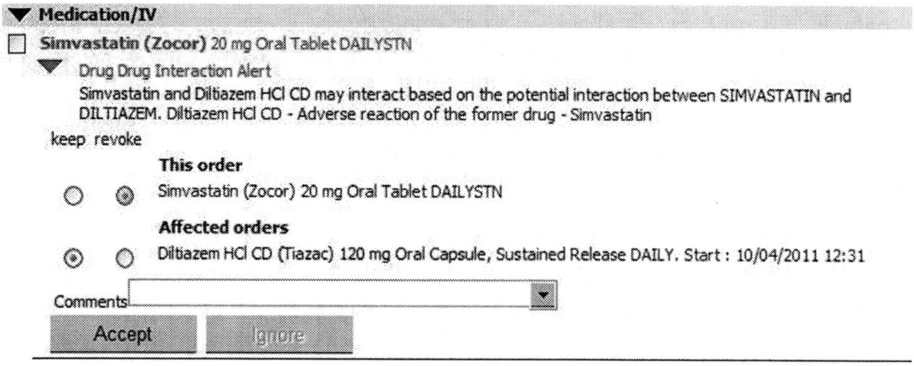

▼ **Medication/IV**

☐ **Simvastatin (Zocor)** 20 mg Oral Tablet DAILYSTN

   ▼ Drug Drug Interaction Alert

      Simvastatin and Diltiazem HCl CD may interact based on the potential interaction between SIMVASTATIN and
      DILTIAZEM. Diltiazem HCl CD - Adverse reaction of the former drug - Simvastatin

  keep revoke

         This order

  ○ ◉   Simvastatin (Zocor) 20 mg Oral Tablet DAILYSTN

         Affected orders

  ◉ ○   Diltiazem HCl CD (Tiazac) 120 mg Oral Capsule, Sustained Release DAILY. Start : 10/04/2011 12:31

  Comments

[**Accept**] [Ignore]

Source: Siemens Soarian® at Main Line Health

Several studies have questioned the impact of CPOE on quality of care and, in some cases, demonstrated a deterioration of care. However, the majority of studies demonstrate a positive effect on quality of care for properly implemented CPOE systems[2,3] and, at this point, we can consider CPOE the state of the art for hospital-based health care. Studies also show that CPOE decreases the turnaround time for laboratory and radiology tests as well as administration of urgent medications.[4] The most important obstacle in implementing CPOE systems is their tendency to increase the time it takes the physician to write orders.[5]

CPOE reduces errors at the point of order writing (approximately 40 percent of medication errors).[6] Barcode medication administration (BCMA) reduces errors at the point of administration. For hospital-based care, these errors account for approximately 30 percent of medication errors.[6] In BCMA systems, the nurse scans two barcodes—one on the medication to be given and one on the patient's arm band. The information system checks the "five rights"—i.e., the right medication for the right patient, at the right time, with the right dose and route of administration. If an error is detected, the system alerts the nurse to avoid the potential error.

The ARRA HITECH program has prompted many hospitals to implement CPOE systems. At present, approximately 23.5 percent of U.S. hospitals have CPOE systems in place. Eleven percent use closed-loop medication administration wherein the entire process—ordering through dispensing—is automated, thus avoiding errors due to handwriting or transcription at any point.[7]

A final category of systems that help providers at the point of care is clinical decision support (CDS) systems. One might consider CDS the holy grail of health informatics—the vision of smart computer systems looking over the provider's shoulder, making appropriate suggestions, and helping to avoid mistakes without being annoying or pointing out the obvious. Despite many years of research and development, it is still a vision.

Most health care information systems use some level of CDS in the form of alerts and reminders to guide users toward the best therapy. Examples include: suggestions for deep vein thrombosis (DVT) prophylaxis, angiotensin-converting enzyme (ACE) inhibitors for patients with congestive heart failure or beta blocker therapy for patients with an acute myocardial infarction (AMI); vaccination reminders; and screening test reminders. Garg's analysis of CDS systems[8] demonstrates that robust and ubiquitous CDS remains a future goal but that current CDS systems help improve outcomes, especially systems that are well-integrated into the user's workflow. As more providers switch from paper-based to computer-based care, opportunities for fitting reminders into the workflow will increase, as will the effectiveness of existing CDS tools.

When alerts and reminders are not well-integrated into the clinicians' workflow, or when the alerts are not sufficiently relevant or important to interrupt workflow, users become annoyed with alerts and begin to ignore them–a condition known as "alert fatigue."[9] Once clinicians begin to ignore alerts, they ignore all of them–including those with high clinical significance.

To avoid alert fatigue, CDS systems must be set up so that interruptions are minimal, and only for very important and significant situations. For instance, a clinician should not be alerted that a pneumovax vaccination is due when the patient is in a life-threatening situation. Setting up systems to deliver only the most important alerts at the right point in the workflow is difficult, and most health systems are still in the early phases of effective use of CDS.

Another obstacle to the widespread implementation of CDS lies in defining the knowledge base. At its core, each CDS system has a "knowledge base"–a set of rules, algorithms, decision tables, or expert systems that determine when to send an alert to a clinician and what message is sent. Event monitors, components in the system that "listen" for specific events, trigger the execution of a rule and generate an alert. For example, when a physician enters an order for the anticoagulant, Warfarin, a rule can retrieve from the database the patient's last three prothrombin time values and the last three doses of Warfarin and display this information to help the physician determine the best next dose. (Figure 2) The building and maintenance of these knowledge bases and sets of rules are difficult and time-consuming. One cannot expect that every health system in the U.S. or in the world will be able to do this.

Figure 2. Warfarin order shows recent INR values

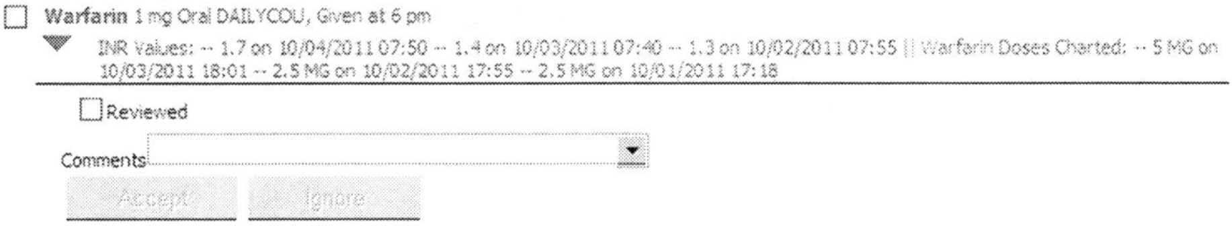

☐ Warfarin 1 mg Oral DAILYCOU, Given at 6 pm
▼ INR Values: -- 1.7 on 10/04/2011 07:50 -- 1.4 on 10/03/2011 07:40 -- 1.3 on 10/02/2011 07:55 ‖ Warfarin Doses Charted: -- 5 MG on 10/03/2011 18:01 -- 2.5 MG on 10/02/2011 17:55 -- 2.5 MG on 10/01/2011 17:18

☐ Reviewed

Comments

Accept   Ignore

Source: Siemens Soarian® at Main Line Health

The Arden Syntax standard [10,11] is a standard language for clinical decision rules that many commercial EMRs support. The idea behind this standard is that rules can be shared among health systems without making modifications to incorporate them. Although the standard has been available for many years, there is no significant exchange of rules among health systems, and there are no online or open source sets of rules written in the Arden Syntax.

In a renewed effort to increase the use of CDS, several efforts, such as the Clinical Decision Support Consortium[12] and the OpenCDS effort,[13] aim not to make the rules portable but rather to make incorporation of knowledge bases easier by standardizing both the request to and the subsequent reply from the knowledge base. A standard query/response mechanism would allow health systems to include knowledge from multiple, disparate sources in their CDS flow without having to re-create and maintain the knowledge itself. This standard is in the early phases of development, and the next few years of work will demonstrate whether it can achieve mass-deployment of CDS.

Outcomes Analysis

As more data become available in structured format, the opportunity to use these data for analysis and measurement increases. Until recently, the only data widely used for outcomes analysis were the claims data used by insurers to track the performance of physicians and hospitals. With clinical data now captured and stored in EMRs, health systems can use these data to measure and track their own performance, compare different clinical therapies, and track the results of performance improvement initiatives.

Outcomes analysis uses two main categories of measurements: outcome and performance measures. *Outcome measures* determine the end-result of a process, irrespective of how it was achieved: for example, length of stay, mortality, re-admission rate, vaccination rate of a population, or cost of care over a certain period or for a certain procedure. *Performance measures* determine to what extent a certain procedure was (or was not) followed, irrespective of whether or not the goal was achieved;—for example, whether a patient with AMI was given aspirin within 24 hours, the door to balloon time, percentage adherence to a clinical guideline, and percentage usage of the CPOE system.

Generally, it is easier to measure and track performance measures than outcomes measures. For performance measures, one need only track the set of health care providers performing this procedure and determine whether they did or did not follow the procedure. Tracking outcomes is generally more difficult. Because the impact of a specific initiative often is modest, a researcher must track a large set of patients to obtain an appropriate measurement. For example, Garg tracks the impact of CDS systems on the care delivered using mostly performance measures to demonstrate the impact.[8]

The informatics aspect of outcomes analysis deals mostly with preparation of the data before performing an analysis. Data are collected and stored in a variety of systems and brought together in a uniform, comparable manner before they can be analyzed. This process is known as extract-transform-load (ETL):

- *Extract* data from a number of source data systems.
- *Transform* the data to make them comparable and ready for analysis.
- *Load* the data into a structure suitable for large analysis.

The hard work comes in the *transform* phase wherein three critical transformations make it possible to analyze outcomes: 1) data model transformations, 2) code set or terminology transformations, and 3) patient identity transformations.

Data model transformations

EMRs, the main source of clinical data, are built to help deliver care to the patient. The data model underlying EMRs focuses on the patient. For outcomes analysis, the goal is to compare care across many patients, which leads to a data structure optimized for cross-patient analysis. The star-schema data structure is the most common way of organizing data for analysis–with the item to be researched (the "fact") surrounded by a "star" of various elements that may have impacted the fact (the "dimensions"). For example, medication orders/prescriptions could be the central fact-table surrounded by multiple dimensions—the ordering physician, the patient for whom it was ordered, the patient's diagnoses or procedures associated with the prescription, the date and time, the location, and whether or not it was administered.

During the transformation phase, details important for day-to-day patient care can be hidden to make it easier for the outcomes analysis team to see the forest through the trees. For example, in an analysis of insulin prescriptions, there will be many forms and regimens of subcutaneous insulin. If the researcher/analyst is only interested in whether physicians prescribed a sliding scale alone versus a full basal/bolus regimen,[14] exposing the researcher to the raw prescription data would complicate the analysis. A transformation can help label or categorize the prescriptions into a "sliding scale" category and a "basal/bolus" category.

Data transformation changes the format and level of detail from a patient care-centered model into a model suitable for analysis and measurement.

Code Set or Terminology Transformations

For outcomes analysis, it is often necessary to bring together data from multiple systems–one or more EMRs from one or more different hospitals, physician practices, health systems, patient registration systems, billing or claims data, pharmacy data from hospital or retail pharmacy systems, and specialty systems (e.g., cardiology systems, lab systems). Each of these systems may use different terminologies and code sets. For data analysis, these terminologies and codes must be mapped into a common terminology. For example, a patient's height and weight are data fields in most EMRs, but one system may call these elements "Ht" and "Wt", while another system may call them "Height" and "Weight," and a third may actually use the standard Logical Observation Identifiers Names and Codes (LOINC) codes 3137-7 and 3141-9. If tracking weight changes or impact on growth is important, the outcomes analysis database must establish one term for height and weight (preferably the standard LOINC term), and map all source data to that standard term.

Code set and terminology mappings are an important part of the data transformation. They affect patient findings and lab results, diagnoses and procedures, medications, and other fields.

Patient Identity Transformations

Within a health system, patients usually are known by one common identifier. Although the patient may have different account numbers in the pharmacy, lab, and outpatient settings, health systems use master patient index systems (MPI) to keep track of their patients. For outcomes analysis within an organization, one must have access to the MPI system to bring together all data for a single patient.

To analyze data from multiple organizations, one must use an algorithm to determine if Mr. J. Doe in one health system is the same as Mr. John Doe in another health system, and then bring this patient's data together in the analytical database. There are a number of algorithms that allow the merging of patient data from multiple data sources. This patient ID mapping also takes place in the transformation stage.

If the objective of the outcomes database is research by parties outside the health system, the patient IDs will often be hidden from the researchers. The resulting "blinded" data have all protected health information removed, and patients are represented by numbers that cannot be traced back to the person. Blinding is part of the transformation process and can only take place after the patient ID mapping has occurred.

Risk Adjustment and Benchmarking

Risk adjustment and benchmarking are valuable approaches to "level the playing field" and provide "apples to apples" comparisons. Typical risk-adjustment methodologies include calculating observed outcomes (O) versus expected outcomes (E), and using the resulting O/E ratio. Benchmarking involves calculating outcomes for a set of high-performing institutions or physicians.

Once the data are in suitable analytical form, analysts can use them to compare populations of patients (e.g., with/without a certain intervention, or before/after an intervention) and groups of providers (e.g., in various hospitals or within a region) and measure and track key performance indicators.

Amarasingham *et al.*[15] performed a large outcomes analysis to measure the impact of EMRs on the quality and cost of care across a large number of hospitals in Texas. To compare the degree of use of an EMR, they developed a scoring system, the Clinical Information Technology Assessment Tool (CITAT), which reflects the extent of EMR implementation. The study suggests that, even if adjusted for a number of confounding factors such as financial strength or weakness of the organization, EMR implementation has a net positive effect on quality of care (i.e., mortality, complication rate) and on efficiency of care (i.e., cost of hospitalization and length of stay). The findings were most pronounced in patient populations with common diagnoses or procedures, such as AMI, coronary artery bypass graft, heart failure and pneumonia. Typically, these are the areas where CPOE order sets and clinical decision support are developed first and will likely have a more measureable impact.

EMRs as Source of Errors and Unintended Consequences

As with other social phenomena, unintended consequences–including adverse ones–can occur with EMRs. Koppel and colleagues[16] note published studies reporting that CPOE reduces medication errors dramatically (in some cases up to 81 percent) but focus instead on medication errors facilitated by CPOE. Their qualitative and quantitative study of house staff interaction with a CPOE system found that the system facilitated 22 types of medication error risks, including fragmented CPOE displays that prevent a coherent view of patients' medications, pharmacy inventory displays mistaken for dosage guidelines, ignored antibiotic renewal notices placed on paper charts rather than in the CPOE system, separation of functions that facilitate double dosing and incompatible orders, and inflexible ordering formats generating wrong orders. Koppel and colleagues concluded that, "As CPOE systems are implemented, clinicians and hospitals must attend to errors that these systems cause in addition to errors that they prevent."[16]

Similarly, Koppel and another team of researchers[17] developed a typology of clinicians' workarounds when using BCMA systems, and identified the causes and possible consequences of each workaround. The team identified 15 types of workarounds, including affixing patient identification barcodes to computer carts, scanners, doorjambs, or nurses' belt rings and carrying several patients' pre-scanned medications on carts. Also, they identified 31 types of causes of workarounds, including unreadable medication barcodes (e.g., crinkled, smudged, torn, missing, covered by another label), malfunctioning scanners, unreadable or missing patient identification wristbands (e.g., chewed, soaked, missing), non-bar-coded medications, failing batteries, uncertain wireless connectivity, and emergencies. They found that nurses overrode BCMA alerts for 4.2 percent of patients charted and for 10.3 percent of medications charted.

Possible consequences of the workarounds include wrong administration of medications, wrong doses, wrong times, and wrong formulations. Koppel *et al.* conclude that "Shortcomings in BCMAs' design, implementation, and workflow integration encourage workarounds... Integrating BCMAs within real-world clinical workflows requires attention to *in situ* use to ensure safety features' correct use."[17]

While Ash,[18] Koppel,[16] and others point to the risk of unintended consequences for EMR implementations, they and most health informatics leaders agree that unintended consequences should not stop health providers from implementing EMRs with all point of care decision support methods. Instead, they caution health care providers not to rely on information systems blindly, to thoroughly and continuously test for these scenarios, and to create a structure within the organization to deal with unintended consequences, minimize the impact, and prevent them from happening where possible. Strong organizational governance is paramount, with well-defined procedures for implementing EMR components, introducing new order sets, training physicians and nurses, and developing an overall awareness of both the positive and the potentially negative implications.

In many cases, the EMR system will not be the single root cause of a patient safety event, but rather a contributing factor in combination with one or more other events—the "Swiss cheese" model wherein all holes line up to let an error through. One of the case studies at the end of this chapter illustrates the role of information systems as a contributing factor to patient safety events.

Access to Health Information for Patients and Their Families

The fourth and most recent development in health informatics is access to health information for patients and their families. New tools (i.e., Internet, portals, personal health records, mobile applications) make this access possible, and the ARRA HITECH stimulus package supports it by making patient and family access part of the Meaningful Use requirements.

Patients and families have always had access to their medical information. They could go to the medical records department and get copies of their charts—large stacks of paper, much of it difficult to read and interpret. Now that more and more data are available electronically, the mechanisms for giving patients access to this information are changing.

ARRA stipulates that patients can obtain an electronic copy of their health information and discharge instructions upon request. It does not specify the method; it could be given to the patient on a CD or a USB drive, via secure email, or by giving the patient access to a secure web portal. All methods will exist, and more.

In addition to having access to their own medical information, it has become much easier for patients and families to interpret the meaning of the data by researching the information available on the Internet—either by consulting Internet-based information resources or by using social networks such as "Patients Like Me"[19] to learn from other patients with similar conditions how to treat or live with their condition.

Patients can store and maintain their personal health information in personal health records (PHRs). Some PHRs are components of a health provider's portal—for example, Kaiser Permanente's "My Health Manager," powered by Epic's MyChart® (www.kaiserpermanente.org), or the Veterans Administration's "My

HealtheVet" (www.myhealth.va.gov). Patients can use these portals to schedule tests and appointments, to see their lab results, to communicate with their physicians, and to track and manage their health data. Importantly, they can pull up these data when they visit different physicians—in a way, carrying their health data with them wherever they go. PHRs that are "tethered" to health system portals are popular and widely used—approximately 30 percent of Kaiser's three million patients have used their personal health record.[20]

Other PHRs are independent of a health care provider (e.g., Microsoft HealthVault. Patients can enter and maintain their health data, and health providers can offer electronic data interfaces into these PHRs. Google Health was a promising independent PHR until Google decided to discontinue it. Was that move indicative of the future of independent PHRs? In all probability, there will be other providers of PHRs; however, it does highlight a challenge in the movement toward PHRs. That is, those who need them the most—the chronically ill with many health care interactions—are least able to use them, and those who are able to use them may not need PHRs for the management of their care.

As more and more data move to "the cloud," and as health information systems get better in communicating data between systems, we will see more patients store their personal data in PHRs and use them to provide continuity of care by making their data available to their providers. Tethered PHRs have shown more early success thanks to the combination of tracking personal health data and enabling transactions with the provider—e.g. scheduling tests and refilling prescriptions. Whatever the model, the trend toward patient control and ownership, enabled by the Internet and information systems, is irreversible.

Health Information Exchange (HIE)

All players in the health care data flow are implementing EMRs, urged on by ARRA stimulus money. Physician offices and hospitals implement EMRs; insurance companies have automated their businesses for a long time; retail and mail order pharmacies operate electronically. However, none of these players has the "full picture" of a patient. Each has its particular slice of patient data—the inpatient slice, the insurance slice, or the medication slice—but no one has the complete data set.

HIE is the concept of linking the various participants electronically to exchange data. There are many public and private initiatives in which data are exchanged within a region, a community, or a health system. For an excellent review of the history, background, current state and challenges of HIE see work by Kuperman.[21]

Challenges/obstacles for HIE include the following:

- Governance; that is, who "owns" the HIE, who pays for it, and how we can make it financially sustainable.
- Bridging various information systems and using standards, the key standards being HL7 and CCD/CCR.

- Need for Record Locator Service—to know where Mrs. Jones has information.
- Security/Privacy.[21]

> **Government Initiatives in Health IT**
>
> The government recognizes the power of Health IT to improve quality, safety, and efficiency of care. A number of governmental agencies strongly promote the adoption and implementation of health information systems.
>
> - American Recovery and Reinvestment Act (ARRA)–with the concept of "Meaningful Use" of EMRs, the ARRA will be the driver of health IT in the U.S. for the next five years and will dramatically increase the use of EMRs. The program provides incentive payments to hospitals and physician practices, rewarding them for implementing and using EMRs. The Meaningful Use criteria are built in three stages, each stage increasing the use and the potential impact and benefit of the information systems to care delivery. The criteria are divided into five categories: Quality and safety, engaging patients and families in their care, coordination of care between participants, public health, and privacy and security. For a detailed description of and current status information on the ARRA Meaningful Use program, refer to the portal website of the HHS Office of the National Coordinator of Health Information Technology: http://healthit.hhs.gov.
>
> - The role of IT in new health care models is defined in the Healthcare Reform Act, specifically accountable care organizations (ACOs) and patient-centered medical home (PCMH). Both rely heavily on key IT functions for coordinating care between the various providers, for tools to deliver the best care possible in the most efficient way and to prevent re-admissions, and for measuring the quality of care. The ACO model of care delivery relies on a sophisticated set of information systems that cover the patient's care over the long term and connect all settings where patients receive care. For detail on the ACO model and the impact on information infrastructure, see DeVore and Champion.[22]

Standards in Health IT

The world of Health IT consists of many systems, each with its own purpose, and data flows from one system to another. Different organizations use different systems made by different companies, and data can flow from one organization to another. For outcomes analysis across organizations, data from many disparate organizations need to come together into one database, with a uniformity that makes analysis possible. At each of these boundaries where data cross from one system to another, or from one organization to another, there is an opportunity for mismatches. Health IT standards are necessary to make these boundary crossings possible.

The key health IT activities where standards play a role are:

- *HIE:* passing a patient's data from the hospital to a physician practice, or from one health enterprise to another.

- *Outcomes Analysis:* bringing data from multiple systems together into one database, and creating uniformity to allow for reporting and analysis.

- *Clinical Decision Support:* applying decision rules to help guide physicians and nurses to the best care possible—which relies on the data that are available for the patient and requires a standard format.

Three main categories of miscommunication exist and, for each of them, there are one or more standards available to help bridge the gap. Each of these standards is managed and maintained by standards development organizations, which serve the health IT industry as well as health care providers by enabling different systems to talk to each other and share data.

Transaction Formats

A laboratory system sends lab results to a hospital's or practice's EMR system, which receives and files them in the patient's record. A practice sends an electronic test order to a lab or an electronic prescription to a pharmacy. A patient is discharged from the hospital, and the hospital wants to send the discharge summary to the patient's primary care physician. In order for all participating systems to send and receive these transactions, there is a standard set of transactions with standard formats. In the U.S. as well as in many other countries, the most widely used transaction format standard is Health Level 7 (HL7). While HL7 offers a comprehensive set of standard transaction formats, there still are significant differences in the ways by which systems communicate. HL7 has made the gap smaller but hasn't fully eliminated it.

Vocabulary and Terminology Standards

Even when the transaction formats match, systems need to use the same vocabulary or terminology to be able to communicate. If the lab system calls the hemoglobin result "Hb" but the receiving EMR has hemoglobin results filed under "Hemoglobin" or "12345," the systems can't communicate. The standard terminology for results and observations is LOINC; while it is the only standard in this domain, it is not yet used by all lab systems and EMRs. Although there are several other medication terminologies, the standard terminology for medications is RxNorm. The standard vocabulary for diagnoses and procedures is Systematized Nomenclature of Medicine-Clinical Terms (SNOMED-CT); however, many organizations also use ICD9 and ICD10 codes. To resolve the issue that systems use different standards and that many organizations still use home-grown, nonstandard terminologies, mapping from one terminology to another is a common step in health information exchanges and for outcomes analysis purposes.

Common Identifiers

Finally, one needs common identifiers—patient identifiers and provider identifiers—to be able to communicate. Efforts to create a common patient identifier have failed because of security and privacy concerns. Instead, most HIEs use matching algorithms to determine if Mr. Doe in the hospital database is also Mr. Doe in the physician office.

Conclusion

Driven by the ARRA Meaningful Use incentives, the health information infrastructure in the U.S. is developing rapidly. Hospitals are implementing information systems to help physicians and nurses provide safe, high-quality care. Physician offices and clinics implement information systems to provide care for their patients and to track patient populations to help manage patients with chronic diseases. These hospital and physician office EMRs open the door to easier access for patients and their families to their health data—through portals, PHRs, and other methods. The increase in EMRs also causes a surge in HIE, the sharing of patient information via public or private exchanges between the various participants in care, and allowing better coordination of the care for their patients.

Health informatics is not just about information technology. Information systems require standards to help them communicate and exchange data. They need governance structures and teams to oversee their development and implementation. They need training and support staff. Information systems become part of the culture of the organization, and they determine how people work. In the words of Dr. David Blumenthal, the National Coordinator for Health IT from 2009 to 2011: *"Information is the life blood of health care, and the information systems are the circulatory system that moves this information to where it needs to be."*[23]

Study and Discussion Questions

1. Health care is complex. List and discuss some of the complexities in health care that converge on information and that make health care IT such a shifting field.

2. How will health care change if the majority of hospitals implement EMRs and meet Meaningful Use requirements? And how about EPs (eligible providers—in other words, physicians in their practices)?

3. What are the most important benefits of CPOE systems? Why are they such an important Meaningful Use requirement? And what are some of the unintended consequences of CPOE systems? Do any of these unintended consequences outweigh the benefits, and might they cause a hospital to stop implementation?

4. Health information exchange aims to connect all players to give everyone access to a complete set of patient data. PHRs would make the patient's record the one place where all data come together. Do you favor one approach over the other? Can you predict which method will become dominant?

5. In what ways do "Health 2.0" applications empower customers to determine the care they receive? Could this affect the health care business model?

Case Studies

Case Study 1: Information Systems as Contributing Factor to Patient Safety Events

This case study illustrates how many small factors line up together, like holes in the proverbial Swiss cheese, to allow a medical error to slip through. Because the error is caused by many factors lining up, the fix doesn't consist of a single change, but rather a series of fixes to eliminate or reduce the risk for each of the contributing factors.

A patient is admitted on the medical unit. The medical admission order sets all have a deep vein thrombosis (DVT) prophylaxis section, and the physician orders low molecular weight heparin (LMWH), at the appropriate dose, to be given once a day at 6PM–the standard administration time for LMWH for *medical* patients.

Three days later, the patient needs a surgical procedure, and at the end of the procedure, the surgeon enters post-op orders for the patient. The post-op orders include DVT prophylaxis. The surgeon fails to see that the patient is already on DVT Prophylaxis, and orders LMWH again–to be given at 6AM, which is the standard for *surgical* patients, in order to meet Surgical Care Improvement Project (SCIP) guidelines, which require that DVT prophylaxis be started within 24 hours of a procedure.

Even though our patient is already on LMWH, the surgeon does not get a duplicate medication alert–since all these alerts were turned off. They were turned off in response to alert overload, and physicians were simply clicking through all duplicate alerts without paying attention.

Also, the physician didn't notice that the patient had two active orders for LMWH, because the list of active orders was sorted in reverse chronological order—so the original order from three days ago was much lower on the list.

The pharmacy team did receive a medication duplicate alert, but didn't act on it, for an unknown reason.

The nursing team didn't receive a duplicate medication alert, because the time window for duplicate administrations was set to 10 hours, and this administration occurred 12 hours after the previous administration.

The patient received two daily doses of LMWH, and suffered a hemorrhagic stroke.

In order to prevent this type of medication error, many changes need to be made—some simple, some more involved:

- Change the sort-order for active medications from chronological to alphabetical, allowing physicians and nurses to see duplicate medications.
- Standardize administration times for anticoagulation medications–either everyone at 6PM or everyone at 6AM, so that a patient crossing over from one group to another would not run the risk of over- or under-medication.
- Turn on duplicate medication checking alerts for selected, high-risk medications, but not for routine, less harmful medications.
- Set the window for nursing administration checks to include duplicate medications for high-risk medications.
- Implement a strong system for medication reconciliation at key transition events: transfers in or out of the operating room or critical care unit—forcing the medical staff to review the patient's medications thoroughly at these transitions.

Lesson learned from this case study: implementation of clinical information systems requires the services of strong informaticians to detect the role information systems play in patient safety events, and to implement measures to prevent and reduce the likelihood and risk for these events.

Case Study 2: Health Information Exchange—How Do Hospitals and Physician Offices Exchange Data Electronically?

The infrastructure to send patient data from hospital to practice, or from practice to practice, or between health care providers, is called health information exchange (HIE).[19] There are a number of public HIEs and a growing number of private HIEs that are usually owned and operated by health systems—also known as enterprise HIEs.

An HIE usually starts with the simplest data to send between participants: lab results and transcribed reports (e.g., radiology, discharge summaries). The HIE system needs to do three things with these data:

1. *Route* the right data to the right practice—so it must keep track of which patient has a relationship with specific physicians.

2. *Transform* the transaction into a format that the receiving EMR will accept. Although all EMRs use HL7, there usually are variations, and the HIE needs to format the transaction in a way that the receiving EMR can process it.

3. *Map* terminology to the receiving EMR's coding system (e.g., the codes for lab results and report codes).

This initial level of exchange is typically one-way (results from the lab/radiology to the practice), and the data are "pushed" into the EMR of the practice receiving the results.

Once this initial level is in place, the next logical step is to implement two-way traffic: orders for lab tests, imaging studies, etc. from the practices to the health system and results back. Also, in this phase practices begin to send and receive referrals.

Under one of the ARRA Meaningful Use criteria, care providers will exchange continuity of care documents (CCD). A CCD is a structured, summarized list of the patient's clinical history and status, including demographics, allergies, problems, medications, and recent results. Because one cannot know when the patient will see another care provider and which provider they will see next, one cannot "push" these CCDs to the next recipient. Instead, CCDs typically are stored in a central database on the HIE and "pulled" as needed when the patient has another encounter.

To pull a CCD, HIEs use a concept called "record locator service" to locate and retrieve a patient's most recent CCD from any of the participants in the HIE.

HIEs begin with simple "push" transactions between the connected participants and, over time, evolve into complex "push and pull" data exchange systems. They enable health care providers to share data about the patients they see, thus avoiding duplication of care; saving time looking for information; and making better, more informed decisions.

Suggested Readings and Web Sites

AMIA, formerly known as the American Medical Informatics Association. www.amia.org

Association of Medical Directors of Information Systems, AMDIS. www.amdis.org

Health Information Management Systems Society, HIMSS. www.himss.org

International Medical Informatics Association, IMIA. www.imia-medinfo.org

Life as a Healthcare CIO, by John Halamka. http://geekdoctor.blogspot.com/

US Department of Health and Human Services Office of the National Coordinator for Health Information Technology. http://healthit.hhs.gov/

References

1. Kilbridge PM, Classen DC. The informatics opportunities at the intersection of patient safety and clinical informatics. *J Am Med Inform Assoc*, 15(4):397-407, July-Aug. 2008.
2. Kaushal R, Shojania KG, Bates DW. Effects of computerized physician order entry and clinical decision support systems on medication safety: as systematic review. *Arch Intern Med*, 163(12):1409-16, June 23, 2003.
3. Devine EB, Hansen RN, Wilson-Norton JL, *et al*. The impact of computerized physician order entry on medication errors in a multispecialty group practice. *J Am Med Inform Assoc*, 17(1):78-84, Jan.-Feb. 2010.

4. Mekhjian HS, Kumar RR, Kuehn L, *et al.* Immediate benefits realized following implementation of physician order entry at an academic medical center. *J Am Med Inform Assoc*, 9(5):529-39, Sept.-Oct. v2009.

5. Niazkhani Z, Pirnejad H, Berg M, Aarts J. The impact of computerized physician order entry systems on inpatient clinical workflow: a literature review. *J Am Med Inform Assoc*, 16(4):539-49, July-Aug. 2009.

6. Poon EG, Keohane CA, Yoon CS, *et al.* Effect of bar-code technology on the safety of medication administration. *N Engl J Med*, 362(18):1698-707, May 6, 2010.

7. HIMSS Analytics EMR Adoption Model, www.himssanalytics.org. Accessed 10/1/2011.

8. Garg AX, Adhikari NKJ, McDonald H, *et al.* Effects of computerized clinical decision support systems on practitioner performance and patient outcomes: a systematic review. *JAMA*, 293(10):1223-38, Mar. 9, 2005. doi: 10.1001/jama.293.10.

9. Van der Sijs H, Aarts J, Van Gelder T, *et al.* Turning off frequently overridden drug alerts: limited opportunities for doing it safely. *J Am Med Inform Assoc*, 15(4):439-48, July-Aug. 2008.

10. Jenders RA, Hripcsak G, Sideli RV, *et al.* Medical decision support: experience with implementing the Arden Syntax at the Columbia-Presbyterian Medical Center. *Proc Annu Symp Comput Appl Med Care,* 169-73, 1995.

11. Health Level Seven. The Arden Syntax for Medical Logic Systems. Ann Arbor: Health Level Seven, 1999. www.hl7.org.

12. Clinical Decision Support Consortium (CDSC). http://www.partners.org/cird/cdsc/ Accessed 12/2011.

13. OpenCDS. http://www.opencds.org/ Accessed 12/2011.

14. Inzucchi, SE. Management of hyperglycemia in the hospital setting. *N Engl J Med*, 355(18):1903-11, Nov. 2, 2006.

15. Amarasingham R, Plantinga L, Diener-West M, *et al.* Clinical information technologies and inpatient outcomes: a multiple hospital study. *Archives of Internal Medicine*, 169(2):108-14, Jan. 26, 2009.

16. Koppel R, Metlay JP, Cohen A, *et al.* Role of computerized physician order entry systems in facilitating medication errors. *JAMA*, 293(10):1197-203, Mar. 9, 2005.

17. Koppel R, Wetterneck T, Telles JL, Karsh B-T. Workarounds to barcode medication administration systems: their occurrences, causes, and threats to patient safety. *J Am Med Inform Assoc*, 15(4):408-23, July-Aug. 2008. doi: 10.1197/jamia.M2616 PMCID: PMC2442264.

18. Ash JS, Sittig DF, Poon EG, *et al.* The extent and importance of unintended consequences related to computerized provider order entry. *J Am Med Inform Assoc*, 14(4):415-23, July-Aug. 2007.

19. PatientsLikeMe. http://www.patientslikeme.com. Cambridge, MA. Accessed 10/6/2011.

20. Beard L, Schein R, Morra D, *et al.* The challenges in making electronic health records accessible to patients. *J Am Med Inform Assoc*, 19(1):116-20, Jan.-Feb. 2011. doi:10.1136/amiajnl-2011-000261

21. Kuperman G. Health information exchange: why are we doing it, and what are we doing? *J Am Med Inform Assoc*, 18(5):678-82, Sept.-Oct. 2011.

22. DeVore S, Champion RW. Driving population health through accountable care organizations. *Health Affairs*, 30(1): 41-50, Jan. 2011.

23. Blumenthal D. AMIA Symposium Keynote Address, November 2009.

Chapter 20

Changing the Health Care Delivery System

By Donald E. Casey, Jr., MD, MPH, MBA, FACP, FAHA

Executive Summary

The Affordable Care Act of 2010 now serves as the fundamental set of solutions needed to address the current shortcomings of the U.S. health care system. In this chapter, the current challenges and opportunities for significant change are identified as a roadmap to improving the health of patients at lower cost.

Learning Objectives

1. Explain some major factors driving current and future health care reform initiatives.

2. Recognize some of the key organizations influencing and supporting the Affordable Care Act legislation.

3. Describe the basic tenets of various new payment models for value being tested by CMS and other payers.

Key Words: Affordable Care Act, Centers for Medicare and Medicaid Services, Avoidable Readmissions, Variations in Care, Accountable Care Organizations

Introduction

The Affordable Care Act of 2010 (ACA) has set forth a detailed and aggressive roadmap for improving health care quality while simultaneously controlling medical cost inflation. This historic legislation has been driven in large part by widespread variations in health care expenditures and resource use across the United States without corresponding differences in health outcomes.[1]

In this chapter, we will identify and evaluate several systematic quality improvement strategies specified in the ACA law that are currently under consideration by the Centers for Medicare and Medicaid Services (CMS), state governments, commercial insurance payers, hospital systems, physicians, and some employers. Policy makers often reference the conceptual frameworks for these innovations using phrases such as "value-based purchasing," "from volume to value," and "no outcome means no income."

The current variations in health outcomes and associated costs are not newly identified challenges to the U. S. health care delivery system. In fact, these issues have been documented for the past several decades.[2] By analyzing patterns of Medicare claims data for hospitals (Part A) and physicians (Part B), experts from the Dartmouth Atlas project[3] have demonstrated significant regional and local geographic differences in the cost of care delivery for both overall and specific health care diagnoses. Some examples are listed in Table 1.

Table 1. Data from the Dartmouth Atlas of Health Care

(Data are by State for Medicare, 2007)	U.S.	High	Low
Total Mortality: ASR-adjusted % of deaths among Medicare enrollees	4.8	5.7	3.9
Congestive Heart Failure Discharges per 1,000 Medicare Enrollees	19.8	27.6	8.7
COPD Discharges per 1,000 Medicare Enrollees	9.9	21.2	2.7
Percent of Medicare decedents admitted to ICU/CCU during the hospitalization in which death occurred	17.1	23.1	10.9
ICU/CCU charges (Medicare) per decedent during the last six months of life	$9,475	$42,498	$1,888
Average annual percent of Medicare enrollees having at least one ambulatory visit to a primary care clinician	77.6	84.1	58.8
Average percent of female Medicare enrollees age 67-69 having at least one mammogram over a two-year period	63.2	71.7	56.0

The Dartmouth Atlas of Health Care http://www.dartmouthatlas.org/tools/downloads.aspx
Accessed October 29, 2011

Comparisons of the U.S. with other developed countries also have shown that American health care is twice as expensive as health care for its international counterparts—with lower life expectancy (Figure 1).[4] These findings suggest that, in spite of differences in national populations, less costly and more traditional approaches to improving health status and quality of life (e.g., primary and secondary prevention, healthy lifestyles, better end-of-life care) may be more desirable than increasingly sophisticated diagnostic and therapeutic methods and technologies designed to extend life of individuals with chronic illnesses.

Other researchers have demonstrated another major weakness of the U.S. health care system—inconsistent and incomplete coordination of care. One striking example of this inconsistency is the high rate of hospital readmissions within 30 days of discharge. Jencks *et al.* have shown that, on average, between one in four to five Medicare beneficiaries admitted to an inpatient facility returned to the hospital within one month of the initial discharge for additional inpatient care (Figure 2, page 316).[5] What is most remarkable about these findings is that only 50 percent of the patients readmitted within 30 days had made a Part B claim during this period, indicating a lack of follow up with a primary care or specialty physician prior to returning to the hospital (Figure 3, page 316). Additionally, there was significant variation in these readmissions rates by state, ranging from 13.3 to 23.2 percent.

Figure 1. Changes in Survival Rates: 1975 to 2005

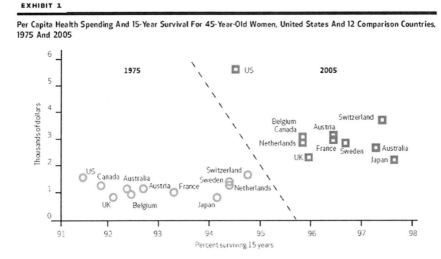

EXHIBIT 1

Per Capita Health Spending And 15-Year Survival For 45-Year-Old Women, United States And 12 Comparison Countries, 1975 And 2005

SOURCE Authors' analysis based on data from the sources described in the text. NOTES The dashed line separates 1975 values (blue circles) and 2005 values (red squares). Values are presented for the percentage of forty-five-year-old women surviving fifteen years.

Meuning PA, Glied SA. What changes in survival rates tell us about U.S. health care. *Health Affairs* 29(11):2105–13, Nov. 2010

Figure 2. Rates of rehospitalization within 30 days after hospital discharge

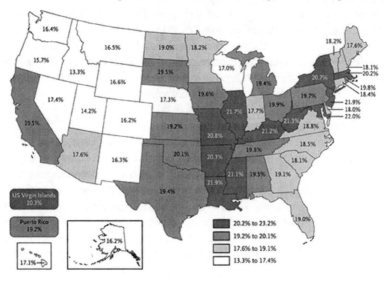

Jencks SF et al. *N Engl J Med* 2009;360:1418-1428

Figure 3. Patients for whom there was no bill for an outpatient physician visit between discharge and rehospitalization

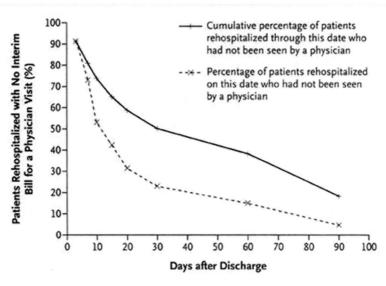

Jencks SF et al. *N Engl J Med* 2009;360:1418-1428

In response to these critical findings, a number of initiatives have emerged on the national front. One important effort is The National Quality Strategy (NQS),[6] which is designed to pursue three broad aims that will be used to guide and assess local, state, and national efforts to improve health and the health care delivery system, namely:

- **Better Care:** Improve overall quality by making health care more patient-centered, accessible, and safe.

- **Healthy People/Healthy Communities:** Improve the health of the U.S. population by supporting proven interventions to address behavioral, social, and environmental determinants of health in addition to delivering higher quality care.

- **Affordable Care:** Reduce the cost of high-quality health care for individuals, families, employers, and government.

To advance these aims, the NQS intends to initially focus on six priorities based on research, input from a broad range of stakeholders, and examples from around the country, which suggests that we have great potential for rapidly improving health outcomes and increasing the value and effectiveness of care for all populations. As the NQS is implemented, stakeholders will create specific quantitative goals and measures for each of these priorities, including:

1. Making care safer by reducing harm caused in the delivery of care.
2. Ensuring that care engages each person and family as partners.
3. Promoting effective communication and coordination of care.
4. Promoting the most effective prevention and treatment practices for the leading causes of mortality, starting with cardiovascular disease.
5. Working with communities to promote wide use of best practices to enable healthy living.
6. Making high-quality care more affordable for individuals, families, employers, and governments by developing and spreading new health care delivery models.

With respect to NQS Goal #3, it should be noted that, under the current system, hospitals and physicians currently receive payments for all services rendered as part of a readmission. Going forward, the ACA has mandated financial penalties via reduction in Medicare Part A payments to hospitals with certain DRG-specific high "avoidable" readmission rates beginning in October 2012. A number of stakeholder organizations, including the National Quality Forum (NQF), the National Priorities Partnership (NPP), the Institute for Healthcare Improvement (IHI), and several medical specialty societies are currently collaborating to identify evidence-based opportunities to reduce unnecessary hospitalizations and improve overall care coordination between various traditional health care "silos" (i.e., hospital, physician office, nursing home, etc.).[7] NQF and NPP have published some important background information on "preferred practices"[8] as well as performance measures for evaluating care coordination effectiveness. These standards are based on a framework that includes the following domains:

Health Care Home[9] Practice Statement

1. The patient shall be provided the opportunity to select the health care home that provides the best and most appropriate opportunities for the patient to develop and maintain a relationship with health care providers. As defined by the NQF-endorsed Framework for Care Coordination, the "health care home" is the usual source of care selected by the patient, such as a large or small medical group, a single practitioner, a community health center, or a hospital outpatient clinic. The health care home should function as the central point for coordinating care around the patient's needs and preferences. In addition, the use of the health care home is relevant for all patients across the continuum of care.

2. The health care home or sponsoring organizations shall be the central point for incorporating strategies for continuity of care.

3. The health care home shall develop infrastructure for managing plans of care that incorporate systems for registering, tracking, measuring, reporting, and improving essential coordinated services.

4. The health care home should have policies, procedures, and accountabilities to support effective collaborations between primary care and specialist providers, including evidence-based referrals and consultations that clearly define roles and responsibilities.

5. The health care home will provide or arrange to provide care coordination services for patients at high risk for adverse health outcomes, high service use, and high costs.

Proactive care plan and follow-up

6. Health care providers and entities should have structured and effective systems, policies, procedures, and practices to create, document, execute, and update a plan of care with every patient.

7. A systematic process of follow-up tests, treatments, or services should be established and be informed by the plan of care.

8. A joint plan of care should be developed and include patient education and support for self-management and resources.

9. The plan of care should include community and nonclinical services as well as health care services that respond to a patient's needs and preferences and contribute to achieving the patient's goals.

10. Health care organizations should utilize cardiac rehabilitation services to assist the health care home in coordinating rehabilitation and preventive care for patients with recent cardiovascular events.

Communication

11. The patient's plan of care should always be made available to the health care home team, the patient, and the patient's designees.

12. All health care home team members, including the patient and his or her designees, should work within the same plan of care and share responsibility for their contributions to the plan of care and for achieving the patient's goals.

13. A program should be used that incorporates a care partner to support family and friends when caring for a hospitalized patient.

14. The provider's perspective of care coordination activities should be assessed and documented.

Information systems

15. Standardized, integrated, interoperable, electronic information systems with functionalities that are essential to care coordination, decision support, quality measurement, and practice improvement should be used.

16. An electronic record system should allow the patient's health information to be accessible to caregivers at all points of care.

17. Regional health information systems, which may be governed by various partnerships, including public/private, state/local agencies, should enable health care home teams to access all patient information.

Transitions

18. Decision making and planning for transitions of care should involve the patient and, according to patient preferences, family and caregivers (including the health care home team). Appropriate follow-up protocols should be used to ensure timely understanding and endorsement of the plan for the patient and his or her designees.

19. Patients and their designees should directly participate in determining and preparing for ongoing care during and after transitions.

20. Systematic care transitions programs that engage patients and families in self-management after being transferred home should be used whenever available.

21. For high-risk chronically ill older adults, an evidence-based multidisciplinary, transitional care practice that provides comprehensive in-hospital planning, home-based visits, and telephone follow-up, such as the transitional care model,[10] should be deployed.

22. Health care organizations should develop and implement a standardized communication template for the transitions of care process, including a minimal set of core data elements that are accessible to patients and their designees during care.

23. Health care providers and health care organizations should implement proto-cols/policies for a standardized approach to all transitions of care. Policies and procedures related to transitions and their critical aspects should be included in the standardized approach.

24. Health care providers and health care organizations should have systems in place to clarify, identify, and enhance mutual accountability (complete/con-firmed communication loop) of each party involved in a transition of care.

25. Health care organizations should evaluate the effectiveness of transition pro-tocols, policies, and outcomes.

No doubt, simultaneous achievement of all 25 of these "Practice Statements" is currently far beyond the reach of the U.S. health system, but the statements serve as a necessary vision for achieving the goals of the ACA and all future health care reform initiatives, whether they be federal, regional, statewide, or health system efforts to improve care coordination.

Of growing importance is the need to involve individuals and their loved ones more consistently and directly in their own health care. Evolution of "shared decision mak-ing" between health care providers and patients has recently emerged as an important approach to ensuring that beliefs and preferences for choosing specific medical and surgical treatments are effectively balanced with realistic and data-driven expecta-tions for clinical outcomes. The evolving focus by HHS, AHRQ, and the National Institutes of Health (NIH) on providing funding for "comparative effectiveness re-search" (CER) has thus been supported by the American Recovery and Reinvest-ment Act of 2009 (ARRA).[11,12,13,14] Some specific priority areas for funding have been identified with the Institutes of Medicine, including effective treatment strategies for low back pain, pharmacologic and non-pharmacologic treatments for Alzheimer's disease, and different strategies currently used to prevent obesity, diabetes, heart dis-ease, and hypertension.[15]

The major goals of CER include systematic evaluation of scientifically published evidence that directly or indirectly compares outcomes between different therapies for the same disease or condition, with the anticipation that such evaluation can yield important information to facilitate more effective, patient-centered, shared decision making as to the best course of treatment (including the option of no treatment). Organizations such as the Institute for Clinical and Economic Review (ICER) have begun to generate and publish CER appraisals online (on topics such as options for management of low-risk prostate cancer) with a goal of engaging health care consumers, physicians, commercial and public insurers, employers, and state governments to facilitate more widespread use of decision-making aids.[16]

Another goal of health care reform is ensuring that every individual's perceptions of the friendliness and accessibility of the delivery system is optimal. For many years, hospitals have evaluated themselves on the satisfaction of patients who receive in-patient care and outpatient services. Recently, more valid and rigorous methods of measuring the "patient experience"—similar to those used by commercial insurers (e.g., Consumer Assessment of Health Providers and Systems,[17] or "CAHPS")—

have been developed and implemented. Results from these surveys show major gaps,[18] suggesting that a more comprehensive method of assessing patient-centered care coordination over the care continuum is sorely needed (Figure 4).

Figure 4. Mean Percentage of Most Positive Responses on HCAHPS Measures for Hospitals Participating in March 2008 and March 2009

	March 2008	March 2009	Difference
Nurse communication	72.7%	73.1%	0.4****
Doctor communication	79.1	79.0	-0.1
Responsiveness of hospital staff[a]	59.9	60.8	0.9****
Pain management[b]	67.1	67.5	0.4****
Communication about medicines[c]	57.5	58.0	0.5****
Cleanliness of hospital environment	67.9	68.3	0.4****
Quietness of hospital environment	53.6	54.5	0.8****
Discharge information	79.1	79.9	0.8****
Recommendation	67.1	67.4	0.3**

SOURCE Data from the Hospital Consumer Assessment of Healthcare Providers and Systems (HCAHPS) survey, October 2006–June 2008. NOTES N = 2,774 hospitals submitting data qualifying them to report their results publicly in both March 2008 and March 2009. As explained in the text, the most positive response option is "always" for the first seven categories above. For discharge information, it is "yes," and for recommendation it is "yes, definitely." [a]Item asked of patients who reported summoning a hospital staff member. [b]Item asked of patients who were prescribed medication for pain management. [c]Item asked of patients who received a new medication. **p < 0.05 ****p < 0.001

Elliott MN, Lehrman WG, Goldstein EH, et al. Hospital survey shows improvement in patient experience. *Health Affairs* 29 (11): 2061–7, Nov. 2010.

Most sobering for American patients are the serious gaps in the delivery of evidence-based interventions necessary to improve their health status and sustain life. For example, in a 2003 study by McGlynn,[19] more than 400 quality measures were evaluated in terms of national performance, with quality varying substantially according to the particular medical condition, with a mean of 54.9 percent and ranging from 78.7 percent of recommended care for senile cataract care to 10.5 percent of recommended care for alcohol dependence.

Fortunately, standardized quality measures have been developed and used with increasing frequency over the past decade, thanks largely to wide-scale cooperative efforts between CMS, NQF, The Joint Commission, the Agency for Healthcare Quality and Research (AHRQ), physician organizations such as the Physician Consortium for Performance Improvement ("PCPI", led by the American Medical Association and its specialty society partners), the National Committee for Quality Assurance ("NCQA", the commercial health plan measure developer), The Leapfrog Group, and commercial private and for-profit health care insurers.

At present, NQF has several hundred standardized quality measures readily available for use by health care providers and their patients—measures designed for accountability through public reporting and quality improvement initiatives at the care delivery level.[20] However, many challenges and barriers to successful implementation remain. For example, the IMPROVE HF study has shown that practicing cardiologists, on average, deliver less than 50 percent of recommended care as specified in the clinical practice guidelines for heart failure developed by the American College of Cardiology and the American Heart Association (Figure 5, page 322).[21] The ACA includes a roadmap (The National Quality Strategy[22]) for creating incentives for clinicians and motivating health care organizations to use quality measurement to improve care at both the individual patient and health system levels.

Figure 5. National Cardiologist Clinical Performance for Heart Failure

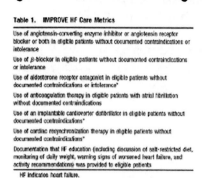

Table 1. IMPROVE HF Care Metrics

Use of angiotensin-converting enzyme inhibitor or angiotensin receptor blocker or both in eligible patients without documented contraindications or intolerance

Use of β-blocker in eligible patients without documented contraindications or intolerance

Use of aldosterone receptor antagonist in eligible patients without documented contraindications or intolerance*

Use of anticoagulation therapy in eligible patients with atrial fibrillation without documented contraindications

Use of an implantable cardioverter defibrillator in eligible patients without documented contraindications*

Use of cardiac resynchronization therapy in eligible patients without documented contraindications*

Documentation that HF education (including discussion of salt-restricted diet, monitoring of daily weight, warning signs of worsened heart failure, and activity recommendations) was provided to eligible patients

HF indicates heart failure.

*These metrics are not American College of Cardiology/American Heart Association performance measures for outpatients with HF.

Fonarow et al   Variation in Heart Failure Care   *101*

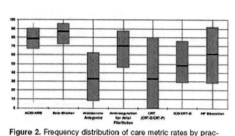

Figure 2. Frequency distribution of care metric rates by practice. Box plots represent median, 10th, and 90th percentiles, and lines for minimum and maximum conformity rates across practices.

Summary Measure	Mean/Median	Low (Bottom Decile)	High (Top Decile)
Composite	68.5%/68.9%	58.3%	78.5%
All or None	27.5%/27.2%	11.8%	45.3%

(Circ Heart Fail. 2008;1:98-106.)

Fonarow GC, Yancy CW, Albert NM, *et al.* Heart failure care in the outpatient cardiology practice setting: findings from IMPROVE HF. *Circ Heart Fail.* 1(2):98-106, July 2008

No doubt the biggest obstacle for current and future health care reform efforts is how best to reduce the overall cost of care. Among the multiple root causes of excessive health care expenses are:

- Inadequate comparative measurement systems of "efficiency."

- Variations in care delivery and local medical practice styles mentioned earlier.

- Dysfunctional traditional payment systems that reward volume (including overuse) rather than value.

- Lack of economic incentive alignments between payers, hospitals, and physicians.

- The rampant practice of "defensive medicine," leading to excess diagnostic testing and unnecessary treatment.[23,24,25]

- Price inelasticity and insensitivity of consumers due to insurance coverage and imperfect publicly available information on quality and cost.[26]

As a starting point to address these issues, the NQF has outlined a model for defining a "patient-centered episode of care" (Figure 6, page 324) that can be used by stakeholders to better evaluate the cost and efficiency of care for specific disease categories.[27] Additionally, the RAND Corporation recently published an elegant summary of several payment incentive models that are currently being tested through many pilots and demonstration initiatives, some of which have served as a critical backdrop to the newer models of reimbursement recommended in the ACA.[28]

Table 2. Analysis of Models and Performance Measurement

Attributes

Model	Performance Measured for a Population	Performance Measured for an Episode of Care	Performance Measured Across More Than One Type of Delivery Organization	Fee-for-Service Payment Applied to One or More Newly Specified Services
Model 1: Global Payment	√√	√	√√	
Model 2: ACO Shared Savings program	√√	√	√√	
Model 3: Medical home	√√	√	√	√
Model 4: Bundled payment	√	√√	√√	√
Model 5: Hospital-physician gainsharing	√	√	√	
Model 6: Payment for coordination	√	√	√	√√
Model 7: Hospital P4P		√		
Model 8: Payment adjustment for readmissions		√	√	
Model 9: Payment adjustment for hospital-acquired conditions		√		
Model 10: Physician P4P		√		
Model 11: Payment for shared decisionmaking		√		√√

Schneider EC, Hussey PS, Schnyer C. Technical report (RAND). Payment reform: Analysis of models and performance measurement implications.

Figure 6. Generic Episode of Care

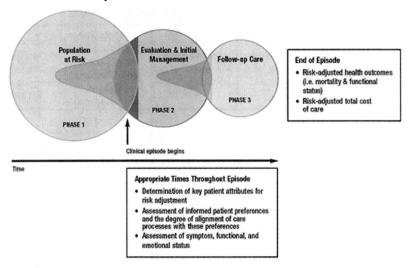

Schneider EC, Hussey PS, Schnyer C. Technical report (RAND). Payment reform: Analysis of models and performance measurement implications. 2011, National Quality Forum

One of the most exciting—and contentious—innovations delineated in the ACA is the concept of the accountable care organization (ACO). At the time of this writing, two pathways for ACO development have been specified by CMS.[29,30] Central to these ACO models is a golden opportunity to achieve better and more effective alignment between hospitals and physicians by moving from a "volume" to a "value" mindset. While the ACO rules give fairly clear direction as to the goals (i.e., achievement of consistently improved clinical outcomes at an overall lower cost of care), they remain ambiguous in the near term as to how best to accomplish these goals.

Conceptually, successful implementation of an ACO depends on a governance structure designed to internally motivate its stakeholders to trust one other and cooperate more closely than ever before. Success also requires a combination of organizational design, ability and experience to measure, report, and improve quality and patient experience results; manage financial and actuarial risk; reduce avoidable rehospitalizations; rely on shared decision making; effectively use interoperable health information systems and other technologies; and provide successful care coordination resources—a robust skill set lacking in most health care providers (especially hospital systems and physician practices).

On a positive note, several ACO-like health system organizations, such as Geisinger (Pennsylvania) and Advocate (Chicago, IL) health systems, have invested in the infrastructure and organizational architecture necessary to demonstrate a positive track record with the strategies as outlined by CMS in its recently published final rule.[31] Additionally, there is legacy experience within CMS from past demonstration projects, including the Physician Group Practice Demonstration, the

Physician Hospital Gainsharing Demonstration, and the Hospital Quality Demonstration Program (developed in collaboration with Premier, Inc., a hospital group purchasing organization).[32] Newer methods, including a Patient-Centered Medical Home Demonstration and another project evaluating "bundled care" payments for coronary artery bypass graft and total joint replacement surgeries, are also under way through the newly established Center for Medicare and Medicaid Innovation.[33] To date, empiric evidence supports the opportunity for these methods to be directly incorporated into the ACO model as it evolves. Commercial health insurance companies are rapidly following suit with similar payment models as the CMS ACO model is launched in the real world of everyday health care.

For the past decade, hospitals have borne the brunt of CMS's payment reform efforts. The focus of newer reform projects has shifted to include physicians. Perhaps the thorniest problem for physicians has been their ability and/or willingness to accept changes in the payment system. It is well documented that physician satisfaction with the practice of medicine has seriously declined over the past 20 years.[34] Much of this chronic unhappiness has been related to factors such as:

• Perceptions of underpayment for professional services.

• Increasing (and at times aggressive) demands of patients for more personalized attention to their care that can lead to overuse.

• Growing fear of malpractice suits.

• Increasing external demands for better and more transparent accountability.

Most health policy experts believe that any health care reform efforts will likely collapse without physician "buy-in," i.e., addressing these issues directly with the profession. Luckily, effective physician leadership has emerged at the grass roots and national levels to help guide these reforms to ensure success. Through national efforts such as the AMA PCPI, expansion of physician organization infrastructure to develop and disseminate better and more credible clinical practice guidelines and corresponding quality measures incorporating systematic reviews of published evidence are more abundant than ever.[35]

Further, the American Board of Medical Specialties (ABMS) now serves as the central guidepost for linking almost all of the physician board-certifying organizations to promote professionalism, with the explicit expectation that quality measurement and improvement will be a part of every physician's day-to-day medical practice.[36] Such expectations serve as an important framework for ensuring that medical students and residents in training clearly understand their roles in evaluating and enhancing the quality of care as a critical expectation of their professional development. Theoretically, by the time they enter practice they will be much better equipped than their predecessors with the understanding, experience, tools, and motivation to actively participate in modern reform efforts such as value-based purchasing. The ACA supports these emerging paradigms as critical success factors for payment reform, and the Federation of State Medical Boards (FSMB) is expected to follow suit with a similar process for state licensure requirements.[37]

The ACA legislation itself is evidence that "physician buy-in" has been achieved to at least some extent. Clearly, Congress and President Obama could not have succeeded in passing this law without the direct involvement of physicians, including several key physician legislators such as Sen. Tom Coburn (R-OK), Former Sen. William Frist (R-TN), and Rep. Jim McDermott (D-WA). Health care reform efforts have signaled a commitment to ensuring that evidence-based care is delivered properly and effectively to all patients through better incentives, support, and commitment of physicians to achieve this end.

Like previous national physician payment reforms, a healthy degree of skepticism remains among some health care providers, politicians, and patients as to whether the federal government can be trusted to achieve its goals.[38] The 2012 U.S. presidential and congressional election campaigns are already under way, with the viability of the ACA as a centerpiece for extensive political debate. The next two years will be, perhaps, the most interesting in the history of the American health care system.

Study and Discussion Questions

1. As a thought experiment, consider what the survey results might be if patients readmitted to a hospital within 30 days of discharge because of inadequate care coordination were asked, "How satisfied were you with your care?" What might be some reasons to consider a given patient's dissatisfaction?

2. Study Figures 2 through 6. Given the current high rates of re-hospitalization, lack of consistent follow up with physicians post hospital discharge, current patient experience scores, and low usage of evidence-based care, how might the Generic Episode of Care model illustrated in Figure 6 serve to address these issues?

3. Review one or two of the current Medicare Demonstration projects listed on the website link provided in Reference 17. What will be some potential obstacles to achieving successful results of improved quality and lower cost? What are some innovative strategies to overcome some or all of these potential obstacles?

4. Read Atul Gawande's article cited in Reference 2. What strategic advice and support could be given to the CEO of the McAllen Medical Center to address the issues raised in this article?

References

1. Obama B. The Affordable Care Act.http://www.whitehouse.gov/healthreform/health-care-overview. Accessed October 22, 2011.

2. Gawande A. The cost conundrum. *The New Yorker*, June 1, 2009.

3. Fisher ES, Bynum JP, Skinner JS. Slowing the growth of health care costs—lessons from regional variation. *N Engl J Med,* 360 (9):849-852, Feb. 26, 2009.

4. Meuning PA, Glied SA. What changes in survival rates tell us about U.S. health care. *Health Affairs,* 29(11): 2105–13, 2 Nov. 010.

5. Jencks SF, Williams MV, Coleman EA. Rehospitalizations among patients in the Medicare fee-for-service program. *N Engl J Med,* 360(14):1418-28, Apr. 2, 2009.

6. US Department of Health and Human Services. National Strategy for Quality Improvement in Healthcare. March, 2011. http://www.healthcare.gov/law/resources/reports/nationalqualitystrategy032011.pdf. Accessed December 8, 2011.

7. National Priorities Partnership.http://www.nationalprioritiespartnership.org/. Accessed October 22, 2011.

8. National Quality Forum. Preferred practices and performance measures for measuring and reporting care coordination, a consensus report. http://www.qualityforum.org/Publications/2010/10/Preferred_Practices_and_Performance_Measures_for_Measuring_and_Reporting_Care_Coordination.aspx. Accessed October 29, 2011.

9. National Quality Forum. Preferred practices and performance measures for measuring and reporting care coordination, a consensus report. http://www.qualityforum.org/Publications/2010/10/Preferred_Practices_and_Performance_Measures_for_Measuring_and_Reporting_Care_Coordination.aspx. Accessed October 29, 2011.

10. Coleman EA, Smith JD, Frank JC, *et al.* Preparing patients and caregivers to participate in care delivered across settings: the Care Transitions intervention. *J Am Geriatr Soc,* 52(11):1817-25, 2004.

11. Wilensky GR. Developing a center for comparative effectiveness research. *Health Affairs,* 25(6):w572–85, Nov.-Dec. 2006. (published online 7 November 2006; 10.1377/hlthaff.25.w572). Accessed October 29, 2011.

12. Orzag P. The case for reform in education and health care. United States Office of Management and Budget.http://www.whitehouse.gov/omb/blog/09/04/20/TheCaseforReforminEducationandHealthCare. Accessed October 29, 2011

13. National Institutes of Health. Comparative effectiveness research (CER) (Also known as patient-centered outcomes research. http://www.nlm.nih.gov/hsrinfo/cer.html. Accessed October 29, 2011.

14. Agency for Healthcare Research and Quality. Effective healthcare program: helping you make better healthcare choices. http://www.effectivehealthcare.ahrq.gov/index.cfm. Accessed October 29, 2011.

15. Greenfield S, Sox H. Report brief: Initial national priorities for comparative effectiveness research. Institute of Medicine, 2009.http://www.iom.edu/~/media/Files/Report%20Files/2009/ComparativeEffectivenessResearchPriorities/CER%20report%20brief%2008-13-09.pdf. Accessed October 29, 2011.

16. Institute for Clinical and Economic Review. Management options for low-risk prostate cancer. http://www.icer-review.org/index.php/Completed-Appraisals/mgmtoptionlrpc.html. Accessed October 29, 2011.

17. Consumer Assessment of Healthcare Providers and Systems (CAHPS). Agency for Healthcare Research and Quality.https://www.cahps.ahrq.gov/default.asp. Accessed October 22, 2011.

18. Elliott MN, Lehrman WG, Goldstein EH, *et al.* Hospital survey shows improvement in patient experience. *Health Affairs,* 29(11):2061-7, Nov. ,2010.

19. McGlynn EA, Asch SM, Adams J, *et al.* The quality of health care delivered to adults in the United States. *N Engl J Med,* 348(26):2635-45, June 26, 2003.

20. National Quality Forum: http://www.qualityforum.org/Measures_List.aspx. Accessed October 22, 2011.

21. Fonarow GC, Yancy CW, Albert NM, *et al.* Heart failure care in the outpatient cardiology practice setting: findings from IMPROVE HF. *Circ Heart Fail*, 1(2):98-106, July 2006.

22. US Department of Health and Human Services. Report to Congress: National Strategy for Quality Improvement in Health Care. http://www.healthcare.gov/law/resources/reports/quality03212011a.html. Accessed October 22, 2011.

23. Studdert DM, Mello MM, Brennan TA. Defensive medicine and tort reform: a wide view. *J Gen Intern Med*, 25(5):380-1, May 2010.

24. Studdert DM, Mello MM, Sage WM, *et al.* Defensive medicine among high-risk specialist physicians in a volatile malpractice environment. *JAMA*, 293(21):2609-17, June 1, 2005.

25. Carrier ER, Reschovsky JD, Mello MM, *et al.* Physicians' fears of malpractice lawsuits not assuaged by tort reforms. *Health Affairs*, 29(9):1585-92, Sept. 2009.

26. Liu S, Chollet D. Price and income elasticity of the demand for health insurance and health care services: A critical review of the literature. Mathematica Policy Inc. http://www.mathematica-mpr.com/publications/pdfs/priceincome.pdf. Accessed October 22, 2011.

27. National Quality Forum. Measurement framework: Evaluating efficiency across patient-focused episodes of care. http://www.qualityforum.org/Publications/2010/01/Measurement_Framework__Evaluating_Efficiency_Across_Patient-Focused_Episodes_of_Care.aspx. Accessed October 23, 2011.

28. Schneider EC, Hussey PS, Schnyer C. Technical report (RAND). Payment reform: Analysis of models and performance measurement implications. 2011. http://www.qualityforum.org/News_And_Resources/Press_Releases/2011/NQF-Commissioned_RAND_Report_Points_Way_to_Using_Health_Performance_Measures_to_Support_Innovative_Payment_Reforms.aspx. Accessed October 23, 2011.

29. Berwick DM. Making good on ACO's promise—The final rule for the Medicare Shared Savings Program. Published online October 20, 2011, at nejm.org. Accessed October 23, 2011.

30. Rosenthal MB, Cutler DM, Feder J. The ACO rules—striking the balance between participation and transformative potential. Published online July 28, 2011 at nejm.org. Accessed October 23, 2011.

31. Department of Health and Human Services, Centers for Medicare and Medicaid Services. Final rule: Medicare shared savings program: Accountable Care Organizations. http://www.ofr.gov/OFRUpload/OFRData/2011-27461_PI.pdf. Accessed October 29, 2011.

32. Medicare Demonstration Projects and Evaluation Reports.Centers for Medicare and Medicaid Services. https://www.cms.gov/DemoProjectsEvalRpts/MD/list.asp. Accessed October 23, 2011.

33. Center for Medicare and Medicaid Innovation: Bundled payments for care improvement. http://innovations.cms.gov/areas-of-focus/patient-care-models/bundled-payments-for-care-improvement.html. Accessed October 23, 2011.

34. Zuger A. Dissatisfaction with medical practice. *N Eng J Med*, 2004; 350:69-75

35. American Medical Association: Physician Consortium for Performance Improvement. http://www.ama-assn.org/ama/pub/physician-resources/clinical-practice-improvement/clinical-quality/physician-consortium-performance-improvement.page. Accessed October 23, 2011.

36. American Board of Medical Specialities.http://www.abms.org/. Accessed October 23, 2011.

37. Chaudry HJ, Rhyne J, Cain FE, *et al.* Maintenance of licensure: Protecting the public, promoting quality health care. *J Med Regulation*, 96(1):1-8, First Quarter 2009.

38. Gawande A. Testing, testing. *The New Yorker*, December 14, 2009.

Chapter 21

Collaboration between Public Health and Health Care Organizations

By Bonnie L. Zell, MD, MPH, Greg D. Randolph, MD, MPH, and Amanda Cornett, MPH

Executive Summary

The ultimate goal of the U.S. health care system is to improve our nation's health. We are far from achieving what is possible given our knowledge and resources. Many efforts are under way to improve health care services; however, improvements in the personal health care system alone will not be sufficient to achieve a healthy population.

This chapter focuses on how public health and health care organizations increasingly will need to collaborate to improve the population's health. The chapter summarizes some of the origins of the historical division of public health and health care, outlines numerous recent changes in policy and practice that serve to facilitate collaboration between public health and health care organizations, highlights several examples of collaborations among public health and health care organizations that have improved health outcomes, and proposes several future opportunities to expand public health and health care collaboration and its impact.

Learning Objectives

1. Understand that health of individuals and populations is the ultimate goal of the health care delivery system.

2. Understand the importance of bringing community context into health care encounters.

3. Understand opportunities and the need for health care, public health, and key community stakeholders to collaborate for individual and population health.

4. List opportunities for elements of the health care delivery system to serve as models and leaders to improve population health.

5. List the social determinants of health and describe how they impact overall health.

Key Words: Collaboration, Context, Determinants of Health, Quality Improvement, Health Care, Public Health, Population Health, Community Health, Triple Aim

Introduction

The ultimate goal of the U.S. health care system is to improve our nation's health; however, we are far from achieving what is possible given our knowledge and resources. It is widely recognized that the quality of health care services is highly variable and generally substandard.[1,2] Although many efforts are under way to improve health care services, health care system improvements alone will not be enough to achieve a healthy population.[3]

Health care cannot dramatically improve population health because it is only one of five domains that influence health—these are often called the *determinants of health.* The other four determinants are genetics, social circumstances, environmental exposures, and behavioral patterns.[3-5] At least 40 percent of deaths in the U.S. can be linked to behavioral factors, with another 20 percent attributable to social circumstances and environmental factors.[6] To address this challenge more fully, many emerging efforts to improve the health of individuals and populations take into account where those individuals spend their time—at home, at work, at school, and in their communities.

Interest in broadening the focus of national health improvement efforts to include population health improvement is growing. Population health has been defined as "an approach to health that seeks to step beyond the individual-level focus of traditional clinical and preventive medicine by addressing a broad range of factors that impact health on a population-level."[7] Population health strategies seek to foster health and wellness and to prevent (rather than simply treat) injury, illness, and disability. Population health considers the context and circumstances of people, both as individuals and as members of groups and communities, and seeks to implement evidence-based interventions to address these multiple factors to improve outcomes.

A common public health framework, the Social Ecological Model, is a useful way to illustrate how these determinants interact to impact health on multiple levels, from the individual to community and societal levels (Figure 1, page 333).[8] Cultural beliefs, social norms, economic circumstances, and policies modified by each individual's values and behaviors have a significant impact on overall health. Where one works, learns, plays, and shops—influenced by level of education, income, and employment—all play important roles. Further, health is determined by access to healthy food, safe environments, and available transportation as well as health care services.

Figure 1. Social Ecological Model[8]

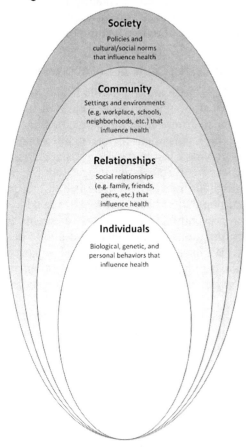

From McLeroy KR, Bibeau D, Steckler A, Glanz K. An ecological perspective on health promotion programs. *Health Education & Behavior.* 15(4):351-77, Dec. 1988.

With these concepts in mind, this chapter will focus on how public health and health care organizations will increasingly need to collaborate to improve the population's health. First, we will list a few definitions that should help readers make the most of this topic.

- *Public health* has been defined as "what we, as a society, do collectively to assure the conditions in which people can be healthy"[9]

- The *public health system* refers to all public, private, and voluntary entities that contribute to the delivery of public health services within a given area, including hospitals and physician practices. Public health systems are networks of entities with differing roles, relationships, and interactions that contribute to the health and well-being of the community or state.[10]

- The term *public health organizations* (a subset of the public health system) includes both local and state governmental agencies plus other not-for-profit entities whose missions include the provision of public health services or the development and advocacy of public health policy.

Historical Context and Current State of Collaboration

For the past century, U.S. medicine and public health have functioned as parallel operations. Since publication of the Flexner Report in 1910, U.S. medical education and practice has been grounded in the biomedical model and mechanisms of disease, focusing on individual patient-physician interactions.[11,12] After the Welch-Rose Report (1915) provided justification for separate schools of medicine and public health, the Rockefeller Foundation began funding numerous new schools of public health throughout the U.S.[13] Public health has been primarily focused on epidemiology and population-based approaches to address health issues, with a major emphasis on prevention.[11] These historical events created distinct frameworks and education programs for medicine and public health—and their "silo" effects persist today. We have two separate sets of organizations that address the public's health– public health organizations (largely reliant on limited public funding) and health care organizations (largely reliant on generous private funding).[14]

Though public health and health care organizations evolved to serve as separate components of our public health system, these organizations have nonetheless managed to collaborate. For example:

- A community hospital may work with a local health department to identify community health needs through an assessment and identify ways to jointly address these needs.

- A physician practice may work with a local health department as well as state or federal public health agencies to address an infectious disease outbreak.

- A state public health agency may collaborate with local hospitals to share data and coordinate resources during a natural disaster.

As these examples illustrate, collaboration between public health and health care organizations typically varies from community to community and is often reactive rather than proactive and strategic.

Recent Changes

Numerous recent changes in law and practice serve as catalysts for more strategic collaboration between public health and health care organizations. Below, we describe several of the most important developments.

Greater emphasis on improving population health to lower health care costs

One of the biggest drivers of health care policy in recent years has been the unabated increase in health care costs. With our aging population, powerful demographic trends are likely to drive up costs further.[15] The increasing focus on improving population health is, in large part, driven by the argument, "If our population is sicker, health care costs will rise even more."

The growing impact of the Triple Aim Initiative is a good example of the increasing focus on population health by health care organizations and the ensuing collaboration with public health organizations. The three aims of this Institute for Healthcare Improvement (IHI) initiative are to: 1) improve population health, 2) reduce health care costs, and 3) improve the patient experience of care.[16] Due in part to IHI's far-reaching influence, the Triple Aim Initiative framework has already been embedded into many aspects of federal policy, such as the National Prevention Strategy—an important set of recommendations required by the Affordable Care Act (ACA) designed to move the U.S. from "a system of sick care to one based on wellness and prevention."[17]

Increasingly, hospitals and public health agencies across the nation are working together to improve population health and lower health care costs through the Triple Aim Initiative. For instance, a Centers for Disease Control and Prevention (CDC) National Public Health Improvement Initiative site in North Carolina is encouraging local health departments across the state to lead Triple Aim projects that will provide greater focus on the population health improvement portion of the framework.[18]

Another example of greater focus on population health by the federal government is the work of the National Priorities Partnership (NPP), a multi-stakeholder group convened by the National Quality Forum, a not-for-profit organization whose mission is to improve the quality of American health care. The NPP collaborative group of stakeholders provides support to the U.S. Department of Health and Human Services (HHS) in setting priorities for its National Quality Strategy. Population health is one of the six national priority areas in which the NPP offers strategies whereby health care and public health can work together—e.g., improving the delivery of evidence-based clinical preventive services.[19]

Greater focus on health care's role in measuring and improving the health of communities

A notable change brought about by the ACA is a new requirement for 501(c)(3) not-for-profit hospitals to assess and improve their communities' health. This designation applies to more than 66 percent of U.S. hospitals.[20] The new regulations require not-for-profit hospitals to conduct a community health needs assessment every three years and to adopt an implementation strategy to meet the identified community health needs.[21] Because many local health departments regularly conduct community health assessments and create action plans to address these needs, this requirement offers an opportunity for hospitals and local health departments to pool resources to efficiently and effectively assess and improve community health.

Another opportunity for health care and public health organizations to collaborate on community health improvement is through the rapidly expanding availability of health data. A positive step in this direction is that health outcome and health determinant data are now available for every county in the U.S. The Robert Wood Johnson Foundation and the University of Wisconsin Population Health Institute have developed county health rankings for each state that are published annually through the Mobilizing Action Toward Community Health (MATCH) initiative.[22] These data can be used by communities as a "call to action" to stimulate health care, public health, and other community organizations to identify and deploy strategies designed to address their communities' health needs.

Any effort to improve health in a community must be guided by timely data to promptly learn if the strategies are having their desired effect.[23] Although MATCH data can be helpful in identifying areas that need improvement, most of these data are not timely enough to guide such improvement efforts. Fortunately, the rapid expansion of health information technology (HIT) and health information exchanges (HIEs) is providing more timely data for communities to identify health problems and guide improvement efforts addressing them. For example, the Beacon Community Program, funded by the American Recovery and Reinvestment Act, is currently accelerating the availability of timely, meaningful HIT through several large pilot projects aimed at HIE capabilities.[24] HIEs allow health and health care data to be shared across multiple organizations; e.g., a physician practice could access influenza vaccination data from a patient's last visit to a local health department through an exchange. Connecting and integrating pertinent health-related data on a regional basis from health care organizations, public health organizations, and other governmental agencies affords an opportunity to translate raw data into actionable information. In turn, this enables the alignment of aims, measures, and interventions across sectors and institutions for the greatest impact on improving individual and community health.

Additionally, the Centers for Medicare and Medicaid Services now provides substantial incentive payments to eligible health care professionals, hospitals, and critical access hospitals as they adopt, implement, upgrade, or meaningfully use electronic health records (EHRs). These incentives are greatly increasing the adoption of EHRs and the availability of data that can be gleaned from these systems through HIEs, which presents new opportunities to use timely health data for improvement.[25] For example, if most pediatricians in a state are using EHRs and are able to participate in an HIE, the state can generate estimates of the average BMI for children at the state, county, and township levels that could be reported regularly (e.g., quarterly) to help monitor the impact of public health interventions to reduce obesity.

Greater focus on applying quality improvement (QI) methods to improve health

Both the health care sector and, more recently, the public health sector are increasing their focus on using QI methods and tools to improve outcomes. In public health, the CDC recently launched the National Public Health Improvement Initiative, which aims to help local health departments and state public health agencies across the country dramatically improve the quality and effectiveness of public health services.[17] In addition, public health has launched a new national accreditation program (via the Public Health Accreditation Board) that is specifically designed to stimulate QI in all local health departments and state public health agencies.[26] In 2008, the HHS Office of Public Health and Science convened the Public Health Quality Forum, which developed a Consensus Statement on Quality in the Public Health System to frame quality in the public health system. They identified nine aims to guide public health improvements across the entire system: population-centered, equitable, proactive, health-promoting, risk-reducing, vigilant, transparent, effective, and efficient.[27]

In health care, numerous programs have been implemented over the past decade to stimulate adoption of QI, including: recent American Board of Medical Specialties board recertification QI requirements; new Residency Review Committees QI requirements for residents; "pay-for-performance" programs whereby payers use financial incentives based on health care outcomes to drive investment in improvement; and improvement collaboratives that bring together groups of health care organizations to combine QI methods and evidence-based practices to address serious gaps in performance for health conditions.[28]

As the public health and health care workforces become more savvy about QI methods and tools and as they begin to use HIT to collect data to drive improvements, a largely untapped opportunity is opening up for health care and public health organizations to work collaboratively on improvement projects that benefit the health of individual patients and the general public.

Future Opportunities

Using context to customize care and increase its effectiveness

As clinicians, we tend to view our assessments, recommendations, and approaches through the lens of the health care delivery system. Although health care is critical when acute needs arise, most factors that influence health are within the social, political, and economic context of each person's life. For clinicians to have a more comprehensive picture of health, we need to incorporate information about the communities in which our patients live and work. We need to build systems for health that incorporate those realities, bringing context into the health care encounter. Broadening our lens gives us a comprehensive, hence more accurate, view of health for individuals and populations within their communities.

Incorporating contextual information in health care delivery system encounters is critical to ensure that assessments, recommendations, and approaches are relevant and feasible. In fact, a study conducted by the U.S. Department of Veterans Affairs suggests that not doing so can be seen as a contextual error—a failure to individualize care—that leads to treatment and management errors that are akin to biomedical errors.[29] For example, when answering the question, "What is the best thing for this patient at this time?" tailoring the intervention to a patient's individual circumstances is critical. Intensifying a medication regimen for uncontrolled hypertension will not be effective if the individual is unable to afford any medications. Thus, in addition to clinical data, contextual data must be collected, integrated, and analyzed to guide resource allocation accordingly. In many cases, this will require greater collaboration with public health organizations.

Collocation of health care services in the community

Community sites where individuals spend their time—e.g., schools, businesses, grocery stores, pharmacies, churches—offer abundant, often untapped, opportunities to address needed clinical preventive services, provide health promotion information and support, and ensure linkages to complementary community resources such as housing, transportation, and social services. Collocation of health care services in communities enhances their ability to impact communities, especially where the prevalence of specific diseases or risk factors is high.

Catholic Healthcare West (CHW), which covers 22 million lives, uses community-level data to design community initiatives, many of which involve collocation of health care services in high-risk communities. In partnership with Thomson Reuters, CHW developed a Community Need Index (CNI) in 2002. This standardized community assessment is based on evidence that socioeconomic barriers, including lower income, lower levels of education, being uninsured, culture/language challenges, and/or substandard housing, puts residents at higher risk of poor health and increased utilization of health care services. The CNI provides a standardized score by zip codes.[30]

Noticing that the CNI score in one service area zip code was in the highest quintile, a hospital in Stockton, California, collaborated with other community organizations to conduct a more in-depth analysis of the data. The data showed that 48 percent of children in this zip code were living in single-parent homes in poverty. Further study found that 52 percent of the children in that zip code were part of the federal free lunch program at school. The hospital revised its mobile van route to include regular stops at the elementary schools in this area, providing free health screenings and immunizations.

In Sacramento, California, the CNI confirmed the need for a community health clinic in an underserved area. Within zip codes for this community, as many as 30 percent of residents lacked health insurance, and up to 43 percent of households were headed by single parents living in poverty. To meet that area's health needs, the CHW hospital partnered with a number of community groups to invest an estimated $300,000 for a community clinic at a local school. Between 2008 and 2010, CHW hospitals invested in preventive and disease management programs for almost 9,000 patients who had been deemed at risk for hospitalization for asthma, diabetes, or congestive heart failure, yielding an 86 percent reduction in admissions.[30]

California Hospital Medical Center, Los Angeles, developed a chronic disease self-management program in multiple sites located throughout its local community. One-year post-intervention, participant utilization of inpatient services decreased 82 percent and emergency department use plummeted from 20 days to one day. Similarly, programs run by community health workers housed throughout the community (e.g., churches, barber shops) demonstrate increased engagement and success with self-management programs for lowering blood sugar in diabetics and blood pressure in those with hypertension because of improved medication adherence and other self-management techniques.[31]

Worksite wellness programs are another example of the power of collocation opportunities. Johnson & Johnson shared financial results of a four-year worksite wellness program involving 18,331 employees that demonstrated an overall savings of $8.5 million annually in reduced health care costs. This translated to a savings of $225 per employee per year.[32]

In addition to reducing costs, companies benefit from implementing worksite wellness programs in terms of increased employee morale, improved employee health, reductions in workers' compensation claims, reductions in absenteeism, lower employee turnover rates, and increases in productivity.[33] A review of published studies on worksite wellness found that the return on investment is $3.48:1 due to reduced medical costs and $5.82:1 due to reduced absenteeism.[34,35]

Applying population strategies to patient populations

Integrating population-level strategies into health care settings (e.g., targeting specific health-related information to patient populations within a practice or a health care system) is another important strategy that should be applied more often in the future.[36] For example, a physician practice could query its EHR to assess, "How many of the individuals we care for with persistent asthma have had a planned asthma visit in the past three to four months?" Those who have not had a visit could be targeted for notification that they are overdue for asthma care. Adding contextual information about the homes and home environments for asthma patients would enable additional analyses of a practice's asthma population. The results may inform actions to address conditions in the community the practice serves, such as health education campaigns related to smoking indoors.

Community health assessments and community benefits

For not-for-profit hospitals, recent requirements related to assessing community health and accounting for how community benefit dollars are invested will offer significant opportunity to utilize health care delivery system influence, expertise, and resources for community health improvement efforts. Ideally, this will lead to the recognition that no one sector can provide all necessary services or health-promoting conditions to address all determinants of health. This, in turn, could facilitate the creation of models for shared accountability. Further, developing funds for shared accountability between health care (e.g., using community benefit dollars from not-for-profit hospitals), public health organizations, and their community stakeholders' could facilitate more effective, aligned action.

Breaking down educational silos

The longstanding educational divide dating back to the early 1900s should be bridged in the future. Joint educational opportunities for health care (e.g., physicians, nurses, pharmacists) and public health professionals can help build a more effective foundation of understanding of how sectors can work jointly to promote health across communities. Opportunities for joint leadership training programs as well as QI training are particularly good targets because these educational needs cut across all disciplines.

Health care organizations modeling the way for improved population health

There are numerous ways that health care organizations can serve as important role models for other community organizations in improving population health. Often, health care organizations are large employers within communities. As such, they can provide and promote the availability of healthy food and onsite exercise programs for their employees through wellness programs and ensure that their benefit packages incentivize healthy behaviors.

The following case study is an example of how health care organizations can help catalyze improvements in population health by serving as role models. Further, it demonstrates other important concepts previously outlined, such as applying evidence-based strategies to impact population health on multiple levels and the role of health care in improving the health of communities.

Case Study

The North Carolina Restaurant and Bar Smoking Ban: Collaborating to Change Behavior, Policy and Health Outcomes

Over the past 20 years, North Carolina has reduced the adult smoking rate by almost 25 percent. How has one of the nation's largest tobacco-producing states achieved this? The answer is through the relentless collaborative efforts of state-wide advocates, businesses, communities, politicians, legal experts, and public health and health care organizations. For two decades, these partners have implemented multi-level evidence-based interventions that have increased knowledge and changed social norms about the harms of tobacco use via mass media campaigns, provided access to cessation resources (e.g., Quitline NC), and promoted adoption of policies and laws to eliminate exposure to secondhand smoke.

The latest breakthrough in North Carolina's efforts to reduce tobacco use and exposure was the passage of a law to prohibit smoking in restaurants, bars, and lodging establishments. The passage of this law represented a major shift for North Carolina regarding tobacco policy; as recently as 1993, the state had a law that required all state and local government buildings to *allow* smoking.[37]

In 2006, a U.S. Surgeon General's report indicated that there was *"no risk-free level of exposure to secondhand smoke"* and recommended eliminating indoor smoking to protect non-smokers from secondhand smoke.[38] Advocates in North

Carolina used this information to increase knowledge of the harms of tobacco and to gain support to pass stricter tobacco regulations—including laws that prohibited smoking in state and local government buildings.

Prior to the passage of these laws, community and statewide advocates launched the tobacco-free schools movement, which was successful in helping all 115 state school districts to adopt a tobacco-free policy.[39] The success of this campaign swayed the social norms concerning tobacco use and helped influence other community partners (including hospitals) to enact tobacco-free policies.[40] In 2006, the Duke Endowment, NC Prevention Partners, and the North Carolina Hospital Association launched the Healthy Hospital Initiative to improve the health of hospital employees and visitors by promoting tobacco-free campuses. By July 2009, all acute care hospitals in the state had established a tobacco-free policy.[41] The hospitals' policy provided an opportunity to model non-smoking behaviors, educate staff and patients about tobacco use, and create access and referral to cessation resources. The success of hospitals further swayed social norms regarding tobacco use in North Carolina and increased interest among businesses and governmental organizations to consider pilot testing similar policies.[41] Evidence from these successful pilot sites coupled with that of the tobacco-free school and hospital campaigns provided the needed information for advocates to lobby and gain support for the Restaurant and Bar law, which was signed into law in May 2009.[42] Since implementation of this law, the average weekly rates of emergency room visits for heart attacks in North Carolina has declined by 21 percent, which represents an estimated $3.3 to $4.8 million in health care cost savings.[43]

Henry Ford once said, "If everyone is moving forward together, then success takes care of itself." This is certainly true for North Carolina's effort to prevent and control tobacco use. The collaborative efforts of hospitals, public health organizations, and other public health system partners played an important role in achieving policy change to reduce the exposure to secondhand smoke—a change that many thought impossible.

Conclusion

Ultimately, all health is local. It is determined at both the individual and population level and is largely influenced by context. While health care usually asks, "How do I treat this patient with this problem at this time?" there are two other important questions:

- "What population-level circumstances are underlying causes of this disease?"
- "What needs to be addressed to keep other people like this person from getting this disease?"

Health care and public health organizations must work together on answering these questions to optimally promote better health for all in the future. As outlined in this chapter, many recent changes in policy and practice are laying a solid foundation for greater collaboration, and there are abundant opportunities for such collaboration to improve health in the U.S.

References

1. Institute of Medicine of the National Academies. Crossing the quality chasm: The IOM health care quality initiative. http://www.iom.edu/Global/News%20Announce-ments/Crossing-the-Quality-Chasm-The-IOM-Health-Care-Quality-Initiative.aspx. Updated 2011. Accessed October 29, 2011.

2. Institute of Medicine of the National Academies. To err is human: Building a safer health system. http://www.nap.edu/openbook.php?record_id=9728&page=R1. Updated 2011. Accessed October 29, 2011.

3. Schroeder SA. Shattuck lecture: We can do better—improving the health of the American people. *New Engl J Med.* 357(12):1221-8, Sept. 20, 2007.

4. McGinnis JM, Williams-Russo P, Knickman JR. The case for more active policy attention to health promotion. *Health Aff.* 2002;21(2):78-93, Mar.-Apr. 2002.

5. McGinnis JM, Foege WH. Actual causes of death in the United States. *JAMA.* 270(18):2207-2212, Nov. 10, 1993.

6. Kindig DA, Asada Y, Booske B. A population health framework for setting national and state health goals. *JAMA,* 299(17):2081-3, May 7, 2008.

7. University of Wisconsin School of Medicine and Public Health. What is population health and public health? http://www.pophealth.wisc.edu/Prospective-Students/PopHealth-PublicHealth. Updated 2011. Accessed October 15, 2010.

8. McLeroy KR, Bibeau D, Steckler A, Glanz K. An ecological perspective on health promotion programs. *Health Education & Behavior,* 15(4):351-77, Winter 1988.

9. Institute of Medicine of the National Academies. The future of public health. http://www.nap.edu/openbook.php?record_id=1091&page=1. Updated 2011. Accessed October 29, 2011.

10. Centers for Disease Control and Prevention. National public health performance standards program: User guide. http://www.cdc.gov/nphpsp/PDF/UserGuide.pdf. Updated 2007. Accessed October 29, 2011.

11. Beitsch LM, Brooks RG, Glasser JH, Coble YD. The medicine and public health initiative: Ten years later. *Am J Prev Med.* 29(2):149-53, Aug. 2005.

12. Poses RM. Money and mission? addressing the barriers to evidence-based medicine. *J Gen Intern Med.* 14(4):262-4, Apr. 1999.

13. Fineberg HV, Green GM, Ware JH, Anderson BL. Changing public health training needs: Professional education and the paradigm of public health. *Annu Rev Publ Health.* 15: 237-57, 1994.

14. Trust for America's Health: Preventing Epidemics. Protecting People. Shortchanging America's health. Healthy Americans Web site. http://healthyamericans.org/report/61/shortchanging09. Updated 2009. Accessed October 29, 2011.

15. Oberlander J. Health care policy in an age of austerity. http://www.nejm.org/doi/full/10.1056/NEJMp1109352. Updated 2011. Accessed September 12, 2011.

16. Institute for Healthcare Improvement. The IHI triple aim: Better care for individuals, better health for populations, and lower per capita costs. Institute for Healthcare Improvement Web site. http://www.ihi.org/offerings/Initiatives/TripleAim/Pages/Approach.aspx. Updated 2011. Accessed September 12, 2011.

17. Centers for Disease Control and Prevention. Sebelius announces $42.5 million for public health improvement programs through the Affordable Care Act. http://www.cdc.gov/media/pressrel/2010/r100920.htm. Updated 2010. Accessed October 15, 2011.

18. Harrison LM. Personal communication, 2011.

19. National Priorities Partnership. About the national priorities partnership. http://www.nationalprioritiespartnership.org/AboutNPP.aspx. Accessed October 29, 2011.

20. Congress of United States Congressional Budget Office. Nonprofit hospitals and the provision of community benefits. http://www.cbo.gov/ftpdocs/76xx/doc7695/12-06-Nonprofit.pdf. Updated 2006. Accessed October 29, 2011.

21. Internal Revenue Service (IRS). Notice and request for comments regarding the community health needs assessment requirements for tax-exempt hospitals. http://www.irs.gov/pub/irs-drop/n-11-52.pdf. Updated 2011. Accessed October 29, 2011.

22. County Health Rankings. Ranking methods. http://www.countyhealthrankings.org/ranking-methods. Updated 2011. Accessed October 15, 2011.

23. Randolph GD, Lea CS. Quality improvement in public health: Moving from knowing the path to walking the path. *Journal of Public Health Management and Practice.* 18(1):4-8, Jan.-Feb. 2012.

24. Department of Health and Human Services. HHS Secretary Sebelius announces plans to establish health IT "Beacon communities". HHS Web site. http://www.hhs.gov/news/press/2009pres/12/20091202a.html. Updated 2011. Accessed October 5, 2011.

25. United States Department of Health and Human Services. The official web site for the medicare and medicaid electronic health records (EHR) incentive programs. http://www.cms.gov/ehrincentiveprograms/. Updated 2011. Accessed October 5, 2011.

26. Public Health Accreditation Board. About PHAB. http://www.phaboard.org/about-phab/. Updated 2011. Accessed October 15, 2011.

27. Consensus statement on quality in the public health system. Waashington, DC: U.S. Department of Health and Human Services. Aug. 2008. http://www.hhs.gov/ash/initiatives/quality/quality/phqf-consensus-statement.html.

28. McLaughlin CP, Kaluzny AD, eds. *Continuous Quality Improvement in Health Care.* Vol 408. 4th ed. Burlington, MA: Jones and Bartlett Publishers, Inc; 2013, pp. 578-86.

29. Weiner SJ, Schwartz A, Weaver F, *et al.* Contextual errors and failures in individualizing patient care: A multicenter study. *Ann Intern Med.* 153(2):69-75, July 20, 20010.

30. Catholic Healthcare West. Nationwide maps guide community health planning. Catholic Healthcare West Web site. http://www.chwhealth.org/CHW_Information/Press_Center/213422. Published February 16, 2011. Updated 2011. Accessed October 3, 2011.

31. Lorig K, Stewart A, Ritter P, *et al. Outcome Measures for Health Education and Other Health Care Interventions.* Vol 1. Newbury Park, CA: Sage Publications, Inc.; 1996.

32. The Health & Economic Implications of Worksite Wellness Programs. Farmington Hills, MI: American Institute for Preventive Medicine Wellness, 2010, White Paper.

33. Center for Prevention and Health Services: Best Practices:. Wellness program evaluation: Getting the best return on your investment. National Business Group on Health Web site. http://www.businessgrouphealth.org/pdfs/Wellness%20Program%20Evaluation%20Getting%20the%20Best%20Return%20on%20Your%20Investment%20Final%20PDF%203.25.09.pdf. Updated 2009. Accessed October 29, 2011.

34. Aldana S. Financial impact of health promotion programs: A comprehensive review of the literature. *Am J Health Promot.* 15(5):296-320, May-June 2001.

35. Chapman LS. Meta-evaluation of worksite health promotion economic return studies: 2005 update. *Am J Health Promot.* 19(6):1-11, July-Aug. 2005.

36. Nash DB, Reifsnyder J, Fabius R, Pracilio VP. *Population Health: Creating a Culture of Wellness.* Burlington, MA: Jones & Bartlett Learning, LLC, 2010.

37. Wall A. Smoking in public places: Recent changes in state law. http://sogpubs.unc.edu/electronicversions/pdfs/hlb90.pdf. Updated May 2009. Accessed September 15, 2011.

38. *The Health Consequences of Involuntary Exposure to Tobacco Smoke: A Report of the Surgeon General.* Washington, DC: U.S. Department of Health and Human Services, 2006.

39. NC Department of Health and Human Services: NC Division of Public Health. NC tobacco free schools. http://www.nctobaccofreeschools.org/. Updated 2011. Accessed September 15, 2011.

40. Shah V, Malek SH, Brown T, Moeykens B. Reducing tobacco use in tobacco country: North Carolina's success story in lowering tobacco use among youth. *NC Med J.* 71(1):81-2, Jan.-Feb. 2010.

41. Okun MF, Thornhill A, and Molloy M. Hospital. Heal thyself: North Carolina hospitals make prevention a priority to support health of their workforce, patients, and communities. *NC Med J.* 71(1):96-100, Jan.-Feb. 2010.

42. Seamans P. The long road to success: Advocating for public policy change. *NC Med J.* 71(1):79-83, Jan.-Feb 2010.

43. NC Division of Public Health: NC Tobacco Prevention and Control Branch Epidemiology and Evaluation Unit. The North Carolina smoke free restaurants and bars law and emergency department admissions for acute myocardial infarction. http://tobaccopreventionandcontrol.ncdhhs.gov/smokefreenc/docs/TPCB-2011SFNCReport-SHD.pdf. Published November 4, 2011. Updated 2011. Accessed November 9, 2011.

Chapter 22

Changing the Culture of Health Care Education

By Peter J. Katsufrakis, MD, MBA

Executive Summary

This chapter reviews aspects of health professions educational culture that pose threats to quality and patient safety, describes a model for transformational change, and provides examples of small- and large-scale interventions to improve the culture of health care education. Manifestations of culture in this context include faculty and student attitudes and behaviors; systems—or their absence—to prepare and support faculty; standards and regulations governing health care and educational institutions; and structural aspects of these institutions. John Kotter's eight-step model for organizational transformation as described in *Leading Change* is presented as an approach to guide thinking about cultural change.

A proposed taxonomy to categorize problems with health care education is based on four different levels at which interventions to improve quality could be targeted as described in *Crossing the Quality Chasm*. Subsequently, specific problems are summarized along with potential strategies for improvement.

The chapter concludes with examples of culture change at health care and educational institutions that illustrate different types of interventions. The examples highlight key success factors, diverse types of outcomes, and varied ways by which the impact of culture change interventions can be measured.

Learning Objectives

1. Identify factors that influence the culture of health professions educational institutions.

2. List Kotter's eight steps for transforming organizations.

3. Describe attributes of current health professions education that adversely affect patient safety.

4. Describe changes to health professions education that would enhance quality and patient safety.

Key Words: Change, Culture, Health Professional Education, Interprofessional, Medical Education, Nursing Education, Organization Culture, Pharmacy Education

Introduction

> *To improve is to change. To be perfect is to change often.*
> —Sir Winston Churchill

In order to institutionalize patient safety practices in an enduring manner, we will need to change the way we teach physicians, nurses, pharmacists, and other health professionals—in effect, by transforming the lessons learned during formative educational experiences. As sites for much of health professions education, our inpatient and ambulatory centers of care provide opportunities to model the best precepts of patient safety—or to thwart the best efforts of determined faculty. Changing care systems in our teaching centers will be a prerequisite to changing learners' experiences and training. We must also look at the culture of health care education—specifically at what is taught and how it is taught—to ensure that curricula are aligned with evolving notions of patient safety.

The authors of *Crossing the Quality Chasm*[1] note that change in our health care system is needed at four levels in order to support enhanced patient safety: at the level of patients' experiences; within the microsystems that actually provide care; in the organizations made up of these microsystems; and in the environment of laws, rules, payment, accreditation, and professional training that reward, constrain, and influence organizations. Inherent in the shift from the status quo to an envisioned future that teaches, embraces, and ensures optimal quality and safety for all patients is the need to undertake significant change, with transformation needed at each of these four levels of our health care system.

What should be our vision for a changed system of health professions education? A national committee[2] convened in response to the *Quality Chasm* report identified five competencies that, regardless of discipline, all health professionals should possess. These are the ability to: 1) provide patient-centered care, 2) work effectively in interdisciplinary teams, 3) employ evidence-based practice, 4) apply quality improvement practices, and 5) utilize informatics. This chapter expands on these themes, moving from aspirational principles to training changes. The chapter begins with a working definition of culture and a description of Kotter's eight stages in transformational organization change. Next considered are elements of current health professions education that constitute areas of concern, organized around a taxonomy that mirrors the four levels of intervention to enhance patient safety described above. The chapter concludes with examples of interventions to improve educational culture at the individual and organizational levels.

Proposed changes will focus on interventions that are particular to educational practices, while recognizing that clinical education is inextricably linked to sites and systems of clinical care. Changes needed for clinical care sites and systems that relate primarily to patient care are addressed elsewhere in this text and thus will not be reiterated here, except to note that such changes are a crucial part of changing the culture of health professions education. This chapter will focus on changes that are specific to health care education.

Definition of "culture"

For the purposes of this discussion, "health care education" will emphasize the educational programs that train physicians, nurses, and pharmacists, though the issues raised will often apply more generally to education of physician assistants, occupational therapists, medical social workers, and the numerous other professionals providing health care services. In this context, "culture" refers to traditional definitions that encompass prevalent shared attitudes, values, beliefs, goals, and practices that characterize health professional education in the United States. Manifestations of culture include explicit statements of values; behavioral norms; rituals and celebrations; expressions of explicit and/or implicit values modeled by senior colleagues and tutors; shared metaphors, meanings, skills, and symbols; and both formal and informal systems of rewards and punishments.[3]

Medical education has been described as having a "culture of no culture,"[4] a process by which students are taught to extract medically relevant information from patients' stories and organize it into a format and substance consistent with their instructors' predominant expectations. This characterization of medicine as cultureless denies the reality of a very strong, pervasive culture, and such denial may pose a barrier to frank assessment and intervention. The first step to change culture must be to recognize that the culture exists.

General principles of culture change

Organizational change is inevitably difficult and often resisted until crisis demands action. In the spectrum of potential kinds of organizational change, one of the most daunting is changing organizational culture.[5]

Individuals have devoted their lives to studying organizational change and identifying strategies that succeed–and fail. In his book *Leading Change,* John P. Kotter outlines eight steps for implementing organizational transformation. Below, each step is described briefly along with a description of common problems that can arise and undermine change efforts:

1. Establish a sense of urgency.

To overcome pervasive resistance, the case in support of change must be framed as both vital and urgent. If the reasons put forward justifying change are deemed insufficiently important, associated change activities may not receive the resources, attention, and priority necessary for success. Similarly, if a need for change is recognized as important but not felt to be urgent, other less controversial activities may take precedence and the change effort dwindles. To drive change in an organization, Kotter stipulates that 75 percent of leadership must believe that the status quo is no longer tenable.

2. Form a powerful guiding coalition.

While change efforts may begin with one or two people, to be sustained and effective the effort will need to attract a significant number of individuals with power and position who share a commitment to change. This coalition will often draw on senior leadership, though it is not uncommon for some senior leaders not to be part of the coalition. Structure and activities outside the established hierarchy may help strengthen the coalition; e.g., an ad hoc team that engages in a several-day retreat to refine vision and strategy.

3. Create a vision.

In order to motivate people who need to change and sustain those intending to change, leaders must communicate a clear, concise, compelling vision of a future state that corrects the problems identified as the basis for change. A vision that is unfocused, confusing, or not easily understood will not survive careful scrutiny and will not sustain significant change.

4. Communicate the vision.

Leaders who develop an exceptional vision for the future and then keep it secret should have saved the effort of developing a vision, for the net effect will be the same. Circulating a white paper that describes the vision, posting the vision statement on an organization's intranet, and including the vision as a theme in the CEO's annual address are by themselves almost worthless. While each is a potentially worthwhile element of a communications strategy, communication should be so frequent, consistent, and pervasive that those who will be responsible for implementing the change can finish the leader's sentences when discussing the vision. Perhaps even more important are the actions that accompany statements of the vision. Leaders must ensure that their actions reinforce, and not contradict, desired changes.

5. Empower others to act on the vision.

This precept embodies two elements: 1) affording others opportunities to try out new ideas with support in the form of time and resources, and 2) providing protection from people, systems, and traditions that impede progress. Individuals and groups undertaking change will inevitably encounter resistance, and they must either have authority and power, or be able to harness these in order to carry through the desired transformation.

6. Plan for and create short-term wins.

Significant organizational change, in particular change in culture, generally requires years to implement, stabilize, and sustain. Few people will have the wherewithal to sustain the effort needed without interim rewards and markers of success. One of the early steps in planning for change should be to identify outcomes that will be visible, reasonably significant, and fairly certain to be achievable, often termed the low-hanging fruit. Such outcomes will demonstrate that change is possible and can reinforce the wisdom of continuing along the path of change.

7. Consolidate improvements and produce still more change.

Once the change process has begun to produce results, advocates for change and the "persuadable middle" will be heartened by their effect. They may also be fatigued by the additional effort change demands. In this setting, a tendency to celebrate success by relaxing efforts in support of change may be embraced by those who still resist change, thereby creating conditions for arrest of progress and backsliding. Easy wins must be characterized and recognized as early markers along the road, and not confused with achieving the final goal.

8. Institutionalize new approaches.

The final phases of a change process involve ensuring that what was previously viewed as "change" has become the status quo. The extent of the change must pervade the organization's culture. Whereas the initial efforts may have been tied to a charismatic leader or dynamic group of change champions, sustained change must be woven into the fabric of an organization and endure despite the departure of its champions.

Overview of current health professions education

Nursing education

Nursing education programs can be hospital- or university-based, and can lead to a nursing diploma (hospital-based) or an associate, baccalaureate, masters, or doctoral degree. Advanced degrees prepare nurses for an academic career and/or for a career providing independent clinical care. Scope of practice is determined by education, training, and statute within the licensing jurisdiction. Taught by experienced nurses and other professionals, courses focus on preparing students for patient care and other professional duties. Training has evolved from an apprenticeship model, designed to support a physician's practice, to a model that prepares nursing students to draw on nursing science and practice to make independent contributions to patient care.

A significant difference between nurse education culture and medicine education culture is the tendency in the latter for established clinicians to assume responsibility for educating students and physicians-in-training. While many practicing physicians volunteer time to teach medical students and residents, nursing students are more likely to be perceived as the responsibility of their university faculty.[6]

Medical education

Typically, medical students complete a baccalaureate degree that encompasses prerequisite science education before beginning four years of medical school; this model is prevalent in North America, while other models exist elsewhere. Physicians attend an allopathic or an osteopathic medical school and earn a medical doctor (MD) or doctor of osteopathy (DO) degree, respectively. Medical schools are almost always associated with a university, in accordance with the recommendations of Abraham Flexner promulgated in the early 20th century, and include both classroom and clinical instruction. Following medical school, three or more years of residency (and/or fellowship) training are required for specialty (and subspecialty) board certification, although a single year of residency training is sufficient to obtain a license to practice medicine in some states.

Pharmacy education

The doctor of pharmacy (PharmD) degree is required to work as a pharmacist. Many pharmacy schools require completion of some undergraduate courses prior to application, but an undergraduate degree is not typically a prerequisite. PharmD programs that combine traditional coursework with clinical training usually take four years to complete. Like nurses and physicians, pharmacists must take one or more licensing examinations to become licensed to practice.

A recent report on the status of pharmacy education describes efforts under way to enhance pharmacy education in a variety of ways, including defining competency outcomes necessary at various stages of education and methods of promoting interprofessional education.[7] The report notes that, in addition to a need for ensuring that graduates keep pace with societal needs and are able to provide patient-centered care on high-functioning interprofessional teams, it is necessary to ensure that faculty members are prepared to implement needed curricular changes to support these goals.

Efforts to promote interprofessional education notwithstanding, these and most other health professions teach their professional groups in isolation from the others. While medical students and nursing students may work in the same area of a hospital and care for the same patients, the formal and informal instruction is typically provided separately to the different types of health professions students.

Problems with current health professions education culture

The four levels at which interventions could be targeted as described in *Chasm Report*[8] may also be used to categorize some of the problems that arise in health professions education.

- Level A, problems of individual learners or teachers *(the experience of patients and communities)*.

- Level B, problems of ward teams *(small units of care delivery or "microsystems")*.

- Level C, problems of schools, hospitals, and clinics *(health care organizations)*.
- Level D, problems of the health care environment.

Such taxonomy is useful when considering where problems exist, how interactions at different levels may support or thwart change efforts, and how best to institute cultural change to support enhanced patient safety. Changing educational culture to ensure patient safety will almost certainly require change at each of these levels. Examples of problems that have been identified are summarized in Table 1 along with the corresponding taxonomy levels.

Table 1. Taxonomy of Problems in Health Professions Education

Level	Problem
A	Student entitlement
A	Faculty attitudinal or skill deficits (authoritarian, antiquated pedagogy)
A	Faculty unprepared to teach systems management
B	Students unaware of systems and resources to report safety problems
B	Dependence on other learners as de facto faculty for much of clinical training
B, C	Tolerance for less-than-professional and/or disruptive behavior
C	Faculty burnout
C	Weak institutional commitment to ensuring patient safety
C, D	Disjointed education and care systems that do not model ideals
D	Turbulent, changing health care environment

Level A: Problems at the level of individual learners or teachers

Student entitlement has been defined variously as expecting high grades for a modest effort, refusing to accept personal responsibility, assuming a "consumer" mentality, and making excessive excuses for one's failures.[9,10] Attempts to understand student entitlement suggest that this behavior may be a coping strategy for students who experience a decline in grades when confronted with more rigorous university courses and with more capable fellow students. Understanding the basis for such behavior can contribute to effective corrective interventions. Strategies to address incivility include improving communication, providing forums for education and discussion, establishing and modeling norms and policies for expected behavior, and addressing incivility promptly and equitably.

Heightened stress levels among faculty and students accompanied by negative attitudes of faculty superiority and student entitlement increase the potential for incivility in nursing education.[10] Faculty superiority, arrogance, and abuse of authority over students are potentially destructive behaviors. When faculty members exert their position and power over students, assume a "know it all" attitude, and arbitrarily threaten to fail or dismiss students, the possibility for uncivil behavior increases.[11] Knowledge or skills deficits can compound attitudinal problems. For example, some have suggested that pharmacy faculty may lack sufficient preparation to teach systems management.[12]

Even well-intentioned attitudes and beliefs on the part of faculty can be barriers to effective nursing education.[13] Traditional expectations about the faculty's role in relation to learners, their unique access to specialized knowledge, and the need for lock-step progression through a curriculum may actually impede learning and adaptation. These and other outmoded approaches to education run counter to our evolving understanding of effective educational practices and optimal learning.

Level B: Problems at the level of ward teams

The presence of sound, safe systems in educational settings is necessary but not sufficient to ensure good outcomes. One study involving pharmacy, medicine, nursing, and physical therapy students found that, even in settings where systems were in place to promote patient safety, students were often unengaged and unaware of reporting mechanisms. In addition to the students' lack of engagement and awareness, researchers found that staff often was too busy to report—or unclear about what and how to report—potential breaches.[14]

Beyond the problems associated with individual learners and faculty members, there are other systematic differences between an ideal educational system and the status quo. Much clinical education depends on the knowledge, teaching skills, and clinical abilities of individuals with relatively little additional training, i.e., residents with only one year more training and experience than those they are expected to teach and supervise. Inevitably there will be occasions when such teachers are limited in their mastery of content and educational techniques, thus compromising the educational outcomes.

"See one, do one, teach one." This oft-repeated maxim of medical education merits scrutiny. Changes in medical education—i.e., increasing attention to the concepts of competency as a basis for teaching as well as for specific, focused assessment; use of technology such as simulations for procedures and patient management; and other advances in both pedagogy and professionalism—have made the "see one" approach increasingly unnecessary, outdated, and often a violation of safe practice. To the extent that this approach endures, it highlights significant problems that prevail in medical education, including inadequate supervision by well-qualified instructors, lack of transparency with patients regarding a learner's actual training and experience, and perpetuation of time-honored though dangerous traditions in clinical training. One area where tradition has been challenged

relates to patient hand-offs and their potential to compromise patient safety. Yet despite the recognized peril, research into how hand-offs may best be improved is inadequate.[15]

Another problematic tradition is dependence on clinical educators who receive little or no formal instruction in sound educational practice. Many clinical educators merely employ the same teaching techniques they were exposed to as students. Techniques that include public belittlement, patient deception or misrepresentation, tolerance for suboptimal patient outcomes in the name of physician education, or other departures from ethical ideals create conditions that are ripe for compromising patient safety as well as demeaning participants in the educational process.[16]

Level C: Problems at the level of schools, hospitals, and clinics

While unprofessional behavior manifests at the level of individual or small group interactions, its impact can be widely felt. Disruptive behavior by health professionals is so pervasive and problematic that, in 2008, The Joint Commission issued a sentinel event alert regarding the consequences of disruptive behaviors on the part of health care providers and their effects on patient care.[17] This publication summarizes research describing the kinds of behaviors that can lead to staff burnout, medical errors, patient dissatisfaction, and adverse outcomes; the involvement (as perpetrators and as victims) of physicians, nurses, pharmacists, therapists, support staff, and administrators; and the root causes and contributing factors that initiate and perpetuate unsafe practices. The Joint Commission's power as an accrediting agency provides the leverage to enforce its demand for the preventive and corrective actions outlined in its report and to influence culture to proscribe such behavior.

Even when the faculty is actively involved in teaching, systemic problems may hamper its effectiveness. Demands on clinical faculty to publish research, provide patient care, and participate in organizational management or governance can compromise the time and effort devoted to teaching. Almost half of medical faculty may experience burnout,[18] a problem with the potential to manifest multiple undesirable consequences—e.g., diminished teaching effectiveness, shortcuts in clinical care, and unprofessional attitudes that can adversely affect patient outcomes.

As has been pointed out by others,[19] few national organizations express the level of commitment to patient safety that might be expected by the public. Rather than being willing to "ensure," "require," or "demand" safe and effective care, the mission statements of national organizations are more likely to *"advance[e] our profession to improve health"* (American Nurses Association), *"promote … the betterment of public health"* (American Medical Association), or *"advance patient care"* (American Pharmacists Association). Enhancing the commitment of national leaders of the professions—and the language that communicates that commitment—may be an important element of a strategy to change educational culture.

Compounding these problems is the lack of curricula focused on patient safety. A survey of U.S. and Canadian medical schools published almost 10 years after the *Chasm* report found that only 25 percent of responding schools had explicit patient safety curricula.[20] Furthermore, quality improvement curricula—where they exist—may exhibit significant deficiencies.[21]

Other researchers have cited a dearth of leaders trained to advance the science and practice of quality and safety.[22] This may be a particularly pernicious problem, because leadership engagement in change to support patient safety has been routinely cited as critical for success.[23,24,25]

Level D: Problems at the level of the health care environment

Much of current health professions education takes place in care systems that are inherently and seriously flawed from the standpoint of best safety practices. Such settings can reinforce, explicitly or implicitly, practices that are antithetical to good care and cause learners to replicate inadequate approaches to patient safety after they have completed their training and assumed independent practice. Ideally, care systems will change to model best practices for learners. At minimum, learners should not be exposed to—and training should not take place in—systems that perpetuate unsafe or poor quality practices.

One challenge to the development of professionals who think systemically in their approach to ensuring patient safety is the fragmented, disjointed experience of many educational programs. Although disciplines of basic science form the foundation of medicine, nursing, and pharmacy practice, instruction is generally separated from the clinical application of this scientific knowledge. Also, despite great overlap in core principles of anatomy, physiology, pharmacology, and molecular biology, instruction is rarely integrated across health professions boundaries. Frequently, the different professional students separately receive similar instruction while seated in different rooms of the same building.

When patient safety principles are taught, they are often taught in a way that does not facilitate improvement in care outcomes; i.e., classroom instruction may not produce effective behaviors in the clinical setting.[26] Care is routinely rendered in groups organized around a single profession; effective cross-discipline integration of students in one team is a rare exception. Even within a single discipline (e.g., medicine), an individual patient with cardiac disease admitted for hip replacement who develops a fever will routinely see at least three or four different groups of specialists who demonstrate little evidence of communicating effectively with one other. When different types of health professionals fail to communicate and coordinate care effectively, the potential for adverse outcomes increases; conversely, learning in settings that promote interprofessional interaction enhances individual learners' appreciation of the roles played by each of the different health professionals.

Despite problems noted above, the practice environment *is* changing. Significant changes include increased awareness of preventable medical errors; changing demographics and patterns of disease; new technologies; changes in health care delivery; increasing consumerism, patient empowerment, and autonomy; an emphasis on effectiveness and efficiency; and changing professional roles. Many of these changes, if pursued to their optimal outcomes, hold the promise of improving both patient safety and clinical care—e.g., technological advances in imaging, diagnostic tools, and clinical decision aids. However, even favorable change has the potential to be destabilizing if the pace and nature of change compromise safety. While change is necessary, the change process must be managed to ensure patient safety and optimize outcomes.

Nature and types of changes desired

Hippocrates advanced the principle of "*primum non nocere*," or "*first do no harm*" almost 2500 years ago. Yet, as demonstrated in *To Err is Human*,[27] it seems we fail this simple test routinely. This Hippocratic value may have persisted for millennia, but it is not uniformly manifest in current practice.

Changing culture is perhaps the most difficult type of change an organization can undertake. Changing the culture that guides an entire profession's educational processes and programs, or that would reshape multiple professions, requires modifications that may be staggering in scope and magnitude. However, it seems certain that fundamental change will be needed in order to reshape health professions education so that it ensures safe patient outcomes. As Churchill points out in the quote at this chapter's beginning, change is the process by which we strive for perfection.

What should be our goal in changing the culture of health care education? Creating a culture of safety would go a long way toward addressing current problems. Such a culture embodies a commitment to safety that permeates all levels of an organization's hierarchy and manifests as:

- Acknowledgment of the high-risk, error-prone nature of an organization's activities.

- A blame-free environment wherein individuals are able to report errors or close calls without fear of reprimand or punishment.

- An expectation of collaboration across ranks to seek solutions to vulnerabilities.

- A willingness on the part of the organization to direct resources for addressing safety concerns.[28]

The authors of *A Bridge to Quality* developed 10 recommendations to guide change.[2] Proposed actions included developing a common "quality language" across the health professions to achieve consensus on a core set of competencies that includes patient-centered care, interdisciplinary teams, evidence-based practice, quality improvement, and informatics; having accreditation bodies revise their standards so that programs are required to demonstrate through process and outcome measures that they educate students in how to deliver patient care using this core set of competencies; developing and funding regional demonstration learning centers, representing partnerships between practice and education that leverage existing innovative organizations to become state-of-the art training settings focused on teaching and assessing core competencies; and funding experiments that drive health professionals to integrate interdisciplinary approaches into educational or practice settings, with the goal of providing a training ground for students and clinicians that incorporates core quality competencies. Substantial progress on various aspects of these recommendations is described below.

The Accreditation Council for Graduate Medical Education (ACGME) and American Board of Medical Specialties (ABMS) framework of six competencies[29] (medical knowledge, patient care, professionalism, interpersonal and communication skills, systems-based practice, and practice-based learning) incorporate principles of patient safety and quality improvement. Similarly, academic nurses formed a multi-institution coalition funded by the Robert Wood Johnson Foundation to formulate Quality and Safety Education for Nurses (QSEN), a detailed description of the knowledge, skills, and attitudes needed for a different set of six competencies: patient-centered care, teamwork and collaboration, evidence-based practice, quality improvement, safety, and informatics.[30]

In 2011 an expert panel comprised of representatives from the American Association of Colleges of Nursing, American Association of Colleges of Osteopathic Medicine, American Association of Colleges of Pharmacy, American Dental Education Association, Association of American Medical Colleges, and the Association of Schools of Public Health produced a report on "Core Competencies for Interprofessional Collaborative Practice."[31] This work defines four domains for collaborative practice: 1) values/ethics for interprofessional practice, 2) roles/responsibilities, 3) interprofessional communication, and 4) teams and teamwork. Within each domain, the authors provide specific behavioral competencies to be developed as well as a framework for developmental growth and assessment. While not specifically addressing cultural change, this work provides substance and direction to support such change.

Some accrediting organizations for health professions schools have incorporated changes to their standards to support these principles. Both pharmacy and nursing school accreditation standards reflect explicit expectations that curricula will address quality and patient safety.[32,33]

Change principles have also been proposed for individual professions. One model advanced for changing nursing culture, fundamentally similar to Kotter's model, involves six steps: 1) conduct an inventory of institutional resources and needs; 2) create the infrastructure (information and people) necessary to advance change; 3) engage the leadership hierarchy in implementing changed processes; 4) educate involved individuals to enable adoption of changes; 5) integrate changes into routine practice; and 6) reflect expected changes in formal policy.[34] Additionally, some have called for other specific types of change to support enhanced patient safety and quality. In nursing, reports of unprofessional or disruptive behavior on the part of students or faculty have engendered calls for academic nurse leaders to address this problem.[35]

Some specific tools have been proposed to enhance patient safety and initiate the cultural shift necessary to revolutionize health professions education. Assessment tools designed to measure students' mastery of safety principles serve the dual purpose of communicating important concepts to learners and providing a measure of the learner's progress. In one example, using a checklist tool[36] facilitated the assessment of a patient's immediate environment for threats to safety and simultaneously structured the interview with a patient to elicit threats to and/or breaches of safety.

Student progress can be guided by tools that measure achievement of developmental milestones, e.g., tools being developed for physician resident training by the ACGME in its Outcome Project that focus on developing specialty-specific milestones. Similar methodology applied in nursing education[37] can be readily adapted to support safety education.

Appreciative inquiry has been described as "the art and practice of asking questions that strengthen a system's capacity to apprehend, anticipate, and heighten positive potential."[38] In practical terms, this means shifting thought patterns from a focus on identifying and solving problems to identifying and building on successes. In addition to being proposed as a strategy for leaders in nursing education as they undertake transformational change generally,[39] appreciative inquiry has demonstrated utility both in facilitating transformation of departmental structures and in enhancing the quality of and satisfaction with nursing leadership. As described in the examples section below,[33] appreciative inquiry has also been employed effectively in changing medical school culture at Indiana University.

Institution-focused strategies can effect change in nursing education. While not specifically designed to change an institution's culture, grant funding to develop a new program may have that effect by fostering new ways of collaboration, focusing attention on problems or opportunities ignored previously, and modeling new ways to achieve success that subsequently spread through an organization and produce transformational change.[40]

As mentioned previously, faculty plays a key role in shaping institutional culture as well as in specific lessons taught and learned. Role modeling provides an opportunity to reinforce structured curricular elements and to demonstrate practices that enhance patient safety. Specific strategies include recruiting and retaining individuals who embody professional ideals, robust evaluation and meaningful feedback to reinforce role modeling, rewards and recognition for excellence, and explicit training of faculty members to be role models.[41] While some individuals demonstrate natural skill as role models, this and other educational techniques are strengthened by focused faculty development.[42] Institution-wide involvement of stakeholders may be necessary to achieve maximal impact when attempting to enhance patient safety and improve key clinical outcomes. Factors shown to be important include clinical department chair involvement in safety initiatives.[43]

Before initiating efforts to enhance patient safety, an institution may find it useful to assess the safety orientation of the current culture to help prioritize efforts and to provide a baseline against which the effect of subsequent change can be measured. Nieva *et al.* provide an overview of potential tools as well as a four-step process to guide assessment: 1) involve key stakeholders, 2) select a safety culture assessment tool, 3) collect data, and 4) implement planning and change.[44] As in Kotter's model for organizational transformation, involving key stakeholders is vital. Culture pervades the fabric of an organization. Because it shapes—and is shaped by—the values, attitudes, and behaviors of an organization's members, changing culture requires changes to all of these. Often, the path to successful change efforts begins with identifying the values and attitudes that reflect the desired change and then focuses on promoting the behaviors that embody the desired values and attitudes.[45]

Examples of institutional change

A number of organizations involved in health professions education have begun or completed significant culture change.

The University of North Carolina's (UNC's) participation in the Agency for Healthcare Research and Quality's (AHRQ's) TeamSTEPPS (Strategies and Tools to Enhance Performance and Patient Safety) patient safety initiative is one example of the kinds of changes schools are making in support of enhanced patient safety.[46] Describing culture change in UNC graduate medical education, Kirch and Boysen identify five factors as critical for the success of this endeavor: 1) explicit leadership from the top, 2) early engagement of health professions students, 3) residents teaching others about patient safety, 4) use of health information technology, and 5) promoting teamwork among health professions. Educational leaders play a vital role in shaping an institution's culture.

Like AHRQ, the Institute for Healthcare Improvement (IHI) is committed to improving health care systems by advancing knowledge of how to improve safety and by fostering knowledge dissemination and change efforts. In 2003, IHI convened representatives from 10 medical schools to pilot changes to medical education that would better support enhanced quality and patient safety. Interviews with the deans of these schools[47] identified several success strategies: developing new organizational structures such as a Center for Health Care Quality; recruiting and/ or reassigning faculty with significant interest and expertise in quality and safety; identifying faculty leaders to serve as role models who exemplify principles of safe, high-quality practice; and revising educational practices to span traditional "walls" and promote interprofessional education.

Expanding on the work of IHI, the medical, nursing, and pharmacy schools of the University of Nebraska described success in developing interprofessional curricular materials in support of teamwork, quality, and safety.[48] Four initiatives resulted from this work: 1) an "interprofessional education day" consisting of both didactic and experiential training for students in multiple professions; 2) a service learning project connecting cross-disciplinary teams with community organizations; 3) an interprofessional simulation designed to highlight the critical role of effective team function; and 4) clinical teaching for senior nursing students modeled after national quality and safety standards.

Recognizing that compromised patient safety often results from fragmented systems and attempts at improvement, leadership of the Massachusetts General Hospital rejected quality and safety efforts designed to achieve measurable progress in a few key areas at the expense of producing widespread change. Instead, they drew upon extensive review of internal and external patient safety data to communicate concerns throughout the institution, from the level of hospital trustees down through department leaders to line administrative and clinical staff. Successful interventions included creating an institutional framework to support patient safety that integrated previously separated activities, processes, and structures; incorporating patient safety and improvement into the routine of daily activities; sharing pertinent information widely and transparently with staff and leadership; and maintaining an institution-wide focus.[25]

Planned curricular change at the Indiana University School of Medicine led to a Relationship Centered Care Initiative designed to better align the informal and formal curricula.[49] Principles guiding these efforts included "emergent design" to allow immediate next steps to be shaped by the preceding results; appreciative inquiry to share successes; and attending to interactions and behavior on a small scale as the means by which to influence large-scale change. The multi-year intervention contributed to increased institutional buy-in and satisfaction with the initiative, pervasive institutional change in the value of relationships, and significant changes in student satisfaction measures.

Crisis is often the catalyst that initiates significant cultural change. Following a failed merger attempt, the Penn State Hershey academic health center undertook structural changes to address barriers to organizational progress arising from insularity and goal conflicts associated with traditional departments and academic units.[50] The leadership created teams organized around missions and resources, and tasked teams to work with existing management structures in a manner that transcended traditional departmental and academic unit barriers. Using teams to address the organization's challenges, leadership identified the following important success factors: 1) involvement of experts in team function to plan implementation and address emergent dysfunction; 2) selection of team members whose roles and personal characteristics would contribute to the team's success; 3) broad representation of staff and faculty, with team membership turnover to increase opportunities for involvement; 4) support by academic department chairs; and 5) effective communication and collaboration between teams and the organization's managers.

Change in academic health center culture that is unrelated to safety may prove useful when considering changes to enhance patient safety. To address under-representation of women and minority faculty, five schools formed a collaborative with private and governmental grant support to study and change institutional characteristics that contributed to this under-representation.[51] Approaches employed in this work that may apply to other types of culture change include: using individuals' or teams' understanding of the basis of problems to identify institutional character-istics that foster or alleviate these problems; self-study to understand the specific issues that are most important in a given institution; and creation of an inter-institu-tional network to share understanding of failures and successes. Although focused on culture change in academic health centers, this work in progress may provide future support for the changes needed to increase patient safety.

Curricular change presents a natural opportunity to—and may be an essential ele-ment of—change in support of patient safety. Whether by incorporating problem-based methodology or merely by reorienting didactic experiences toward a patient focus, reshaping a traditional, discipline-based curriculum into patient-centered learning provides a clear opportunity to integrate patient safety principles into the curriculum.[52]

While curricular change typically takes place at the level of a single institution, change can also span multiple institutions. In 1999, the U.S. Department of Veter-ans Affairs established the National Center for Patient Safety to "develop and nur-ture a culture of safety throughout the Veterans Health Administration."[53] In 2011, the VA established five Centers of Excellence in Primary Care Education[54] ex-pressly "to develop and test innovative approaches to prepare physician residents and students, advanced practice nurse and undergraduate nursing students, and as-sociated health trainees for primary care practice in the 21st Century." These five centers will explore how to change education and clinical training to:

- Foster better coordination between professions.

- Enhance team functioning.

- Improve the quality and safety of patient care.

The VA has complemented its efforts to change institutions with support for de-veloping individual leaders. In collaboration with Dartmouth Medical School, its two-year Veterans Affairs National Quality Scholars Fellowship Program relies on distance learning technologies, face-to-face meetings, local mentorship, and expe-riential projects to prepare physicians to engage in and lead initiatives to improve health care quality and safety.[55]

Although institution-level change may be the basis for changing educational cul-ture, smaller scale efforts also can be effective in promoting a culture that better supports patient safety. Even a one-day lecture-workshop program can produce significant changes in student attitudes and beliefs about patient safety,[56] and suc-cessful programs for students can form a basis for faculty-directed interventions.[57]

Conclusion

In summary, changing the culture of health professions education and the insti-tutions involved in training will be essential to transforming how health care is provided. An important element of this change will be to increase the emphasis on and effectiveness of interprofessional education and training. Although the difficulty associated with changing educational culture—or any culture—is legendary, recent experience shows increasing coalescence around the principles that should guide changes to health care systems, willingness of national organizations to commit resources and leadership to effect change, and a growing number of initiatives to understand and implement improvements in health professions education. Combining this commitment to change with knowledge of critical success factors will enable the transformation necessary for ensuring safe, high-quality outcomes for all patients.

Acknowledgements

The author gratefully acknowledges the editorial assistance and guidance of M. Brownell Anderson, and the assistance of Harold Venable with manuscript preparation.

Study and Discussion Questions

1. What are the most problematic aspects of health professions education culture? What impact do these have on patient safety?

2. Considering the principles outlined for implementing successful change, what stakeholders should be convened to form a "powerful guiding coalition" to effect positive change in the culture of health professions education?

3. What barriers exist to implementing effective interprofessional education programs? How might these barriers be overcome?

4. What lessons are demonstrated by successful programs to change educational culture?

Suggested Readings

Burke WW. *Organization Change.* Thousand Oaks, CA: Sage Publications, 2011.

Greiner AC, Knebel E, eds. *Health Professions Education: A Bridge to Quality.* Washington, DC: National Academies Press, 2003.

Heath C and Heath D. *Made to Stick.* New York, NY: Random House, 2007.

Kotter J. *Leading Change.* Boston, MA: Harvard Business School Press, 1996.

Kouzes JM and Posner BZ. *The Truth about Leadership.* San Francisco, CA: Jossey-Bass, 2010.

Suggested Web Sites

AAMC "Best Practices for Better Care" web site. https://www.aamc.org/initiatives/best-practices/. Accessed July 14, 2011.

The Agency for Healthcare Research and Quality (AHRQ), Education Opportunities for Health Professionals web site [section on "Quality & Patient Safety"]. http://www.ahrq.gov/clinic/eduopps.htm. Accessed July 14, 2011.

The Institute for Healthcare Improvement (IHI) web site. http://www.ihi.org/about/pages/default.aspx. Accessed July 14, 2011.

Interprofessional Education Collaborative Expert Panel. *Core competencies for interprofessional collaborative practice: Report of an expert panel.* Washington, D.C.: Interprofessional Education Collaborative; 2011. https://www.aamc.org/download/186750/data/core_competencies.pdf . Accessed July 14, 2011.

MedlinePlus, the National Institutes of Health's web site produced by the National Library of Medicine [for patients] http://www.nlm.nih.gov/medlineplus/patientsafety.html. Accessed July 14, 2011.

Quality and Safety Education for Nurses (QSEN) web site. http://www.qsen.org/. Accessed July 14, 2011.

References

1. Institute of Medicine. Committee on Quality of Health Care in America. *Crossing the Quality Chasm: A New Health System for the 21st Century.* Washington, DC: National Academies Press, 2001.

2. Greiner A, Knebel E. *Health Professions Education: a Bridge to Quality.* Washington, DC: Institute of Medicine, 2003.

3. Schein EH. *Organizational Culture and Leadership.* San Francisco, CA: Jossey-Bass, 2010.

4. Taylor JS. Confronting "culture" in medicine's "culture of no culture." *Acad Med.* 78(6):555-9, June 2003.

5. Swenk J. Planning failures: decision cultural clashes. *Rev High Educ.* 23(1):1-21, 1999.

6. Dobson PM. Changing the culture in nursing—a strategy. *Contemp Nurse.* 9(3-4):261-2, Sept.-Dec. 2000.

7. Maine LL. Pharmacy education redux. *Pharmacotherapy.* 24(5):682-4, May 2004.

8. Berwick DM. A user's manual for the IOM's "Quality Chasm" report. *Health Affairs (Project Hope).* 21(3):80-90, May-June 2002.

9. Greenberger E, Lessard J, Chen C, Farruggia S. Self-Entitled College Students: Contributions of Personality, Parenting, and Motivational Factors. *J Youth Adolescence.* 37(10):1193-204, 2008.

10. Clark C. The dance of incivility in nursing education as described by nursing faculty and students. *Adv Nurs Sci.* 31(4):E37-E54, Oct.-Dec. 2008.

11. Clark C. Student perspectives on faculty incivility in nursing education: An application of the concept of rankism. *Nurs Outlook.* 56(1):4-8, Jan.-Feb. 2008.

12. Di Benedetto LM, Droege M. Pharmacy education: a student's perspective. *Am J Pharm Educ.* 70(3):72, June 15, 2006.

13. Hegge MJ, Hallman PA. Changing nursing culture to welcome second-degree students: Herding and corralling sacred cows. *J Nurs Educ.* 47(12):552-6, Dec. 2008.

14. Pearson P, Steven A, Howe A, *et al.* Learning about patient safety: Organizational context and culture in the education of health care professionals. *J Health Serv Res Policy.* 15(suppl. 1):4-10, Jan. 2010.

15. Riesenberg LA, Leitzsch J, Massucci JL, *et al*. Residents and attending physicians handoffs: a systematic review of the literature. *Acad Med*. 84(12):1775-87, Dec. 2009.

16. Stern DT. *Measuring Medical Professionalism*. New York, NY: Oxford University Press, 2006.

17. The Joint Commission. Behaviors that undermine a culture of safety. *The Joint Commission Web site* http://www.jointcommission.org/assets/1/18/SEA_40.PDF.

18. Shanafelt TD, Sloan JA, Habermann TM. The well-being of physicians. *Am J Med*. 114(6):513-9, Apr. 15, 2003.

19. Jorm C, Kam P. Does medical culture limit doctors' adoption of quality improvement? Lessons from Camelot. *J Health Serv Res Policy*. 9(4):248-51, Oct. 2004.

20. Alper E, Rosenberg EI, Obrien KE, *et al*. Patient safety education at U.S. and Canadian medical schools: results from the 2006 clerkship directors in internal medicine survey. *Acad Med*. 84(12):1672-6, Dec. 2009.

21. Windish DM, Reed DA, Boonyasai RT, *et al*. Methodological rigor of quality improvement curricula for physician trainees: A systematic review and recommendations for change. *Acad Med*. 84(12):1677-92, Dec. 2009.

22. Pronovost PJ, Miller MR, Wachter RM, Meyer GS. Perspective: Physician leadership in quality. *Acad Med*. 84(12):1651-6, Dec. 2009.

23. Jenson HB, Dorner D, Hinchey K, *et al*. Integrating quality improvement and residency education: insights from the AIAMC national initiative about the roles of the designated institutional official and program director. *Acad Med*. 84(12):1749-56, Dec. 2009.

24. Nedza SM. Commentary: A call to leadership: the role of the academic medical center in driving sustainable health system improvement through performance measurement. *Acad Med*. 84(12):1645-7, Dec. 2009.

25. Bohmer RMJ, Bloom JD, Mort EA, *et al*. Restructuring within an academic health center to support quality and safety: The development of the Center for Quality and Safety at the Massachusetts General Hospital. *Acad Med*. 84(12):1663-71, Dec. 2009.

26. Ferguson KE, Jinks AM. Integrating what is taught with what is practised in the nursing curriculum: a multi-dimensional model. *J Adv Nurs*. 20(4):687-95, Oct. 1994.

27. Kohn LT, Corrigan J, Donaldson MS. *To Err Is Human: Building a Safer Health System*. Washington, DC: National Academies Press, 2000.

28. Glossary – Safety Culture. *AHRQ Patient Safety Network Web site* http://www.psnet.ahrq.gov/popup_glossary.aspx?name=safetyculture.

29. OutcomeProject. The General Competencies. *ACGME Web site* http://www.acgme.org/outcome/comp/refList.asp.

30. Cronenwett L, Sherwood G, Barnsteiner J, *et al*. Quality and safety education for nurses. *Nurs Outlook*. 55(3):122-31, May-June 2007.

31. IECEP. Core competencies for interprofessional collaborative practice: Report of an expert panel. *Association of American Medical Colleges Web site* https://www.aamc.org/download/186750/data/core_competencies.pdf.

32. Accreditation Standards and Guidelines for the Professional Program in Pharmacy Leading to the Doctor of Pharmacy Degree. *Accreditation Council for Pharmacy Education Web site* http://www.acpe-accredit.org/pdf/S2007Guidelines2.0_ChangesIdentifiedInRed.pdf. Accessed March 6, 2011

33. NLNAC 2008 Standards and Criteria. *National League for Nursing Accrediting Commission, Inc. Web site* http://www.nlnac.org/manuals/SC2008.htm. Accessed March 6, 2011.

34. Ogiehor-Enoma G, Taqueban L, Anosike A. 6 steps for transforming organizational EBP culture. *Nurs Manag.* 41(5):14-17, May 2010.

35. Clark CM, Springer PJ. Academic nurse leaders' role in fostering a culture of civility in nursing education. *J Nurs Educ.* 49(6):319-25, June 2010.

36. Girdley D, Johnsen C, Kwekkeboom K. Facilitating a culture of safety and patient-centered care through use of a clinical assessment tool in undergraduate nursing education. *J Nurs Educ.* 48(12):702-5, Dec. 2009.

37. Cooper E. Creating a culture of professional development: a milestone pathway tool for registered nurses. *J Contin Educ Nurse.* 40(11):501-8, Nov. 2009.

38. Cooperrider DL, Sorensen PF, Whitney D, Yaeger TF. *Appreciative Inquiry: Rethinking Human Organization Toward a Positive Theory of Change.* Champaign, IL.: Stipes Pub., 2000.

39. Moody RC, Horton-Deutsch S, Pesut DJ. Appreciative inquiry for leading in complex systems: supporting the transformation of academic nursing culture. *J Nurs Educ.* 46(7):319-24, July 2007.

40. Lange JW, Ingersoll G, Novotny JM. Transforming the organizational culture of a school of nursing through innovative program development. *J Prof Nurs.* 24(6):371-7, Nov.-Dec. 2008.

41. Maudsley RF. Role models and the learning environment: essential elements in effective medical education. *Acad Med.* 76(5):432-4, May 2004.

42. Steinert Y, Mann KV. Faculty development: principles and practices. *J Vet Med Educ.* 33(3):317-324, Fall 2006.

43. Behal R, Finn J. Understanding and improving inpatient mortality in academic medical centers. *Acad Med.* 84(12):1657-62, Dec. 2009.

44. Nieva VF, Sorra J. Safety culture assessment: a tool for improving patient safety in healthcare organizations. *Qual Saf Health Care.* 12(suppl 2):17-23,Dec. 2003.

45. Burke WW. *Organization Change: Theory and Practice.* Los Angeles, CA: Sage Publications, 2008.

46. Kirch DG, Boysen PG. Changing the culture in medical education to teach patient safety. *Health Affairs (Project Hope).* 29(9):1600-4, Sept. 2010.

47. Griner PF. Leadership strategies of medical school deans to promote quality and safety. *Joint Comm J Qual Pat Safe.* 33(2):63-72, Feb. 2007.

48. Thompson SA, Tilden VP. Embracing quality and safety education for the 21st century: building interprofessional education. *J Nurs Educ.* 48(12):698-701, Dec. 2009.

49. Cottingham AH, Litzelman DK, Frankel RM, *et al.* Enhancing the informal curriculum of a medical school: A case study in organizational culture change. *J Gen Intern Med.* 23(6):715-22, June 2008.

50. Grigsby RK, Kirch DG. Faculty and staff teams: a tool for unifying the academic health center and improving mission performance. *Acad Med.* 81(8):688-95, Aug. 2006.

51. Powell D, Scott JL, Rosenblatt M, *et al.* Commentary: A call for culture change in academic medicine. *Acad Med.* 85(4):586-7, Apr. 2010.

52. Christianson CE, McBride RB, Vari RC, *et al.* From traditional to patient-centered learning: curriculum change as an intervention for changing institutional culture and promoting professionalism in undergraduate medical education. *Acad Med.* 82(11):1079-88, Nov. 2007.

53. VA National Center for Patient Safety home page. *US Department of Veterans Affairs Web site* http://www.patientsafety.gov/.

54. VA Centers of Excellence in Primary Care Education. *US Department of Veterans Affairs Web site* http://www.va.gov/oaa/rfp_coe.asp.

55. Splaine ME, Ogrinc G, Gilman SC, *et al.* The Department of Veterans Affairs National Quality Scholars Fellowship Program: Experience from 10 years of training quality scholars. *Acad Med.* 84(12):1741-8, Dec. 2009.

56. Moskowitz E, Veloski JJ, Fields SK, Nash DB. Development and evaluation of a 1-day interclerkship program for medical students on medical errors and patient safety. *Am J Med Qual.* 22(1):13-7, Jan.-Feb. 2007.

57. Meiris DC, Clarke JL, Nash DB. Culture change at the source: a medical school tackles patient safety. *Am J Med Qual.* 21(1):9-12, Jan.-Feb. 2006.

Clinical Reflection

By John W. Caruso, MD, FACP

As a fledgling house officer in August of 1991, I experienced a seminal event that all medical trainees must—my first patient died unexpectedly. I had experienced patient deaths before, especially since my previous rotation had been in an intensive care unit where multiple patients were critically ill. However, the deaths there had been expected or at least "explainable" based on patients' terminal diagnoses or recent clinical events. This man's case was different, and its circumstances are ones I still remember some 20 years later because this patient's demise was another first—it was the first time I believed that our team's actions directly contributed to a patient's death.

In his 60s and unknown to our institution, Mr. X was brought to the emergency department (ED) of our university hospital on a Saturday night. His family reported that he had a change in mental status. They also noted that, while his abdomen was not large, it was more distended than normal. They now were unable to care for him at home. He was seen by multiple physicians in the emergency department—including specialists in emergency medicine, internal medicine, and gastroenterology—who noted that he was jaundiced with mild hepatic enzyme elevations, but his remaining clinical and laboratory findings were not consistent with hepatic encephalopathy. When Mr. X admitted to drinking alcohol daily, it was surmised that he had developed acute alcoholic hepatitis. The ED team thought that he was also withdrawing from alcohol and that this explained his delirium. It was decided that he would be admitted to the inpatient setting for a comprehensive evaluation and treatment of alcohol withdrawal.

The resident who met me at Mr. X's room was hurrying in after supervising another intern on different admission. The time was just after midnight. Because on weekends interns were supervised by residents who covered multiple intern teams, it was the first time I had met this resident. After brief introductions, the resident and I went to see Mr. X.

Our patient was in obvious distress, and looked much older than his chronological age. He also was gaunt and appeared malnourished. He offered only brief responses to our questions, and we could gather no useful information that helped us identify a "unifying" diagnosis. No longer with him, his family could not be reached because no one in the ED had recorded their contact information. With limited information available, we discussed the case with the attending physician who was supervising us that evening from home. As a team, we decided to begin the supportive care recommended for patients with malnutrition and chronic alcohol use, and sent additional blood tests for other liver diseases that could have been contributing to his condition. We also prescribed prophylactic benzodiazepines, assuming that alcohol withdrawal was contributing to his delirium. Since additional information was not obtainable, we continued on the path that was set in the ED and that was based on partial findings.

The remainder of the evening was marked by continued deterioration in Mr. X's status. His delirium worsened and his vital signs became unstable. His blood pressure was steadily dropping, and we had no satisfying explanation. We sent additional blood for culture and more advanced chemistries. He was started empirically on antibiotics on the assumption that he was "septic," even though he had no fever or elevation in his white blood cell count. His intravenous fluids were accelerated and, after a time, his blood pressure stabilized.

In the morning, our patient continued to deteriorate. We anxiously awaited our attending's and gastroenterology consultant's evaluations in hopes that these senior clinicians could identify what was causing our patient's worsening status and guide our management. The ward attending typically saw only outpatients at another institution, attended only once or twice a year, and covered some weekends. He was unfamiliar with the hospital coverage teams and had difficulty locating us to discuss the case. When he did find us, the hurried suggestions he offered were not helpful to our team.

After seeing the patient at noon, the gastroenterology team called with suggestions. One of their most prominent recommendations was to perform a diagnostic paracentesis as soon as possible, based on the ascites suspected in the ED. It was now 1pm, and my "covering" resident had gone home, leaving the Sunday team to supervise me. I had never done a paracentesis before, and I needed the help and supervision of a resident for this invasive procedure. Finally, after several calls, I found the resident who was designated to supervise me.

When he arrived, the resident was resentful that this procedure was now his responsibility. I assumed that he had a list of patients to be admitted, and my request was pulling him away from the Sunday interns on call. I still recall him telling me, "You should just do this yourself—this is a ward patient after all." When we started the procedure, it became clear that the reason for his reticence went beyond a preoccupation with his other duties. In fact, he was as inexperienced with this procedure as I was, and I would not have the guidance I had hoped for.

A resident was expected to know the paracentesis procedure well, so he agreed to supervise me without disclosing his lack of experience. As I continued the procedure, I found myself questioning his every instruction and becoming fully conflicted with every step of the process. After several attempts at placing a needle in the peritoneal space, no fluid was obtained and we decided to end the procedure. In most cases, the procedure would be terminated with the assumption that there was no fluid to be obtained. In this case, we wondered if we had placed the needle in the correct location, if we had used the correct syringe, and even if we had positioned the patient correctly.

It was now after 3pm, and I was exhausted. I had begun this shift at 7am on Saturday. I had less than one hour of sleep, and even that was interrupted by calls about the patients I was covering. The patient looked worse, and we had no further information on which to act. While I was waiting for the call back from the gastroenterology team, a nurse ran into the conference room where I was writing my post procedure note. Mr. X had become unresponsive and hypotensive without a pulse, and a "code" was called. I was not on the code team, but I ran to the room to provide the senior residents and fellows on the team with whatever information I could. Despite a prolonged attempt at resuscitation, Mr. X died.

During the resuscitation efforts, we noticed a hematoma growing on his flank, corresponding to where the resident and I had attempted the paracentesis. This was obviously distressing to me, and the sensation was only heightened when the senior residents all aggressively questioned us as to why we chose the location we did for this procedure. This location was too close to the spleen, and therefore a risky choice. I was personally devastated, and remember thinking, "This is simply not the way things should happen in a modern university hospital."

At the time, I focused only on my actions—I ordered the procedure, and I held the needle. Most of all, I feared that I should have recognized the problem before the patient was in a cardiac arrest. Over time, with the help of mentors and colleagues alike, I broadened my focus to include all clinicians who cared for Mr. X. At first, this change in viewpoint was merely comforting, but it proved to be transformative in the long run. I became interested in patient safety and how it could be improved.

As I learned more about patient safety principles, this case became another first. It was the index case for me in illustrating how adverse events typically occur—multiple systems failures, developing over time, were as important in this patient's outcome as my failed procedure. Moreover, the failures in this case were demonstrative of risks and challenges to patient safety that were all too common in training programs of that era.

I can see where the care should have been improved. First, the "handoff" between the residents in the ED and our team was non-existent. Such a conversation would have reinforced all the important findings, including the ascites that was identified by his family and gastroenterology fellow. If this had been noted sooner, he may have had the paracentesis 12 hours sooner, supervised by an entirely different resident, although even this is uncertain because the resident who supervised me was overseeing more patients and more interns than would now be allowed by residency accreditation bodies. The supervising attending's unfamiliarity with the hospital environment would now be distinctly unusual in the era of dedicated "hospitalists". My inexperience in a critical procedure would now be identified before I started internship, and I would have learned this procedure in a clinical skills center before ever performing it on an actual patient.

I hope that these lessons, learned over time, have improved the care of many of my subsequent patients. However, I also believe strongly that these lessons could have been learned before the incident. Since these events, the Institute of Medicine and the Accreditation Council for Graduate Medical Education have begun to revolutionize how residents are trained. Twenty years ago, it was assumed that if you received training at a good school, and had done well there, you would be a safe physician. Unfortunately, the ability to ensure patient safety takes more than experiencing a science curriculum intended to produce a knowledgeable and skilled physician.

While we have made progress in teaching our students and residents safety principles, we need to go further. Our curricula need to prominently include training on care systems, how they fail, and how to improve them. This includes sessions during clinical rotations and not just lectures on principles of safety and quality early in the undergraduate curriculum. To be successful, we must develop a culture wherein an inexperienced intern would be expected to recognize a potentially dangerous situation before it happened. I am not sure we are fully there yet even though it has been 20 years since Mr. X presented to a university hospital ED, and died within 24 hours.

Nursing Education Perspective

By Mary Lou Manning, PhD, CRNP

There is nothing more difficult to take in hand, more perilous to conduct, or more uncertain in its success than to take the lead in the introduction of a new order of things. Because the innovator has for enemies all those who have done well under the old conditions, and lukewarm defenders in those who may do well under the new.

—The Prince by Niccolo Machiavelli

Introduction

There are more than three million registered nurses in the U.S., representing the largest sector of health care professionals. Almost 90 percent of new nursing graduates are employed in hospital-based practice for their first position, but increasing numbers are migrating to non-acute care settings.[1] Currently, about 60 percent of all nurses practice in hospitals while the remainder practice in non-acute settings such as schools, private homes, retail health clinics, long-term care facilities, employee workplaces, and community and public health centers.[2] Over a quarter million nurses are advanced practice registered nurses (APRNs) who have earned master's or doctoral degrees and have passed national certification examinations. Nurse practitioners, clinical nurse specialists, nurse anesthetists, and nurse midwives are licensed as APRNs. Regardless of the setting, nurses' regular, close proximity to patients and substantial knowledge of care processes across the continuum of care make them more likely than any other health professional to recognize, interrupt, and correct health care errors.[2-4]

The work environments of nurses are increasingly complex and hazardous. Burgeoning information, the plethora of new technologies, and the demands for evidence-based practice challenge even the most experienced nurse. Care is further complicated by changing patient demographics; emerging new health care needs; multiple treatment regimens; numerous providers; shifts in patient care, recovery and management to the home and community settings; and relentless social, economic, and political pressures. Faced with expanding regulatory, accreditation, and quality performance standards, as well as measures and mandates focused on health care quality and patient safety, today's nurses must have an expansive world view and function as leaders and stewards. The rapid pace of change in health care has fueled significant changes in nursing practice and the need for nurses with advanced competencies.[2,3] Profound changes in nursing call for a radical transformation in how nurses are educated. The next generation of nurses must have the capacity to practice safely, accurately, and compassionately, in varied settings, where knowledge and innovation increase at an astonishing rate.

Calls to Action

During the past decade, the Institute of Medicine (IOM) has repeatedly highlighted the lack of preparation of health professionals in interdisciplinary teamwork, systems thinking, use of information systems, patient-centered care, and quality improvement. After the IOM report, *Crossing the Quality Chasm: A New Health System for the 21st Century*,[5] drew focused attention to patient safety and emphasized the importance of patient-centered care provided by effective interdisciplinary teams, academic institutions were called on to educate health professionals to work collaboratively.

Finding health professionals' education in need of major reform, the authors of *Health Professions Education: A Bridge to Quality* [6] proposed five core competencies beyond the command of knowledge and facts that all health care providers should possess. Another report, *Keeping Patients Safe: Transforming the Work Environment of Nurses* concluded that the typical work environment of nurses is characterized by many serious threats to patient safety, and noted that "how well we are cared for by nurses affects our health, and sometimes can be a matter of life or death...nurses are indispensable to our safety."[7] This report stressed that safe care requires a nursing workforce appropriate in size and expertise as well as the adoption of transformational leadership and evidence-based care.

Nursing education was the focus of two major reports in 2010:

1. *Educating Nurses: A Call for Radical Transformation*,[2] by the Carnegie Foundation, concluded that, while nursing education has been effective in forming professional identity and ethical comportment and in providing powerful clinical practice learning experiences, a challenge remains in anticipating the changing demands of practice through strengthening of scientific education (e.g., nursing science, natural sciences, social sciences, technology, and humanities) and integration of classroom and clinical teaching.[2,8] The authors found that the current climate rewards short-term focus, efficiency, and cost-savings that can compromise the quality of nursing education and patient care, and identified the redesign of nursing education as an urgent societal agenda.

2. *The Future of Nursing, Leading Change, Advancing Health*[3], from the Robert Wood Johnson Foundation (RWJF) Initiative on the Future of Nursing at the IOM, provides a vision of a future health care system that would make high-quality care accessible to all, promote wellness and disease prevention, improve health outcomes, and provide compassionate care throughout a person's lifespan.[9] The issues raised by the report should not be viewed merely

as "nursing" issues, but rather as health care, health system, and health reform issues. This report is a potential catalyst for all health professions to find significant opportunities for collaboration among health professions and, by playing to each profession's strengths, to advance high-quality health care for all citizens. Consequently, the report's authors have been communicating their recommendations to other health care providers and to interprofessional groups.[10]

The report contains four key messages and eight recommendations that serve as "the building blocks required to expand innovative models of care, as well as improve the quality, accessibiltiy, and value of care, through nursing."[3] Two of the four key messages relate to nursing education; namely, nurses should achieve higher levels of education and training through an improved education system that promotes seamless academic progression, and nurses should be full partners with physicians and other health professionals in redesigning health care in the U.S. Recommendations included: increasing the proportion of nurses with a baccalaureate degree to 80 percent by 2010, doubling the number of nurses with a doctorate by 2010, ensure that nurses are lifelong learners, and preparing and enabling nurses to lead change to advance health.

Finally, building on the widespread national interest to transform health professions education, six national associations of health professions schools, including the American Association of Colleges of Nursing, formed the Interprofessional Education Collaborative and, in May 2011, released a consensus report entitled *Core Competencies for Interprofessional Collaborative Practice*.[11] The competencies are congruent with those identified by the IOM, the Carnegie Foundation, and the RWJF.

Nursing Profession Response

Both the American Association of Colleges of Nursing (AACN) and the National League for Nurses (NLN) agree that nursing education is in need of transformation and support the change to competency-based nursing education. Rather than the one-size-fits-all curriculum, competency-based education allows for a highly individualized learning process.[8]

In 2004, members of the AACN endorsed the *Position Statement on the Practice Doctorate in Nursing*, and subsequently voted to move the current level of preparation necessary for advanced nursing practice from the master's level to the doctorate level by 2015.[12] *Essentials of the Doctoral Education for Advanced Practice Nursing* identifies the foundational curriculum content and outcome-based competencies necessary for all students pursuing the DNP.[13] Competency based education is further promulgated in the AACN's 2008 *Essentials of Baccalaureate Education for Professional Nursing Practice*, and the 2011 *Essentials of Master's Education in Nursing*.[14-16] In 2010 the NLN published an education competency model supporting an inclusive national approach to nursing education.[17]

Quality and Safety Education for Nurses (QSEN), a national initiative funded by the RWJF, is designed to build the will and generate the ideas for transforming nursing education through curricula that support learning of quality and safety competencies.[18-20] The QSEN faculty and national advisory board, with representatives from national nursing organizations, adopted the IOM competencies and outlined six competency domains: patient-centered care, teamwork and collaboration, evidence-based practice, quality improvement, safety, and informatics. Specific knowledge, skills, and attitudes required for nursing students to achieve each of the competencies were defined. The initial QSEN focus was competency development during pre-licensure nursing education, followed by suggested adaptation for graduate and practice doctorate nursing education.[19] QSEN provides the discipline with a consensually validated, concise, and explicit framework for advancing quality and safety across all types of nursing programs.

The RWJF-sponsored *The Future of Nursing, Campaign for Action* is a collaborative effort to implement solutions to the challenges facing the nursing profession and to build upon nurse-based approaches to improving quality and transforming the way Americans receive health care. The campaign's Action Coalitions are important agents of change. To date there are coalitions in 15 states driving change at the local, state, and regional levels.[21]

Today's nursing faculty is faced with the challenge of incorporating and applying the competencies in nursing curricula as they prepare current and future nurses to practice effectively within the complex and ever-changing health care environment.[1,22] Concurrently, the faculty must self-reflect and assess their own knowledge, skills, and abilities to teach these concepts and, as needed, develop their own personal improvement plans. Faculty must harness the curiosity, energy, and passion of those embarking on their nursing careers and help them become indispensable health care professionals and leaders who, working together, can invent, connect, create, and make things happen to realize the vision of a health care system free of patient harm.

Conclusions

This is truly an exciting time in nursing and nursing education. There is a national sense of urgency to change how nurses and other health professionals are educated and significant support within and across the health professions to do so. The days are fading when health professions education can focus solely on the development of individual practitioners who are able to deliver high-quality care within their designated discipline. As Tilden recently wrote, "Nursing, medicine, and other health professions are tightly linked by our social contracts to serve the public good, and we share the urgency of finding different education and care models to do that. As respected colleagues in education and care delivery, let us dismiss outdated suspicions and ride the tides of change."[23]

References

1. Hickey MT, Forbes M, Greenfield M. Integrating the Institute of Medicine competencies in baccalaureate curricular revision: process and strategies. *J Prof Nurs,* 26(4):214-22, July-Aug. 2010.

2. Benner P, Sutphen M, Leonard V, Day L. *Educating Nurses: A Call for Radical Transformation.* San Francisco, CA: Jossey-Bass, 2009.

3. Institute of Medicine. *The Future of Nursing: Leading Change, Advancing Health.* Washington, DC: National Academies Press, 2010.

4. Rothschild JM, Hurley AC, Landrigan CP, Cronin, JW. Recovering from medical errors: The critical care nursing safety net. *Joint Commission J Qual & Pt Safety,* 32(2):63-72, Feb. 2006.

5. Institute of Medicine. *Crossing the Quality Chasm.* Washington, DC: National Academies Press, 2001.

6. Institute of Medicine. *Health Professions Education: A Bridge to Quality.* Washington, DC: National Academies Press, 2003.

7. Institute of Medicine. *Keeping Patients Safe: Transforming the Work Environment of Nurses.* Washington, DC: National Academies Press, 2004.

8. Frenk J, Chen L, Bhutta ZA, *et al.* Health professionals for a new century: transforming education to strengthen health systems in an interdependent world. *Lancet,* 376(9756):1923-58, Dec. 4, 2010.

9. Hassmiller SB. An "action-oriented blueprint" for the future of nursing. *AJN,* 110(12):7, Dec. 2010.

10. Fairman JA, Rowe JW, Hasmiller S, Shalala DE. Broadening the scope of nursing practice. *N Engl J Med,* 364(3):193-6, Jan. 20, 2011.

11. Interprofessional Education Collaborative, Core Competencies for Interprofessional Collaborative Practice 2011. http://www.aacn.nche.edu/Education/pdf/IPECReport.pdf. (accessed July 8, 2011).

12. American Association of Colleges of Nursing. AACN Position Statement on the Practice Doctorate in Nursing October 2004. http://www.aacn.nche.edu/dnp/pdf/DNP.pdf. (Accessed July 8, 2011).

13. American Association of Colleges of Nursing. The essentials of doctoral education for advanced nursing practice 2006. http://www.aacn.nche.edu/dnp/pdf/Essentials.pdf. (Accessed July 8, 2011).

14. American Association of Colleges of Nursing. The essentials of Baccalaureate Education for Professional Nursing Practice 2008. http://www.aacn.nche.edu/Education/pdf/BaccEssentials08.pdf. (Accessed July 8, 2011).

15. American Association of Colleges of Nursing. The essentials of master's education in nursing 2011. http://www.aacn.nche.edu/Education/pdf/DraftMastEssentials.pdf. (Accessed July 8, 2011).

16. American Association of Colleges of Nursing. U.S. Nursing school transform master's education by adopting new standards reflecting contemporary nursing practice. *J Prof Nurs,* 27(3):131-2, May-June 2011.

17. National League for Nursing, Outcomes and competencies for graduates of practical/vocational, diploma, associate degree, baccalaureate, master's, practice doctorate, and research doctorate programs in nursing 2010. http://www.nln.org/facultydevelopment/competencies/index.htm. (Accessed July 8, 2011).

18. Cronenwett L, Sherwood G, Barnsteiner J, *et al*. Quality and safety education for nurses. *Nurs Outlook,* 55(3):122-31, May-June 2007.

19. Cronenwett L, Sherwood G, Pohl J, *et al*. Quality and safety education for advanced nursing practice. *Nurs Outlook,* 57(6):338-48, Nov.-Dec 2009.

20. Cronenwett L, Sherwood, G. and Gelmon SB. Improving quality and safety education: The QSEN Learning Collaborative. *Nurs Outlook*, 57(6):304-12, Nov.-Dec. 2007.

21. Future of Nursing, Campaign for Action. http://www.thefutureofnursing.org/. (Accessed July 8, 2011).

22. Thornlow DK, McGuinn K. A necessary sea change for nurse faculty development: spotlight on quality and safety. *J Prof Nurs,* 26(2):71-81, Mar. 2010.

23. Tilden VP. The tides of change: Are we ready for interprofessional collaboration? *Nurs Outlook,* 59(3):107-8, May-June 2011.

Section VI.

Future Directions for Quality Measurement and Improvement

Chapter 23

Entering the Health Care Crossroads

By Michael Dowling

Unlike any time in the history of the nation's health care system, we are at a crossroad that will likely determine the future of how we provide medical care and improve the health status of Americans for decades to come. With political winds swirling around us, we are crossing the threshold of the status quo into a new era of health care delivery that will require courage, agility, and focus. For the heads of health care organizations, it is an exhilarating time, especially for those who:

- Want to lead, not just follow;

- Believe in change and transformation;

- Believe in carefully managing the present but selectively forgetting the past, and who are not preservers of tradition;

- Believe in creating a new future, not because we are mandated to but because we know it is the right thing to do;

- Understand that the current trajectory of health care usage and spending is unsustainable; and

- Are optimistic and positive.

Negativity does not inspire confidence, yet it is the prevailing attitude at far too many national and state meetings of health care leaders. There's an ancient proverb that reads: "Just when the caterpillar thought the world was over, it became a butterfly." Leaders recognize reality, take risks, inspire, and see a greatly improved future built around the needs and desires of the customer and the patient.

Celebrate Progress

Despite misgivings about the rate and pace of changes in health care delivery, as well as the quality and safety of the services we deliver, we should recognize the enormous progress we have made. We have built significant momentum and a sturdy foundation on which to expand our efforts. Right now, our nation's health care system and consumers are benefitting from:

- Greater acceptance of performance measurement, transparency, and public reporting;

- Improved oversight and regulatory processes instituted by government agencies to monitor and evaluate quality;

- General acceptance that the traditional fee-for-service payment system, in many instances, impedes the quality movement and the introduction of new, innovative payment methodologies; and

- Ongoing restructuring, consolidation, and integration by many hospitals and health systems, making them more viable financially, improving quality outcomes, and enabling them to lead in this new health care environment.

Many good things are happening. Leading organizations have demonstrated sustained improvements. It is almost universally accepted that the delivery of health care must move in a new direction.

Figure 1. A view of the changing landscape

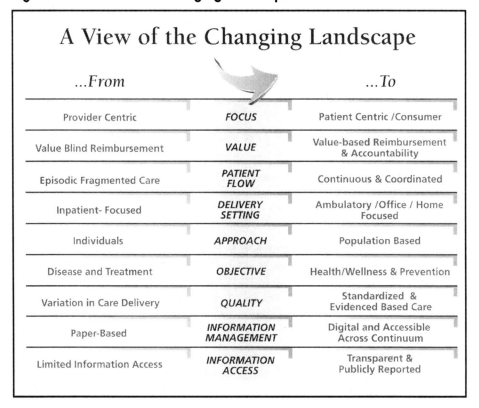

...From		...To
Provider Centric	FOCUS	Patient Centric /Consumer
Value Blind Reimbursement	VALUE	Value-based Reimbursement & Accountability
Episodic Fragmented Care	PATIENT FLOW	Continuous & Coordinated
Inpatient- Focused	DELIVERY SETTING	Ambulatory /Office / Home Focused
Individuals	APPROACH	Population Based
Disease and Treatment	OBJECTIVE	Health/Wellness & Prevention
Variation in Care Delivery	QUALITY	Standardized & Evidenced Based Care
Paper-Based	INFORMATION MANAGEMENT	Digital and Accessible Across Continuum
Limited Information Access	INFORMATION ACCESS	Transparent & Publicly Reported

The trends outlined in Figure 1 are at the core of current policy and legislation, including the federal health reform law—the Patient Protection and Affordable Care Act. They are not totally new or recent—in fact, they have been discussed in policy circles for more than a decade. The good news is that, finally, they are getting universal acceptance and better traction.

The Journey Ahead

Legendary football coach Vince Lombardi once said, "Perfection is not attainable, but if we chase perfection we can catch excellence." The pursuit of excellence in health care has a multiplicity of components, many of which have been adequately discussed in previous chapters. However, we need to focus on, and continue the progress we have made in a number of key areas.

My perspective is shaped by my role as the president and CEO of one of the largest health systems in the U.S. and by my ongoing communications with middle managers, clinicians, nurses, and front-line staff. My views are also guided by my previous role in the New York State government as a policymaker and regulator. Outlined below are several underlying issues that we must address:

Quality Metrics: The Need to Focus

Because of the increased attention dedicated to the quality agenda, an entire subset of health care-related businesses have cropped up over the past decade to rate and compare hospitals, nursing homes, and other health care providers. Companies such as HealthGrades, Hospital Compare, *U.S. News and World Report*, Press Ganey, J.D. Power & Associates, National Research Corporation, and numerous others produce their own versions of hospital report cards and develop their own set of quality measures and oversight procedures. Often, hospitals must enter into marketing agreements with the companies performing these quality assessments in order to promote positive findings.

The lack of an objective source, and the disparities in findings, are confusing to consumers and frustrating for providers. Who should you believe? It is like a soccer game with a dozen referees, each using different rules to officiate the game. As Margaret O'Kane, President of the National Committee for Quality Assurance, once said, "The quality community has become a quality problem in its own right. Confusion is an impediment to progress. As the environment gets more confusing, we're in danger of providers throwing up their hands in frustration." (Figure 2, page 382)

If this is confusing for leaders in the field, imagine the impact on middle management, physicians, and front-line staff. The existence of so many different quality measures can easily lead to distraction, frustration, and "metric fatigue." There is an obvious lack of clarity and standardization. What's needed is a national consensus on a smaller, more manageable number of quality metrics that all parties believe are at the core of good patient care. While the National Quality Forum, the Institute of Medicine and the Centers for Medicare and Medicaid Services, and others have made some progress in developing unified standards on which all providers can be evaluated, much more needs to be done.

Figure 2. The Quality Agenda

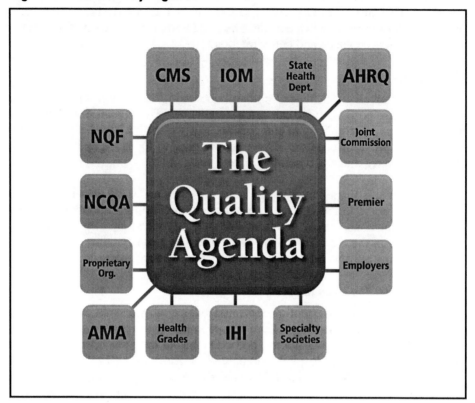

Despite the confusion and pressure to adhere to quality indicators developed by self-proclaimed quality consultants, every hospital and health system needs to stay focused on its own internal pursuit of clinical excellence. My advice is to prioritize by choosing a small number of key impactful areas that drive overall improvement. For our organization, we have chosen mortality, sepsis, and patient readmissions. This focus needs to be ongoing rather than a project of the month. All staff, especially those at the front lines, must be able to understand and describe the organization's quality agenda and relate it to their own work and how they contribute each day. Such focus requires the setting of strategic priorities; the realignment of organization structures; and investments in education, training, and skill development.

Creating a Learning Environment

To advance an organization's strategic and business goals, its leadership must foster growth and continuous learning among employees. Achieving that goal among health care providers requires investments in the workforce that will help transform the organization to meet the demands of the new health care environment. Organizations don't change; people do. Making change happen and breaking down barriers to change requires system-wide commitment, from the corporate suite to the front-line staff, including physicians.

The objective is to build a "learning organization"—the creation of a workforce culture that is grounded in the desire to continually strive to do things better as part of an ongoing pursuit of excellence.

To make it happen, the commitment must be significant and ongoing. Otherwise, meaningful changes and cultural transformations will be unsuccessful. In our organization (North Shore-Long Jewish [North Shore-LIJ]), for example, we established a corporate university called the Center for Learning and Innovation in 2002. Now headquartered in a 45,000-square-foot facility in Lake Success, NY, the Center's goals are to:

- Build a first-class organization of continuous learning.
- Build among employees the knowledge, attitude and skills necessary to support a reform agenda.
- Develop a cadre of leaders throughout the organization.
- Create and promote a culture that is consumer- and patient-centric and dedicated to excellence, teamwork, and continuous change.

Among the steps North Shore-LIJ has taken to achieve those goals are to incorporate courses on "fast-track" decision-making for solving organizational problems, "change acceleration" processes for breaking down barriers to change, and Six-Sigma and LEAN management processes for identifying and correcting errors in existing processes. By integrating these practices in our hospitals and facilities, we've been able to make measurable strides in driving quality, increasing efficiency and improving the environment for both patients and employees.

One of the centerpieces of our corporate university is a Patient Safety Institute that features sophisticated patient simulators with computer-based technology. Faculty in control rooms with one-way mirrors manipulate the patient simulators to mimic diverse medical scenarios found in all areas of health care. The simulation center is a resource for professionals at all clinical levels, and clinical teams from throughout our health system have regularly scheduled sessions. We built it on the premise that there must be a zero-tolerance policy toward medical errors and infections.

Physician Education

Improving quality and care delivery requires rethinking of how physicians are trained. For some time, there was much discussion on the need to reform medical education, but little changed. Most medical schools developed their curricula on principles and practices dating back to the 1890s. For much of the 20th century, medical education outside the classroom involved students accompanying an academic professor in a hospital, where the doctor would analyze, diagnose, and treat patients for however long it took before they were well enough to go home or they died.

Today, a patient's care typically is delivered by a team of clinicians that includes multiple doctors, nurses, social workers, and specialists. Unlike years ago, the vast majority of care is delivered in outpatient settings; if patients do require hospitalization, they're usually there for days rather than weeks.

However, old systems and processes still persist, creating a chasm between what is done and what is required. Excessive specialization, autonomy, and memorization must give way to medical training in which the focus is on teamwork and collaboration. Given the amount of knowledge available as a result of scientific and technological advancement, physicians cannot be the only source of all patient health information. If our true goal is to deliver excellent care, it's imperative for medical students to work with nurses and other patient caregivers—in essence, learning in a collaborative, interdisciplinary team environment.

Students admitted to the Hofstra North Shore-LIJ School of Medicine's first class, in August 2011, are immersed in patient care from the beginning to help them develop an early medical skill set. In lieu of the traditional approach (i.e., one which separates the science from the practice of medicine by keeping students primarily in classes for the first two years and primarily in clinical settings for last two years) our curriculum integrates the clinical and the scientific. Within one month of their arrival, students are trained and certified as emergency medical technicians, and begin working on ambulances, and treating patients in their homes, communities, and medical facilities. By learning first to be EMTs and practicing emergency care from the start of their studies, students are exposed to patients in crisis situations as members of emergency-response teams—working not only with doctors and nurses, but also with police, firefighters, social workers, and other first responders. This reinforces the fact that the best medicine is practiced by caregivers working as a team, not individually. Also, by interacting with patients and their family members early in their education, students develop greater sensitivity and appreciation of patients as real people, with strong emotional and cultural ties to their families and communities.

Partnering with Patients/Consumers

A core value of the Patient-Centered Medical Home (PCMH) is its focus on engaging patients and families in the care process. This is also the subject of a wonderful new book entitled *Your Medical Mind* by Drs. Jerome Groopman and Pamela Hartzband. Discussions around patient engagement have been going on for decades, but health care organizations have not modified their operational or clinical processes, or changed their structures, to make it happen. Engaging patients and their families in the delivery of care is now a central task in the transformed health care landscape. It requires fundamental change in the historic roles of both patient and provider, and in the cultural mindset of the health care industry. Done properly, patient engagement improves the process of care and quality outcomes, has the potential to reduce cost, and promotes wellness and disease self-management. There are successful examples both here and abroad that attest to the benefits. The task is to create the environment in which such a partnership is allowed to blossom.

At the 2011 Institute for Healthcare Improvement (IHI) Annual Meeting, I met a young Swedish nurse. He shared his story of gaining greater autonomy with his kidney dialysis and paving the way for a change in Swedish hospital policy so other patients could follow his lead and receive their dialysis at home. He spoke about how leaders can remove barriers and create cultures in which patient engagement is not just possible but encouraged. Getting providers closely involved enables patients and families to learn how their behaviors affect their health.

Metrics: From Medical Care to Health

One of the overarching strategic imperatives of health reform is to change our primary focus from treating people who are already sick to preventing them from getting sick in the first place by promoting wellness and a healthy lifestyle. In other words, we're shifting from a medical care delivery system to a health promotion system. Most agree that this is necessary and desirable, but it requires a new focus and the adoption of a different set of skills and relationships by hospitals and medical care delivery systems, as well as new forms of reimbursement.

Because medical conditions are primarily determined by environmental factors, lifelong behaviors, and lifestyle choices, this "new" focus is critical if we are to improve the health of individuals. Getting the "best" medical care will not, in and of itself, improve an individual's overall health status, a fact recognized with the formation of the Community Health Center movement in the 1960s. A broad, holistic vision of health, this movement was based on the theory that social, environmental, and economic conditions need to be integrated with medical care.

The focus had been on illness metrics, such as rates of hospital-acquired infections and patient readmissions. This new view raised fundamental issues: How do we measure "health?" What are the metrics and who should be held responsible? If population health is a new domain, we need to develop the measures. How do we know if we're successful? What is the responsibility of individuals? What is health quality? It is not sufficient to say we are reducing readmissions. After finally reaching a general degree of consensus on hospital-based or illness metrics, we now need the same for community and public health.

The Challenge of Information Management

The worlds of health care and information technology (IT) are coming together at a warp speed to create an aligned, integrated galaxy unlike any other in the universe of high-tech businesses. For decades, health care has evolved to feature enhanced technology equaled by few other industries—just observe all the advanced diagnostic equipment, robotic surgical devices, and countless other gadgets used by hospitals and physicians. Technology has advanced our ability to do wondrous things in the treatment of patients and the curing of disease. Yet, health care has lagged behind other industries in the technology that *manages* knowledge, communication, and information.

That's changing now with the advent of sophisticated electronic health record capabilities. The reasons are obvious: the collective goals of enhancing quality, managing patient care, monitoring and influencing population health, and reducing cost growth are unachievable if information cannot be shared, tracked, and used.

While the benefits are well-documented, the implementation is not easy. Bringing the worlds of IT and health care delivery together is much more that than a technical challenge—it requires major cultural change, ongoing training, and structural transformation. But there is a bigger potential problem—data overload. In other words, how do we understand and make intelligent use of all the data at our disposal?

The analytical resources necessary to decipher such growing supplies of data are enormous and costly. Many health care organizations simply do not have the financial wherewithal to manage such a Herculean IT challenge. It is becoming increasingly clear that our ability to collect data is surpassing our ability to absorb and understand the data. Just as we have become overwhelmed in trying to review and respond to all of the paperwork, emails, text messages, phone calls, voicemails, and other communication that preoccupy our personal lives, we are being drowned in the seemingly endless volume of data that gives us the capacity to deliver the highest level of care to our patients. Organizations need to develop the analytical capacity to evaluate and convert all of these data into information that can be understood and used by the practitioners who are diagnosing and treating patients.

Conclusion

The drivers of health care transformation in what promises to be an exciting decade ahead must come from the provider community—the administrators, physicians, nurses and others who understand the uniqueness of health care delivery and its potential better than any distant policy maker. It's their obligation and responsibility to identify and implement solutions. The alternative is a bureaucratically driven and micro-managed scenario that will, over time, stifle innovation and creativity.

My experience working in the regulatory, policymaking, insurance, and provider worlds has provided me with a unique perspective on the issues facing health care. After 16 years on the provider side, I clearly understand the degree of caring, compassion, and professionalism that exists among the thousands of caregivers with whom I regularly interact. It's a reservoir of talent, and, as leaders, it's imperative that we tap into it and let it flow throughout our respective organizations.

Nursing Credentialing — Raising the Bar on Clinical Excellence

By Karen Drenkard, PhD, RN, NEA-BC, FAAN

"Credentialing is a mode of self-regulation in which interests of the professions, industries, academia, or other fields of endeavor band together to establish quality and performance standards for their own constituencies and to measure performance against those standards for the betterment of society."[1]

As a form of self-regulation in a discipline, credentialing offers a means for a profession to set standards for both individuals and organizations and to measure the qualifications, knowledge, skills, and outcomes that indicate excellence. Credentialing is a complicated arena with many laws and requirements of its own. The combination of regulatory requirements and voluntary credentialing services can work together to protect the public and ensure competence of individual practitioners and organizations. In addition, voluntary credentialing can raise the bar on practice by setting standards for excellence. As individuals and organizations work to meet these high standards of practice, patient care and outcomes can improve.

There are several types of credentialing, including licensure, registration, accreditation, certification, recognition, approval, and endorsement.

- *Licensure* is a process by which an agency of a state government grants permission to individuals accountable for the practice of a profession to engage in the practice of that profession and prohibits all others from legally doing so. It permits use of a particular title, and its purpose is to protect the public by ensuring a minimum level of professional competence.

- *Accreditation* is the process by which a voluntary, non-governmental agency or organization appraises and grants accredited status to institutions and/or programs or services that meet predetermined structure, process, and outcome criteria.

- *Certification* is a process by which a non-governmental agency or association certifies that an individual has met certain predetermined standards specified by that profession for specialty practice. Its purpose is to assure various publics that an individual has mastered a body of knowledge and acquired skills in a particular specialty.

- *Recognition* is formal acknowledgement that a program, institution, or service has met a set of criteria promulgated by an official agency.

- *Approval* is a process by which a school and/or a program has met the prescribed minimum standards set by the appropriate regulatory body.

- *Endorsement* is an expression of support or approval by an authority in the field of a product, program, or service.[2,3] Credentialing serves to protect the health, safety or welfare of the public by establishing standards for professional knowledge, skills, and practice and assuring consumers that professionals have met standards of practice.

Benefits of credentialing include meeting the requirements of governmental regulators, advancing the profession, providing a sense of pride and professional accomplishment, and demonstrating commitment to a profession and to life-long learning. Maintaining the credential of a professional certification requires renewal by continuing education, examination, and self-assessment. The nursing profession includes parallel and overlapping systems of both voluntary and mandatory credentialing. In the U.S., there are two types of credentialing—one at the individual level and one at the organizational level. Individual credentialing includes certification of providers, such as nurse practitioners and specialty nurses. Organizational credentialing accredits organizations—for example, educational institutions or health care organizations such as hospitals, long-term care facilities, and other care centers.

Individual credentialing

Within the profession of nursing, individuals receive credentials at the advanced practice and specialty level through examination that validates nurses' skills, knowledge, and abilities. At the American Nurses Credentialing Center (ANCC), a commission of experts and nurse peers constitutes the Commission on Certification. This commission oversees examination eligibility requirements and test parameters that ensure legally defensible and psychometrically sound examinations. Nurses who are deemed eligible may sit for an exam and, upon passing, are conferred the credentials "board certified." At many certifying agencies, such as ANCC, the process, structure, and content of exams are also accredited by external credentialing organizations. The Accreditation Board for Specialty Nursing Certification (ABSNC) is the only accrediting body specifically for nursing certification. ABSNC accreditation is a peer-review mechanism that allows nursing certification organizations to obtain accreditation by demonstrating compliance with the highest quality standards available in the industry. In addition, certification exams and programs can be credentialed by the National Commission for Certifying Agencies (NCCA). The NCCA helps to ensure the health, welfare, and safety of the public through the accreditation of a variety of individual certification programs that assess professional competency. In this way the certification exams being offered are also externally reviewed for high quality and compliance to external standards. NCCA credentials certification exams in any field and is not specific to health care.

Trends in individual credentialing:

In the 1990s, it became clear that the definitions and the coordination between licensure, accreditation of curriculum programs for schools of nursing, and certification eligibility requirements were not aligned. An alliance of over 40 nursing organizations worked collaboratively to represent the stakeholders of licensure, accreditation, certification and education in creating a Consensus Model for APRN Regulation. This transformative model will provide needed uniformity for the advanced practice registered nurse (APRN) profession. The consensus model was designed to align the inter-relationships among licensure, accreditation, certification, and education to create a more uniform practice across the country. The resulting consistency and clarity will take advanced practice nursing to the next level, benefiting individual nurses and enhancing patient care. Full implementation of the consensus model, anticipated in 2015, will require coordination between the involved stakeholders. Key changes include clear alignment of advanced practice nurses into four roles: nurse anesthetist, nurse midwives, nurse practitioners, and clinical nurse specialists. Once roles are determined, populations of study will be aligned, including neonatal, pediatric, adult-gerontology, women's health/ gender-related, family/individual across the lifespan, and psychiatric mental health. Further specification of knowledge would occur at the specialty level (e.g., areas such as oncology, palliative care, and forensics) and would include a focus of practice beyond the role and population linked to the health care needs of individuals.

As a result of the consensus model, changes are happening across regulatory arenas to protect licensure for advanced practice RNs as well as aligning certification exams with educational requirements for these roles and populations. This model will align the interlocking pieces of educational preparation and licensure and certification across the nation, allowing advanced practice nurses to have mobility in their practice and for the public to have assurance that competent, qualified advanced practice nurses are caring for them.

Organizational credentialing

Certifying agencies have the capability to credential health care organizations. While there are credentialing programs that recognize subsets of whole organizations (e.g., the Beacon Program that recognizes critical care units), perhaps the best known organizational credentials in health care are The Joint Commission accreditation and certification programs and the Magnet Recognition Designation program.

As described in previous chapters, The Joint Commission, an independent, not-for-profit organization, accredits and certifies more than 19,000 health care organizations and programs in the U.S. Joint Commission accreditation and certification reflects an organization's commitment to meeting certain performance standards. The accreditation of hospitals and health care organizations by the Joint Commission is also recognized as having met the CMS Standards of Participation by the federal government.

The Magnet Recognition Program, an organizational credentialing program managed by the ANCC and the Commission on Magnet, requires organizations to demonstrate excellence in nursing care and provide written evidence of meeting standards (called sources of evidence) for structures, processes and outcomes of patient satisfaction, nurse satisfaction, and clinical outcome measures of patient care. A rigorous process of review includes a multi-day site visit of the organization to validate, clarify, and amplify the results of the written study. At present, there are almost 400 *Magnet*®-designated hospitals around the world. The designation period is four years, with requirements for interim monitoring and reports. Nearly 98 percent of all magnet-designated organizations work to become re-designated, and several magnet organizations have been re-designated four times, demonstrating their commitment to excellence in nursing and patient care. A growing body of evidence also has linked Magnet designation with improved clinical outcomes.[4,5] The original and ongoing research represents the implementation of evidence-based practice in nursing services and hospital administration. Another organizational credential that is growing in importance is the *Pathway to Excellence*™ designation. This credential recognizes 12 practice standards of a positive practice environment at the organization level.

Issues and trends in organizational credentialing

One of the key areas for future consideration is a growing need for research that links standards for credentialing to improvement in patient outcomes. This relatively new field is growing swiftly, and the ANCC is leading the way by exploring the research questions and providing guidance for methods and analysis. With most credentialing, whether individual or organizational, the designation is voluntary. It is a major challenge to compare credentialed versus non-credentialed variables, because many non-credentialed organizations and individuals share the same characteristics but chose not to go through the credentialing process. Rigorous research methods, sound design, and large enough sample sizes are required to ensure the growth of a scholarly evidence base regarding the merits of credentialing and its link to outcomes of care.

Another area of exploration is the link between credentialing and competency. Does certifying an individual ensure competence? Is there an improvement in patient outcomes? For organizations being credentialed, both for education and practice, does the credential link to improved systems of care that produce competent health care providers and result in improved patient outcomes? For example, individual activity outcomes are evaluated in continuing education for nurses, but few linkages have been made between the educational activity and the outcomes of patient care. The linkage to patient care outcomes is clearly the direction of the future. In terms of both reimbursement and spending on health care infrastructure, there must be a clear return on investment.

When standards are set, organizations and individuals work to meet the standards. If the bar is set high, the level of effort and results will be high as well. Credentialing is a powerful lever to improve patient care knowledge of caregivers, continuing education, and organizational systems. Knowing which standards impact outcomes will be key to improving quality. Future improvements in credentialing science research methodology; analysis of existing data; and conceptual models of competency, quality, and excellence will all contribute to the creation of the best outcomes in patient care.

Suggested Reading

Chappell K, Drenkard K. Credentialing: Achieving quality in continuing nursing education. *J Contin Educ Nurs,* 41(7):2292-3, July 2010.

Gibbs JQ, Reissour SM. Evaluating outcomes: evidence of success. *J Contin Educ Nurs,* 41(11):484-5, Nov. 2010.

Reid, J. Ensuring Quality and Safety. *Radiologic Tech,* 81(5):499-501, May-June 2010.

Drenkard K, Morgan S, Wolf G (ed), *Magnet: The Next Generation.* Silver Spring, MD: American Nurses Credentialing Center, 2011.

Institute of Medicine. *Redesigning Continuing Education in the Health Professions.* Washington, DC: The National Academies Press. 2010.

Smolenski, MC. Credentialing, certification, and competence: issues for new and seasoned nurse practitioners. *J Amer Acad Nurse Practitioners,* 17(6):201-4, June 2005.

Styles MM, Schumann MJ, Bickford C, White KM. Specialization and Credentialing. In *Nursing Revisited: Understanding The Issues, Advancing The Profession.* Silver Spring, MD: American Nurses Association, 2008.

References

1. Jacobs, JA, Glassie, JC. *Certification and Accreditation Law Handbook,* 2nd edition, Washington, DC: American Society of Association Executives, 2004.

2. Hickey JV, Venogoni SL, Ouimette RM (Eds). Practice Credentials: Licensure, Approval to Practice, Certification and Privileging, Advanced Practice Nursing: Roles and Clinical Applications, 2nd ed. Philadelphia, PA: Lippincott, 1999, pp. 66-81.

3. Mickie S. Rops and Associates, "Credentialing, Licensure, Certification, Accreditation, Certificates: What's the difference?", e-answers 1(3), May 2002, www.msrops.com. http://msrops.blogs.com/akac/files/Credentialing_Terminology.pdf. Accessed 11.10.11.

4. Aiken LH, Smith HL, Lake ET. Lower Medicare mortality rates among a set of hospitals known for good nursing care. *Medical Care,* 32(8):771-87, 1994.

5. Aiken LH, Clarke SP, Sloane, M, *et al.* Effects of hospital care environment on patient mortality and nurses outcomes. *J Nurs Adm,* 38(5):223-9, 2May008.

The Future Is Now

By David E. Longnecker, MD, FACP
and Dave Davis, MD, CCFP, FCFP

Perhaps the most important message regarding future directions is the realization that *the future is now*. Never has the health care delivery environment been more dynamic than it is today. Some have described it as "constant whitewater" characterized by rocks, eddies, whirlpools, and waterfalls with labels such as payment reform, risk-based reimbursement, bundled payments, public reporting, accountability, transparency, meaningful use, team-based care, maintenance of certification, maintenance of licensure (MOL), OPPE, FPPE, etc. While we recognize that significant challenges face today's practitioners, we also embrace these changes because we envision a future that is focused on quality as defined by the Institute of Medicine (IOM) (i.e., safe, timely, effective, efficient, equitable, patient-centered) and the Centers for Medicare and Medicaid Services (CMS) (i.e., better health for individuals, better care for populations, and lower costs through improvement). Together, these approaches are facilitating a transformation in care delivery that is unprecedented in American history.

Although the pace may be dizzying for individual providers, the long-term benefits more than justify the effort. Further, we firmly believe that the changes occurring today will continue whether or not the Patient Protection and Affordable Care Act of 2010 is affirmed, rejected, or modified by the pending Supreme Court review. Put simply, the changes now occurring throughout health care have moved beyond the "tipping point"; they have gained so much support and momentum that a return to "business as usual" is simply not feasible. These views are also shared by keen observers of social trends.[1]

For individual practitioners, three major quality themes will be especially prevalent in their future practice: 1) increased collection of quality data ("transparency"), 2) increased assessment of personal competence and practice performance, principally via the American Board of Medical Specialties MOC initiative ("accountability"), and 3) the expectation that any gaps in performance will be corrected ("quality improvement" [QI]). The combined effects of transparency, accountability, and QI can have a profound effect on the quality of care offered by individual providers and by the health care "system" overall. We will address each of these areas below.

Maintenance of Certification

In the U.S., board certification by an American Board of Medical Specialties (ABMS) member board has long been considered the gold standard for documenting physician competence. For most of the 20th century this documentation was achieved by a single examination that resulted in a lifetime certificate. Maintaining that certification and maintaining medical licensure were generally simple, and mostly passive, processes that involved accruing a defined threshold of continuing medical education (CME) credits. CME credits were awarded for attendance at accredited CME courses and other less formal educational activities such as journal clubs, discussions with peers, and personal reading. There was little or no emphasis on actual clinical performance and quality of practice.

Over time, the medical profession began to recognize that knowledge alone did not ensure excellence in performance and that the standard, didactic CME model of passive learning was relatively ineffective.[2] Additional evidence indicated that physicians were generally ineffective at assessing their own learning needs or their clinical care gaps.[3] Thus, in 2000, the ABMS member boards adopted the concept of MOC, which involves four major components:

- Part I requires maintenance of licensure as a prerequisite to certification;

- Part II requires documentation of life-long learning and self-assessment;

- Part III requires a cognitive evaluation (i.e., evidence of current knowledge); and, notably,

- Part IV requires an assessment of actual practice performance, compared to standard norms and other practitioners.

Combined with time-limited certification (approved by all ABMS member boards in 2006), MOC is now the standard for evaluating the continuing competence of board diplomates. However, implementation of Part IV still varies among the ABMS member boards. Although all are working to achieve the desired goal, some (e.g., the boards for internal medicine, pediatrics and family medicine) have rather robust processes whereas others remain in earlier phases of implementation.

The moves to MOC and MOL represent dramatic changes in the way physicians are evaluated, and they provide greater assurance and validity to the board certification process. We believe that these changes are essential for improving the quality of care throughout the U.S., and we support them enthusiastically. The effectiveness of Part IV (practice assessment) depends greatly on the quality, extent, and timeliness of data gathered from physician practices—thus the current emphasis on implementing electronic health records (EHRs) that will facilitate data reporting.

Further, measurement of performance is a necessary, but insufficient, step toward improving performance. If gaps in clinical care are uncovered, clinicians must be competent in the discipline of QI to effectively implement corrective action.

Quality Measurement and QI

Americans have long been fascinated with performance measurement. We evaluate teams based on wins versus losses and athletes based on batting averages, home runs, goals scored, blocked shots, and an endless array of other measures. We evaluate financial performance by measures such as the Dow Jones Industrial Average® and the NASDAQ®. We evaluate thousands of products through rating systems such as Consumer Reports®. In short, we are obsessed with "keeping score," yet performance in health care has been a notable latecomer to this process.

In 2002, the CMS and the Hospital Quality Alliance collaborated to form Hospital Compare, which now provides publicly available quarterly reports on the performance of approximately 4,000 hospitals.[4] Additional legislation, passed in 2006, prescribed the Physician Quality Reporting System (PQRS), which eventually will provide similar information on the performance of individual physicians and/or their group practices. The PQRS initiative is managed by CMS, but its goals are facilitated by policies generated in the Department of Health and Human Services' Office of the National Coordinator of Health Information Technology (ONC), which provides financial incentives to clinicians for implementing health information technology in their practices and for reporting their performance data. Several of these initiatives are aligned to encourage physician quality reporting. For example, physicians who report their data via an EHR can receive additional incentives by also participating in MOC. Although still in the early stages of development, we see this convergence as an important catalyst for what we hope will become the standard of practice—i.e., timely reporting of performance data by all clinicians, with such information widely available to individuals and employers. Almost certainly, shining a light on performance will be a strong stimulus for performance improvement throughout the provider community, and we applaud this approach.

Keeping score alone is not enough. How does an individual clinician, or a group of practitioners, go about improving quality when gaps in clinical care are identified? All clinicians want what is best for their patients, but health care is now a complex process that often involves far more than an individual clinician working in a solo practice. For persons with advanced illness or multiple chronic conditions, the spectrum of providers includes primary care physicians, medical specialists, nurses, pharmacists, social workers, pastoral care workers, home health services, and more! Clearly, one needs an organized approach to manage and improve care in this system of care. Fortunately, there is a ready template for initiating such work—it is called QI.

W. Edwards Deming, PhD, an American statistician and process improvement expert, provided a framework for such efforts and demonstrated its effectiveness through his work in Japan in the 1950s. Japanese manufacturers were in a state of utter collapse following the massive destruction of their infrastructure during WWII. Deming led the redesign and rebuilding of Japanese industry using his now well-established Plan-Do-Study-Act (PDSA) cycle. Using this systematic approach, and incorporating the fundamental principle of team-based engagement, he not only revived Japan's manufacturing but also created a standard of excellence that has served as a model for world-wide industry, including a growing number of health care organizations (e.g., the Virginia Mason Health System, Seattle, WA). But there are caveats to this approach.

Although the PDSA cycle provides a framework for QI, full effectiveness is achieved only when all providers involved in the delivery of care are equally engaged in the design (*plan*) and implementation (*do*) of that care. Further, the subsequent "study" phase must be supported by timely, reliable, and meaningful data. Finally, the resulting *action* must be effectively implemented, whereupon the cycle is continuously repeated. Experience reveals that such a process, taken seriously and with an emphasis on teamwork, leads to the development of a *culture of quality* in an organization that far exceeds the accomplishments achieved by simply expecting each person to "do their job well." Humans are inherently error-prone, and they benefit greatly from the wisdom and watchfulness of engaged colleagues (*the team*) who are constantly checking for errors and opportunities for improvement. Indeed, highly reliable organizations are characterized by such approaches. But how does one learn the quality improvement methodology?

Medical schools and graduate medical education programs are now incorporating QI education and training into their curricula, and this bodes well for the future of the health care improvement initiative. In our experience, students and residents are literally "hungry" for the opportunity to make a difference by improving the quality, safety, timeliness, and efficiency of their practice. However, practitioners who received their training previously may need guidance and continuing education when seeking such knowledge. Several ABMS member boards and specialty societies provide access to online CME to guide the neophyte through this process. Examples include the American Board of Internal Medicine Practice Improvement Modules,[5] the American College of Surgeons Division of Education,[6] and numerous others. The respective ABMS member boards, professional societies, or a local CME provider can provide guidance for both individuals and group practices.

Summary

Beyond the 'whitewater' of health care change, we see a bright future—one not yet fully achieved but one that is based on the principles of safe, high-quality, person-centered, cost effective care delivery, guided by timely data that inform the practitioner and his or her care team of the effectiveness of their care processes based on meaningful quality metrics, and functioning collaboratively in a

QI framework. Selected health care organizations have implemented these approaches successfully, and the incentives for movement in this direction are increasingly attractive. While much remains to be done, the momentum for change suggests there is no turning back. Providers, educators, specialty societies, health insurers (both government and commercial), and the public increasingly expect such improvements and most are unwilling to tolerate the status quo–this alone is a strong impetus for action.

References

1. Abelson R, Harris G, Pear R. Major changes in health care likely to last. *New York Times.* November 15, 2011, p. A1.

2. Forsetlund L, Bjørndal A, Rashidian A, *et al.* Continuing education meetings and workshops: effects on professional practice and health care outcomes. *Cochrane Database of Systematic Reviews,* 2009, Issue 2. Art. No.: CD003030. DOI: 10.1002/14651858. CD003030.pub2.

3. Davis DA, Mazmanian PE, Fordis M, *et al.* Accuracy of physician self-assessment compared with observed measures of competence: a systematic review. *JAMA,* 296(9):1094-102, Sept. 6, 2006.

4. U.S. Department of Health and Human Services Hospital Compare. http://hospitalcompare.hhs.gov/. Updated October 13, 2011. Accessed November 23, 2011.

5. American Board of Internal Medicine Maintenance and Recertification Guide. http://www.abim.org/moc/. Updated March 31, 2011. Accessed November 23, 2011.

6. American College of Surgeons Division of Education. http://www.facs.org/education/index.html. Updated October 11, 2011. Accessed November 23, 2011.

CPSIA information can be obtained at www.ICGtesting.com
Printed in the USA
LVOW10s0850071013

355739LV00001B/4/P